1998
YEAR BOOK OF
UROLOGY®

Statement of Purpose

The YEAR BOOK Service

The YEAR BOOK series was devised in 1901 by practicing health professionals who observed that the literature of medicine and related disciplines had become so voluminous that no one individual could read and place in perspective every potential advance in a major specialty. In the final decade of the 20th century, this recognition is more acutely true than it was in 1901.

More than merely a series of books, YEAR BOOK volumes are the tangible results of a unique service designed to accomplish the following:

- to *survey* a wide range of journals of proven value
- to *select* from those journals papers representing significant advances and statements of important clinical principles
- to provide *abstracts* of those articles that are readable, convenient summaries of their key points
- to provide *commentary* about those articles to place them in perspective

These publications grow out of a unique process that calls on the talents of outstanding authorities in clinical and fundamental disciplines, trained literature specialists, and professional writers, all supported by the resources of Mosby, the world's preeminent publisher for the health professions.

The Literature Base

Mosby and its editors survey approximately 500 journals published worldwide, covering the full range of the health professions. On an annual basis, the publisher examines usage patterns and polls its expert authorities to add new journals to the literature base and to delete journals that are no longer useful as potential YEAR BOOK sources.

The Literature Survey

The publisher's team of literature specialists, all of whom are trained and experienced health professionals, examines every original, peer-reviewed article in each journal issue. More than 250,000 articles per year are scanned systematically, including title, text, illustrations, tables, and references. Each scan is compared, article by article, to the search strategies that the publisher has developed in consultation with the 270 outside experts who form the pool of YEAR BOOK editors. A given article may be reviewed by any number of editors, from one to a dozen or more, regardless of the discipline for which the paper was originally published. In turn, each editor who receives the article reviews it to determine whether the article should be included in the YEAR BOOK. This decision is based on the article's inherent quality, its probable usefulness to readers of that YEAR BOOK, and the editor's goal to represent a balanced picture of a given field in each volume of the YEAR BOOK. In addition, the editor indicates when to include figures and tables from the article to help the YEAR BOOK reader better understand the information.

Of the quarter million articles scanned each year, only 5% are selected for detailed analysis within the YEAR BOOK series, thereby assuring readers of the high value of every selection.

The Abstract

The publisher's abstracting staff is headed by a seasoned medical professional and includes individuals with training in the life sciences, medicine, and other areas, plus extensive experience in writing for the health professions and related industries. Each selected article is assigned to a specific writer on this abstracting staff. The abstracter, guided in many cases by notations supplied by the expert editor, writes a structured, condensed summary designed so that the reader can rapidly acquire the essential information contained in the article.

The Commentary

The YEAR BOOK editorial boards, sometimes assisted by guest commentators, write comments that place each article in perspective for the reader. This provides the reader with the equivalent of a personal consultation with a leading international authority—an opportunity to better understand the value of the article and to benefit from the authority's thought processes in assessing the article.

Additional Editorial Features

The editorial boards of each YEAR BOOK organize the abstracts and comments to provide a logical and satisfying sequence of information. To enhance the organization, editors also provide introductions to sections or individual chapters, comments linking a number of abstracts, citations to additional literature, and other features.

The published YEAR BOOK contains enhanced bibliographic citations for each selected article, including extended listings of multiple authors and identification of author affiliations. Each YEAR BOOK contains a Table of Contents specific to that year's volume. From year to year, the Table of Contents for a given YEAR BOOK will vary depending on developments within the field.

Every YEAR BOOK contains a list of the journals from which papers have been selected. This list represents a subset of approximately 500 journals surveyed by the publisher and occasionally reflects a particularly pertinent article from a journal that is not surveyed on a routine basis.

Finally, each volume contains a comprehensive subject index and an index to authors of each selected paper.

The 1998 Year Book Series

Year Book of Allergy, Asthma, and Clinical Immunology: Drs. Rosenwasser, Borish, Boguniewicz, Nelson, Routes, and Spahn

Year Book of Anesthesiology and Pain Management®: Drs. Tinker, Abram, Chestnut, Roizen, Rothenberg, and Wood

Year Book of Cardiology®: Drs. Schlant, Collins, Gersh, Graham, Kaplan, and Waldo

Year Book of Chiropractic®: Dr. Lawrence

Year Book of Critical Care Medicine®: Drs. Parrillo, Balk, Calvin, Franklin, and Shapiro

Year Book of Dentistry®: Drs. Meskin, Berry, Jeffcoat, Leinfelder, Roser, Summitt, and Zakariasen

Year Book of Dermatologic Surgery®: Drs. Greenway, Barrett, Papadopoulos, and Whitaker

Year Book of Dermatology and Dermatologic Surgery: Drs. Thiers and Lang

Year Book of Diagnostic Radiology®: Drs. Osborn, Groskin, Dalinka, Maynard, Pentecost, Rebner, Ros, Smirniotopoulos, and Young

Year Book of Drug Therapy®: Drs. Lasagna and Weintraub

Year Book of Emergency Medicine®: Drs. Wagner, Dronen, Davidson, King, Niemann, and Roberts

Year Book of Endocrinology®: Drs. Bagdade, Braverman, Horton, Kannan, Landsberg, Molitch, Morley, Nathan, Odell, Poehlman, Rogol, and Ryan

Year Book of Family Practice®: Drs. Berg, Bowman, Davidson, Dexter, and Scherger

Year Book of Gastroenterology: Drs. Aliperti and Fleshman

Year Book of Geriatrics and Gerontology®: Drs. Burton, Beck, Ostwald, Rabins, Reuben, Roth, Shapiro, and Whitehouse

Year Book of Hand Surgery®: Drs. Amadio and Hentz

Year Book of Hematology®: Drs. Spivak, Bell, Ness, Quesenberry, Wiernik, and Horowitz

Year Book of Infectious Diseases: Drs. Keusch, Barza, Bennish, Poutsiaka, Skolnik, and Snydman

Year Book of Medicine®: Drs. Cline, Frishman, Jett, Klahr, Malawista, Mandell, McCallum, and Utiger

Year Book of Neonatal and Perinatal Medicine®: Drs. Fanaroff, Maisels, and Stevenson

Year Book of Nephrology, Hypertension, and Mineral Metabolism: Drs. Schwab, Bennett, Emmett, Hostetter, Kumar, and Toto

Year Book of Neurology and Neurosurgery®: Drs. Bradley and Gibbs

Year Book of Nuclear Medicine®: Drs. Gottschalk, Blaufox, Neumann, Strauss, and Zubal

Year Book of Obstetrics, Gynecology, and Women's Health: Drs. Mishell, Herbst, and Kirschbaum

Year Book of Occupational and Environmental Medicine®: Drs. Emmett, Frank, Gochfeld, and Hessl

Year Book of Oncology®: Drs. Ozols, Eisenberg, Glatstein, Loehrer, and Tallman

Year Book of Ophthalmology®: Drs. Wilson, Augsburger, Cohen, Eagle, Grossman, Laibson, Maguire, Nelson, Penne, Rapuano, Sergott, Spaeth, Tipperman, Ms. Gosfield, and Ms. Salmon

Year Book of Orthopedics®: Drs. Morrey, Beauchamp, Currier, Tolo, Trigg, and Swiontkowski

Year Book of Otolaryngology–Head and Neck Surgery®: Drs. Paparella and Holt

Year Book of Pathology and Laboratory Medicine®: Drs. Raab, Cohen, Olson, Sirgi, and Stanley

Year Book of Pediatrics®: Dr. Stockman

Year Book of Plastic, Reconstructive, and Aesthetic Surgery®: Drs. Miller, Bartlett, Garner, McKinney, Ruberg, Salisbury, and Smith

Year Book of Psychiatry and Applied Mental Health®: Drs. Talbott, Ballenger, Frances, Lydiard, Meltzer, Schowalter, and Tasman

Year Book of Pulmonary Disease®: Drs. Jett, Maurer, Ryu, Strollo, and Wenzel

Year Book of Rheumatology®: Drs. Panush, Hadler, LeRoy, Liang, Reichlin, Simon, and Weinblatt

Year Book of Sports Medicine®: Drs. Shephard, Drinkwater, Eichner, Torg, Alexander, and Mr. George

Year Book of Surgery®: Drs. Copeland, Bland, Deitch, Eberlein, Howard, Luce, Seeger, Souba, and Sugarbaker

Year Book of Thoracic and Cardiovascular Surgery®: Drs. Ginsberg, Wechsler, and Williams

Year Book of Urology®: Drs. Andriole and Coplen

Year Book of Vascular Surgery®: Dr. Porter

1998

The Year Book of UROLOGY®

Editors

Gerald L. Andriole, Jr., M.D.
Professor of Urologic Surgery, Division of Urology, Washington University School of Medicine, St. Louis, Missouri

Douglas E. Coplen, M.D.
Assistant Professor of Urologic Surgery, Director of Pediatric Urology, Division of Urology, Washington University School of Medicine, St. Louis, Missouri

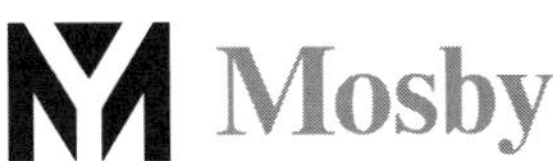

St. Louis Baltimore Boston Carlsbad Naples New York Philadelphia Portland London
Madrid Mexico City Singapore Sydney Tokyo Toronto Wiesbaden

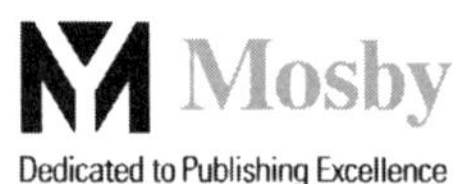

Publisher: Cheryl A. Smart
Managing Editor: Gina G. Byrd
Developmental Editor: Laura C. Berendson
Manager, Periodical Editing: Kirk Swearingen
Production Editor: Pat Costigan
Project Supervisor, Production: Joy Moore
Project Assistant, Production: Laura Bayless
Manager, Literature Services: Idelle L. Winer
Illustrations and Permissions Coordinator: Phyllis K. Thompson

1998 EDITION
Copyright © 1999 by Mosby, Inc.

Printed in the United States of America
Composition by Reed Technology and Information Services, Inc.
Printing/binding by Maple–Vail

Mosby, Inc.
11830 Westline Industrial Drive
St. Louis, MO 63146

International Standard Serial Number: 0084–4071
International Standard Book Number: 0–8151–2548–8

Contributors

Charles L. Bennett, M.D., Ph.D.
Associate Professor of Medicine, Northwestern University Medical School; Senior Research Associate, Veterans Administration Chicago Health Care System, Lakeside Division, Chicago, Illinois

David A. Goldfarb, M.D.
Department of Urology, The Cleveland Clinic Foundation, Cleveland, Ohio

David P. O'Brien III, M.D.
Professor of Surgery (Urology), Section of Urology, The Emory Clinic, Inc., Atlanta, Georgia

Jerry Yuan, M.D.
Assistant Professor of Surgery (Urology), Section of Urology, The Emory Clinic, Inc., Atlanta, Georgia

Table of Contents

Journals Represented

Mosby and its editors survey approximately 500 journals for its abstract and commentary publications. From these journals, the editors select the articles to be abstracted. Journals represented in this YEAR BOOK are listed below.

ASAIO Journal
Acta Obstetricia et Gynecologica Scandinavica
American Journal of Kidney Diseases
American Journal of Obstetrics and Gynecology
American Journal of Pathology
American Journal of Roentgenology
American Surgeon
Annals of Internal Medicine
Annals of Surgical Oncology
Archives of Family Medicine
Archives of Pediatrics and Adolescent Medicine
Archives of Surgery
British Journal of Radiology
British Journal of Surgery
British Journal of Urology
British Medical Journal
Canadian Journal of Surgery
Cancer
Clinical Radiology
European Urology
Fertility and Sterility
Human Reproduction
International Journal of Radiation, Oncology, Biology, and Physics
Journal of Clinical Oncology
Journal of Infectious Diseases
Journal of Pharmacology and Experimental Therapeutics
Journal of Urology
Journal of the American Medical Association
Journal of the National Cancer Institute
Lancet
Nature Genetics
Nature Medicine
New England Journal of Medicine
New Zealand Medical Journal
Pediatric Infectious Disease Journal
Pediatric Nephrology
Radiology
Scandinavian Journal of Urology and Nephrology
Spinal Cord
Transplantation
Transplantation Proceedings
Urology

STANDARD ABBREVIATIONS

The following terms are abbreviated in this edition: acquired immunodeficiency syndrome (AIDS), cardiopulmonary resuscitation (CPR), central nervous system

(CNS), cerebrospinal fluid (CSF), computed tomography (CT), deoxyribonucleic acid (DNA), electrocardiography (ECG), health maintenance organization (HMO), human immunodeficiency virus (HIV), intensive care unit (ICU), intramuscular (IM), intravenous (IV), magnetic resonance (MR) imaging (MRI), ribonucleic acid (RNA), ultrasound (US).

NOTE

The YEAR BOOK OF UROLOGY is a literature survey service providing abstracts of articles published in the professional literature. Every effort is made to assure the accuracy of the information presented in these pages. Neither the editors nor the publisher of the YEAR BOOK OF UROLOGY can be responsible for errors in the original materials. The editors' comments are their own opinions. Mention of specific products within this publication does not constitute endorsement.

To facilitate the use of the YEAR BOOK OF UROLOGY as a reference tool, all illustrations and tables included in this publication are now identified as they appear in the original article. This change is meant to help the reader recognize that any illustration or table appearing in the YEAR BOOK OF UROLOGY may be only one of many in the original article. For this reason, figure and table numbers will often appear to be out of sequence within the YEAR BOOK OF UROLOGY.

Introduction

The 1998 YEAR BOOK OF UROLOGY has been assembled from more than 3,000 articles selected from worldwide, peer-reviewed publications. It represents an attempt to summarize some of the best and most important contributions this year to the specialty of urology. We hope that the reader will find this an easy-to-read update.

New this year is a chapter devoted to evidence-based medicine as well as reviews of the latest American Urological Association Guidelines.

Imaging

Fielding et al. and Remer et al. evaluate and show distinct advantages in the use of non-contrast spiral CT as an alternative to urography and ultrasound in the evaluation of acute flank pain and in the follow-up of those with known urolithiasis. Chemical shift MR imaging is the best test to distinguish adrenocortical adenoma from other pathological adrenal masses (Schwartz et al.).

Calculus Disease

Segura reports the results of the American Urological Association Ureteral Stones Clinical Guidelines Panel. Kopp reviews the identification and treatment of the novel crystals and calculi associated with the new class of protease inhibitors used in the treatment of acquired immunodeficiency.

Transplantation and Renovascular Disease

Dr. David Goldfarb has reviewed abstracts in this expanded section that includes the appropriate evaluation of donors, expansion of the donor pool, and the latest on the evaluation and treatment of rejection episodes.

Urinary Tract Reconstruction

In an important abstract, Stein delineates guidelines and techniques for orthotopic urinary tract reconstruction in females. The Mitrofanoff principle remains the continence mechanism of choice. When the appendix is not available, transverse retubularized ileum is a simply created stoma that is easily catheterized (Gerharz et al.).

Urothelial Cancer

A minority of patients on bladder-preservation protocols survive five years with their bladder in place, as shown by Kachnic et al. and Shipley et al. Radical cystectomy alone is curative in only 50% of patients (Ghoneim et al.), but gemcitabine is a promising new chemotherapeutic agent with a good safety profile that may further improve the outcomes with neoadjuvant and adjuvant therapies.

Benign Prostatic Disease

This chapter abstracts the continued attempt to place the surgical, nonsurgical, and medical treatment of benign prostatic hyperplasia in perspective. Finasteride (McConnell, Marks) and doxazosin (Lepor) have long-term efficacy and safety in appropriately selected men. In a large and well-done study, Cattolica et al. show that transurethral resection is not associated with increased mortality when compared to watchful waiting or open prostatectomy.

Prostate Cancer Screening

This is a must-read chapter with abstracts reviewed by Dr. Charles Bennett. To screen or not to screen for prostate cancer? That is the question that must be addressed by primary care physicians (Austin et al.), families with cancer (Bratt, et al.), and urologists. Preliminary reports from the American Cancer Society (Mettlin et al.), European randomized screening study (Standaert, et al.), and Austria (Reissigl et al.) do not conclusively show a long-term survival benefit to screening, but the Washington University study (Smith et al.) clearly shows the detection of clinically significant localized cancers with screening.

Prostate Cancer

This chapter reflects the refinement in our understanding of the limitations of the various approaches to early-stage prostate cancer. Studies from Scandinavia (Johannsen et al. and Borre et al.) have defined the limits of watchful waiting for men with early-stage disease. Similarly, a relatively new treatment for prostate cancer, ultrasound-guided interstitial 125 brachytherapy, has been reported by Ragde et al. and demonstrates significant PSA control rates at 7 years of follow-up. In contrast, reports by Porter et al. and Pisters et al., question the role of cryosurgical ablation to treat this disease.

Outcomes/Quality of Life

This section is new to the YEAR BOOK OF UROLOGY. The reader will find abstracts discussing the importance of preoperative symptoms, postoperative outcomes, and care pathways in patient perception of quality of life.

Infertility

Reports by Pavlovich et al. and Kolettis et al. show that surgical correction of obstructive azoospermia offers the highest chance of live birth at a lower cost than sperm aspiration and intracytoplasmic injection.

Testis Tumors

In Mead's report, primary mediastinal metastases, visceral metastases, and a markedly elevated lactate dehydrogenase are associated with a lower long-term survival in cisplatin treated tumors. Travis et al. show a 1.4-fold increased incidence of secondary malignancy in testicular cancer survivors.

Vesicoureteral Reflux

Treatment for vesicoureteral reflux based upon peer-reviewed outcomes is presented in the American Urological Association Guidelines (Elder et al.). As discussed by Yeung et al., male neonatal reflux is a distinct entity that is associated with preexisting renal scarring and a high rate of resolution even for high grades of reflux. Renal scarring can occur at any age in the absence of symptoms or reflux (Benador et al. and Vernon et al.).

Gerald L. Andriole, Jr., M.D.

Douglas E. Coplen, M.D.

1 Imaging

Spiral Computerized Tomography in the Evaluation of Acute Flank Pain: A Replacement for Excretory Urography

Fielding JR, Steele G, Fox LA, et al (Brigham and Women's Hosp, Boston)
J Urol 157:2071–2073, 1997
1–1

Introduction.—Excretory urography (IVP), long the test of choice for evaluation of renal colic, has several disadvantages. The patient is exposed to potentially toxic IV contrast agents and significant time is often required to complete IVP. A study of 100 consecutive patients with flank pain examined the diagnostic value of noncontrast enhanced spiral CT in the evaluation of suspected renal colic.

Methods.—The patients were admitted to the emergency department with flank pain with or without hematuria. Excluded were patients who were pregnant and those with apparent sepsis. All patients were studied with CT if the most likely diagnosis was believed to be renal colic. Parameters used included no oral or IV contrast medium, 5 mm slice thickness reconstructed at 5 mm intervals, 120 kVp, and 210 to 280 mAs. Patients were followed at the urology outpatient clinic and/or by telephone interview.

Results.—Ureteral obstruction was demonstrated at CT in 55 of 100 patients. Radiographic signs of hydronephrosis and hydroureter were present in 5 patients who reported recent passage of a stone. Fifty patients had stones, 14 in the proximal, 4 in the mid, and 32 in the distal ureter. The average stone size was 3.7 mm. Eleven patients underwent endoscopic removal of the stones and 2 had extracorporeal shock wave lithotripsy. Spontaneous stone passage was documented in 39 patients. In the group without obstruction, 38 did not pass calculi and 14 had a definite diagnosis based on CT findings. There was 1 false negative study. Overall, clinical follow-up was adequate in 89 cases. In this group, noncontrast enhanced spiral CT yielded a sensitivity of 98%, a specificity of 100%, a positive predictive value of 100%, and a negative predictive value of 97%.

Conclusion.—Unenhanced spiral CT was highly accurate in identifying the size and location of obstructing ureteral stones in patients with flank pain. A disadvantage of this imaging method compared to IVP is the absence of evaluation of renal function and the urothelium. The time

1

required for CT is reduced relative to IVP, but costs of CT may be higher at some institutions.

▶ Non-enhanced spiral CT (5mm cuts) can be performed in less than 5 minutes and avoids contrast reactions associated with IVP. Cost is comparable to an IVP. This and other studies confirm accuracy and reliability in the diagnosis of acute colic.[1, 2] A calculus is definitively diagnosed when it is seen in the ureter. A circumferential rim of soft-tissue ("tissue-rim" sign) surrounding a calculus is useful in differentiating ureteral calculi from extraurinary abdominal or pelvic calcifications though the absence of the rim does not exclude a urinary stone. In these cases, secondary signs of ureteral or collecting system dilatation and perinephric stranding help in diagnosis when a stone is not identified. All of these are indicative of acute inflammation and are helpful in determining whether an identified stone is the cause of flank pain.[2]

D.E. Coplen, M.D.

References

1. Smith RC, Verga M, Dalrymple N, et al: Acute ureteral obstruction: value of secondary signs on helical unenhanced CT. *AJR* 167:1109–1113, 1996.
2. Kawashima A, Sandler CM, Boridy IC, et al: Unenhanced helical CT of ureterolithiasis: value of the tissue rim sign. *AJR* 168:997, 1997.

Spiral Noncontrast CT Versus Combined Plain Radiography and Renal US After Extracorporeal Shock Wave Lithotripsy: Cost-identification Analysis
Remer EM, Herts BR, Streem SB, et al (Cleveland Clinic Found, Ohio)
Radiology 204:33–37, 1997   1–2

Background.—Ultrasound combined with plain radiography is typically used to assess the abdomen for complications after extracorporeal shock wave lithotripsy (ESWL). However, spiral computed tomography (CT) has been shown to identify nephrolithiasis in the renal collecting system and ureters, which makes it a candidate for post-ESWL monitoring also. These authors examined the costs of spiral CT vs. ultrasound plus plain radiography in examining patients after ESWL for stone fragments and possible complications.

Methods.—Twenty-four patients (21 men, 3 women) 25 to 74 years old (mean age 50 years) underwent ESWL. The left ureter was involved in 10 patients, the right in 7, and bilateral ESWL was performed in 7. Approximately 1 month after the procedure, each patient underwent imaging by plain abdominal radiography, renal ultrasound, and spiral CT. Standard imaging protocols were used, and examination times were noted. A procedural-based cost-accounting system was used to calculate the direct technical costs associated with ultrasound plus radiography and with spiral CT.

Findings.—The average elapsed time for spiral CT (15.3 minutes) was significantly shorter than that of the combined ultrasound plus radiography approach (37.2 minutes). Interestingly, the per-minute technologist and equipment costs associated with the 2 approaches did not differ greatly ($1.11/min for ultrasound plus radiography vs. $1.03/min for spiral CT). However, when the direct technical costs were calculated (per-minute cost multiplied by the duration of the procedure, plus any variable costs such as film), spiral CT ($36.86) was substantially less expensive than ultrasound plus radiography ($57.60). Because a large proportion of the costs of these procedures is fixed (film, etc.), even reducing the amount of time spent on ultrasound or radiography would not become cost-equivalent to performing spiral CT.

Conclusions.—Both the elapsed time and the direct technical costs associated with spiral CT are less than those associated with combined ultrasound plus radiography in the assessment of patients post-ESWL. But of course, cost is not the only determinant of which modality to use: The next step is to assess whether spiral CT is as accurate as ultrasound plus radiography in monitoring complications after ESWL.

▶ This is a cost comparison study that does not address clinical outcomes. However, since plain film nephrotomograms are more sensitive than a plain film radiograph in detecting residual fragments after ESWL, spiral CT should similarly be more sensitive. CT would detect other abnormalities such as perinephric hematomas, but the follow-up studies are usually obtained 2 to 4 weeks after the lithotripsy so this would not necessarily be an advantage of CT. The use of more sensitive tests would result in more accurate reporting of ESWL results.

D.E. Coplen, M.D.

Testicular Blood Flow in Boys as Assessed at Color Doppler and Power Doppler Sonography
Bader TR, Kammerhuber F, Herneth AM (Univ of Vienna; Univ of Graz, Austria)
Radiology 202:559–564, 1997   1–3

Introduction.—Testicular torsion must be diagnosed rapidly in order for testicular viability to be preserved. Color Doppler sonography is often used to evaluate the acute scrotum because of its ability to provide information about morphologic abnormalities and blood supply. But in prepubertal boys with acute scrotal pain, the detection of testicular blood flow is quite variable with color Doppler. A prospective study of 86 boys with normal testes sought to determine the age at which testicular blood flow can be demonstrated consistently by color Doppler sonography and power Doppler sonography, a new modality with a higher sensitivity to blood flow.

Methods.—Study participants had been referred for US examinations of the abdomen or urinary tract and were asked to volunteer for US of the testes. Excluded were boys with scrotal pain or any history of testicular disease. Those in the study group ranged in age from 4 days to 15.9 years (mean 7.2 years). Gray-scale US was performed to exclude morphologic abnormalities and obtain longitudinal and transverse maximum diameters. Color Doppler scans were obtained with the lowest flow setting and in multiple orientations. Power Doppler sonography was performed with the same transducer in power Doppler mode and a setting designed for detection of low-volume, low-velocity blood flow.

Results.—Supratesticular vessels and capsular vessels were detected in all boys with both color Doppler and power Doppler sonography. Intratesticular vessels were not consistently seen, however, until age 8 with power Doppler sonography and until age 12 with color Doppler sonography. The same number of vessels was detected in 135 (78%) testes with both modalities. Power Doppler sonography identified vessels in 13 of 51 testes in which color Doppler sonography failed to depict vessels. In no case did color Doppler sonography demonstrate more vessels than power Doppler sonography. Age was more closely correlated than was testicular volume with the number of visible intratesticular vessels.

Conclusion.—In boys aged 4 days to 15 years, and especially those younger than 10, power Doppler sonography was more sensitive to flow than was color Doppler sonography. Power Doppler sonography demonstrated more intratesticular vessels and showed intratesticular blood flow in many testes in which color Doppler sonography failed to depict flow. The use of power Doppler sonography should improve the accuracy of diagnosis of testicular torsion in pediatric patients.

▶ Ultrasound is commonly used to assess boys with testicular pain. Color Doppler is inconsistent in prepubertal boys because of the relatively low blood flow. Power Doppler has higher sensitivity for blood flow but still was unable to detect flow in 33% of boys less than 8 years old and 5% of boys older than 8 years. My experience is that the incidence of patients with nondetectable blood flow is much lower than this, but when it does occur, absence of blood flow in the nonpainful normal testis makes interpretation of the test difficult.

D.E. Coplen, M.D.

Clinical Value of Renovascular Resistive Index Measurement in the Diagnosis of Acute Obstructive Uropathy
Older RA, Stoll HL III, Omary RA, et al (Univ of Virginia, Charlottesville)
J Urol 157:2053–2055, 1997   1–4

Introduction.—The most commonly used studies for the investigation of possible urinary tract obstruction are US and excretory urography (IVP). Gray scale US, however, may not resolve the question of urinary tract obstruction versus a nonobstructive cause of pain. A study of patients with suspected acute urinary tract obstruction was conducted to assess the diagnostic value of the renal resistive index (peak systolic velocity–end diastolic velocity/peak systolic velocity).

Methods.—Between March 1993 and November 1994, attempts were made to measure the resistive index in 54 patients. Excluded were US patients who bypassed IVP and proceeded directly to therapy and patients with negative IVPs. The study sample included the 19 patients with unilateral obstruction documented with excretory urography. All were studied with an Acoustic Imaging 5200S US unit and a 3.5 and/or 5 MHz transducer. One to 5 resistive index measurements were obtained per kidney; values were averaged to determine a mean resistive index for both the obstructed and nonobstructed kidney.

Results.—The US resistive index criteria for obstruction were a resistive index of 0.70 or greater or a difference of 0.10 or greater between a patient's 2 kidneys. The mean resistive index was 0.72 for all obstructed kidneys and 0.66 for all nonobstructed kidneys. Although these values were statistically different, a scattergram of resistive indexes showed wide overlap. Sensitivity of the resistive index for obstruction was 42%, specificity was 79%, and positive and negative predictive values were 67% and 57%, respectively.

Conclusion.—The sensitivity and specificity of the resistive index for urinary obstruction were too low to be clinically useful. Because positive and negative predictive values were also poor, this measurement appears to have no significant value in the examination of patients with renal colic.

▶ Ultrasound relies upon hydronephrosis, hydroureter, and/or an identifiable cause to diagnose obstruction. The use of resistive index as a non-invasive method of diagnosing either acute or chronic obstruction is controversial. Although this study shows a significant difference between the mean resistive index of obstructed and non-obstructed kidneys, the overlap in values limits the utility in individual patients.

D.E. Coplen, M.D.

Comparison of Two Algorithms and Their Associated Charges When Evaluating Adrenal Masses in Patients With Malignancies

Schwartz LH, Panicek DM, Doyle MV, et al (Mem Sloan-Kettering Cancer Ctr, New York; Cornell Univ, New York)
AJR 168:1575–1578, 1997   1–5

Objective.—Magnetic resonance imaging can distinguish benign and malignant solid adrenal masses on the basis of pulse sequences. A comparison was made of the relative charges associated with 2 proposed algorithms for characterizing adrenal masses discovered at MR imaging during staging of neoplasms, with CT-guided adrenal biopsy only when MR findings were not diagnostic.

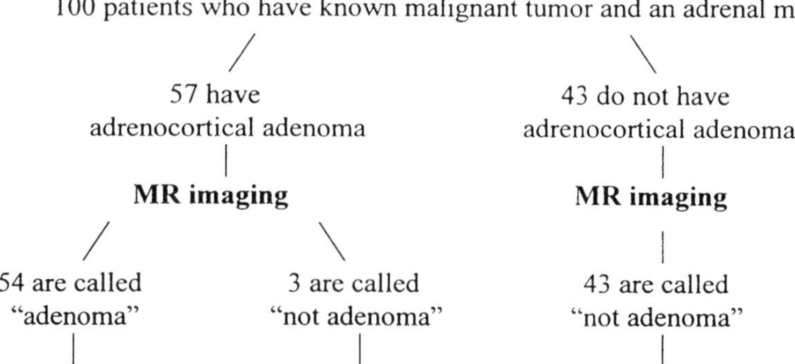

FIGURE 1.—Flowchart shows expected distribution of 100 patients who have known malignant neoplasms and are seen for evaluation of adrenal mass, based on data obtained in this study (57% prevalence of adrenocortical adenoma in this population of patients who have adrenal masses, and sensitivity of 94% and specificity of 100% for revealing adrenocortical adenoma with chemical shift imaging). (Courtesy of Schwartz LH, Panicek DM, Doyle MV, et al: Comparison of two algorithms and their associated charges when evaluating adrenal masses in patients with malignancies. *AJR* 168:1575–1578, 1997.)

Methods.—Between November 1993 and November 1995, MR (chemical shift) imaging was performed on 54 patients with adrenal masses no more than 7 days before CT-guided biopsy with a 22-gauge needle. Associated charges were normalized using national relative-value scale charges and US national conversion factors.

Results.—The MR images were of diagnostic quality in all patients. The average sizes of benign and malignant adrenal masses were 1.8 and 4.1 cm, respectively. Adrenal-spleen signal intensity ratios were 0.30 for adrenal adenomas and 0.78 for adrenal metastases. The sensitivity and specificity of the ratio were 94% and 100%. Computed tomography-guided biopsy was successful in all patients, and 23 were shown to be metastases. There were 2 complications, a pneumothorax in 2 patients. The MRI charges were $1,032 per patient; the CT charges were $1,875 per patient. Chemical shift imaging would be expected to diagnose adrenocortical adenoma correctly in 54% of patients (Fig 1). If all patients had MR imaging and 46% also had a CT-guided biopsy, the per-patient cost would be $1,895, whereas if all patients had CT-guided biopsy only the per-patient cost would be $1,875. Magnetic resonance imaging should be used first because it is noninvasive.

Conclusion.—Chemical shift MR imaging is a sensitive and specific technique for distinguishing between malignant and benign adrenal masses.

▶ This manuscript highlights an evolving consensus that MR imaging with use of chemical shift imaging is the best test to distinguish an adrenocortical adenoma from other pathologic masses in an adrenal gland. As shown in Figure 1, among a hypothetical group of 100 patients who have cancer and an adrenal mass, only about 40% have metastases and these are virtually always correctly identified by this type of MR imaging. Among the 60% of patients who harbor an adrenocortical adenoma, only about 5% will be inappropriately labeled as having a nonadenoma. Therefore, use of this type of MR imaging would result in only 46 CT-guided biopsies to "rule in" adrenal metastases. This strategy may be compared to a strategy of performing CT-guided biopsy in all 100 patients in lieu of MR imaging. When one considers the MR imaging charge of $1,032 per patient and a biopsy charge of $1,875 per patient and the miscellaneous charges that may be associated with biopsy complications, an equivalent amount of money is spent and biopsies are averted on almost half of the patients.

The authors point out, however, that some patients may prefer a biopsy to an MRI scan so that physicians must continue to individualize their approach to these lesions.

G.L. Andriole, Jr., M.D.

MR Differentiation of Phaechromocytoma From Other Adrenal Lesions Based on Qualitative Analysis of T2 Relaxation Times

Varghese JC, Hahn PF, Papanicolaou N, et al (Harvard Med School, Boston)
Clin Radiol 52:603–606, 1997   1–6

Background.—Previous reports have indicated that pheochromocytomas have a higher signal intensity on T2-weighted magnetic resonance (MR) images than do benign adenomas or malignant lesions. Thus, a higher signal intensity is often used to differentiate pheochromocytomas from other lesions. However, because these authors have noted numerous pheochromocytomas with intermediate signal density, they report their experience with the diagnostic accuracy of MR imaging in differentiating these lesions.

Methods.—Retrospective analysis over 4 years identified 65 patients (37 men, 28 women, 29 to 87 years old) with 67 masses (excluding cysts, myelolipomas, and adrenal hemorrhage; average size 3.7 cm). T1- and T2-weighted spin-echo MR images had been obtained for all patients, and these images were reviewed by 3 observers who were blinded to the diagnosis. Masses were categorized as a benign adenoma (signal intensity equal to or slightly higher than that of the liver), malignant lesion (signal intensity greater than that of the liver but less than that of cerebrospinal fluid), or pheochromocytoma (signal intensity equal to that of cerebrospinal fluid).

Findings.—Surgery, biopsy, or computed tomography confirmed that there were 32 benign adenomas, 18 malignant lesions, and 17 pheochromocytomas. Of the 17 pheochromocytomas, 6 (35%) had low signal intensity and were misclassified by observers (5 as malignant lesions, 1 as benign adenoma). Likewise, 6 nonpheochromocytomas (12%) had high signal intensity and were misclassified (3 were actually benign adenoma, 2 were adrenal carcinomas, and 1 was a metastasis). Thus, the sensitivity of MR imaging in detecting pheochromocytomas was 65%, specificity was

88%, the positive predictive value was 65%, and the negative predictive value was 88%.

Conclusions.—In this report, basing the diagnosis of pheochromocytoma on the presence of a hyperintense signal misclassified over one third of these lesions. Likewise, 1 of 10 lesions with a hyperintense signal was misclassified as a pheochromocytoma. Thus, one cannot rely on the MR appearance of a hyperintense signal to confirm pheochromocytoma, and appropriate biochemical screening must be used in patients with suspected pheochromocytoma.

▶ Pheochromocytoma usually exhibits higher signal intensity than do benign adenomas and malignant lesions on T2-weighted imaging. In this series, 35% of pheochromocytomas had short T2 relaxation times (less intense), so biochemical analysis is definitely required in the evaluation of adrenal masses in both the asymptomatic and the hypertensive person.

D.E. Coplen, M.D.

Detection of Urethral Diverticula in Women: Comparison of a High Resolution Fast Spin Echo Technique With Double Balloon Urethrography

Neitlich JD, Foster HE Jr, Glickman MG, et al (Yale Univ, New Haven, Conn)
J Urol 159:408–410, 1998
1–7

Background.—Clinically diagnosing urethral diverticula can be difficult. A rapid high-resolution MRI technique was compared with contrast urethrography in detecting urethral diverticula in women.

Methods.—Thirteen patients with clinically suspected urethral diverticula underwent MRI and contrast urethrography during a 19-month period. Double balloon urethrography was done in 12 patients and voiding cystourethrography in 1. A fast spin echo T2-weighted pulse sequence and a dedicated pelvic multicoil were used. After a sagittal localizer sequence 3 mm thick, axial sections were obtained from the bladder base through the whole urethra. Total time needed for imaging was 15 minutes.

Findings.—Urethrography and MRI were negative for urethral diverticula in 7 patients, and cystourethroscopy was negative in 1. In 1 patient, MRI showed a vaginal inclusion cyst that was confirmed surgically. No other studies or procedures were done in 3 patients. Magentic resonance imaging was positive for urethral diverticula in 6 patients, including 4 with subsequent surgical confirmation of diverticulum, 1 who declined surgery, and 1 lost to follow-up. Double balloon urethrogram was negative in 3 of the 4 patients with surgically confirmed diverticulum.

Conclusions.—Magnetic resonance imaging is a valuable noninvasive method for determining the presence of urethral diverticula and other abnormalities. The sensitivity and negative predictive value of MRI were much higher than double balloon urethrography in this study.

▶ The classic symptoms of urethral diverticula are dyspareunia, dysuria, and dribbling (post-void). In the absence of a palpable mass, the clinical diagnosis is difficult to make. The orifice is usually small and may not be evident on urethroscopy. The double balloon technique was not as useful (25%) as is reported elsewhere in the literature (75%–80%). The MRI helps to define the extent of the diverticulum and also identified other pathology that was the cause of symptoms (vaginal cyst). Transvaginal ultrasound is also a useful imaging modality and can be used intraoperatively.

D.E. Coplen, M.D.

2 Genitourinary Infections

Allergic Nephropathy Associated With Norfloxacin and Ciprofloxacin Therapy: Report of Two Cases and Review of the Literature
Hadimeri H, Almroth G, Cederbrant K, et al (Univ Hosp, Linköping, Sweden)
Scand J Urol Nephrol 31:481–485, 1997   2–1

Introduction.—Acute interstitial nephritis (AIN) is a potential complication of drug therapy. This report describes a case of AIN associated with norfloxacin treatment and another case of AIN associated with ciprofloxacin treatment.

Case 1.—Woman, 68, presented with loin pain, fever, and glucosuria. Norfloxacin treatment was initiated. Symptoms gradually disappeared but recurred on the seventh day. Serum creatinine increased. Renal biopsy revealed edema, acute interstitial inflammation with eosinophils, and a histopathological appearance that was consistent with drug-induced AIN. Norfloxacin was discontinued, and patient gradually improved. No corticosteroid treatment was employed.

Case 2.—Woman, 70, had one course of chemotherapy. The second course was delayed because of fever and angiitis and treated with ciprofloxacin. Serum creatinine, white cell count, ESR, and CCRP became elevated. Renal biopsy revealed histopathologic appearance compatible with drug-induced AIN. Ciprofloxacin was discontinued. Corticosteroid treatment was not employed. The patient gradually improved.

Conclusions.—Clinicians should be aware of the possibility of quinolone-associated acute interstitial nephritis, a rare but potentially serious renal complication.

▶ Although a rare complication, flouroquinolones can be associated with AIN. This is felt to be a delayed hypersensitivity reaction. The clinical features include nonoliguric renal failure, fever, rash, and eosinophilia. No subset of patients appears to be at increased risk. Acute interstitial nephritis usually occurs within 3 weeks of starting therapy and usually resolves after stopping the antibiotic. Treatment with steroids is not useful in most cases. Clinicians should be aware of this potentially dangerous renal complication of quinolone therapy.

D.E. Coplen, M.D.

Prevalence of Penile Human Papillomavirus DNA in Husbands of Women With and Without Cervical Neoplasia: A Study in Spain and Colombia
Castellsagué X, Ghaffari A, Daniel RW, et al (Ciutat Saintària i Universitària de Bellvitge, Barcelona; Johns Hopkins Univ, Baltimore, Md; Internatl Agency for Research on Cancer, Lyon, France)
J Infect Dis 176:353–361, 1997   2–2

Background.—Human papillomavirus (HPV) is a cause of cervical cancer in women, but its effects in men are not as serious. But could men be infected by their female partners, and thereby become carriers of HPV? This study examined the prevalence of HPV DNA in men whose female partners did or did not have HPV infection in an area with a high risk (Colombia) and a low risk (Spain) for cervical cancer.

Methods.—The study included current husbands of 388 women with cervical cancer (cervical intraepithelial neoplasia stage III or with in situ and invasive carcinoma) and 428 current husbands of age-matched controls without cervical cancer. All enrollees provided serum samples and either penile cell or cervical cell samples. All penile and cervical cell samples were analyzed by the ViraPap test, and most (95%) were also analyzed by polymerase chain reaction to identify cellular HPV DNA.

Findings.—β-Globin or HPV DNA was found in 595 of the 816 penile cell samples (77%). The ViraPap test did not reveal differences between HPV DNA prevalences of husband-wife pairs in either country, nor according to husband-case vs. husband-control pairs. Analysis by polymerase chain reaction, however, revealed that HPV DNA prevalences were higher in husbands of cases than in husbands of controls. This prevalence was significantly higher in Spain (17.5% in husbands of cases vs. 3.5% in husbands of controls) but did not achieve statistical significance in Colombia (25.7% vs. 18.9%, respectively). HPV DNA prevalences were 5 times higher in Colombia than in Spain for husbands of controls (18.9% vs. 3.5%, respectively; $p = 0.0001$) and were also slightly higher for husbands of cases (25.5% vs. 17.5%, respectively). Husband-case pairs in which both partners had HPV DNA were more predominant in Colombia (4.9%) than in Spain (0.9%). In Spain, a significant association was seen between the prevalence of HPV DNA and at-risk sexual behavior–related characteristics of the couple. In both countries, husbands of nonmonogamous women had more penile HPV DNA than husbands of monogamous women.

Conclusions.—HPV DNA was found in husbands of controls in both countries (18.9% in Colombia vs. 3.5% in Spain); this 5-fold-higher background male infection rate in Colombia likely helps explain why Colombian women have an 8-fold increased risk of cervical cancer compared with Spanish women. Sexual promiscuity was strongly associated with an increased risk for penile HPV infections in both countries, and was the most important risk factor for penile HPV infection.

▶ A higher incidence of penile HPV DNA is consistent with the higher incidence of cervical cancer. Sexual promiscuity appears to be the most important risk factor for penile HPV infection and cervical carcinogenesis in female sex partners. HPV is associated with male genital malignancy, and there may be an increased incidence of cervical cancer in spouses of men with genital squamous-cell cancer.[1] Partners of men with HPV need to be screened for cervical malignancy on a regular basis.

D.E. Coplen, M.D.

Reference

1. Iverson T, Tretli S, Johansen A, et al: Squamous cell carcinoma of the penis and of the cervix, vulva and vagina in spouses: Is there any relationship? An epidemiological study from Norway, 1960–92. *Br J Cancer* 76:658–660, 1997.

3 Genitourinary Trauma

Preservation of Renal Function After Reconstruction for Trauma: Quantitative Assessment With Radionuclide Scintigraphy
Wessells H, Deirmenjian J, McAninch JW (Univ of California, San Francisco; San Francisco Gen Hosp)
J Urol 157:1583–1586, 1997   3–1

Introduction.—Many patients with major renal injuries can be treated successfully with reconstruction rather than total nephrectomy. At the study institution, an attempt is made to preserve enough renal parenchyma to prevent the need for dialysis should the contralateral renal unit ever be lost. A review of the records of patients who underwent renal reconstruction for trauma sought to quantify the effectiveness of reconstruction in preserving renal function.

Methods.—Between 1977 and 1995, 283 of 2,935 patients with traumatic renal injuries underwent renal reconstruction at San Francisco General Hospital. In 52 cases, radionuclide renal scintigraphy was performed postoperatively. Records of these 52 patients were reviewed for mechanism of injury, blood pressure and heart rate at admission, associated injuries, severity of injury, nature of renal reconstruction, operative variables, and outcome. Preservation of renal function was judged adequate if more than one third of the injured kidney was preserved (25% differential function). Reconstructed kidneys with 25% function or less were considered to have inadequate preservation.

Results.—The patient group had a mean age of 29 years and a mean of 2.33 associated injuries per patient. Penetrating injuries were present in 75%, 62% were in shock at admission, and 21% had vascular injuries. Renal scans were performed at a mean of 11.4 days after reconstruction. Mean renal function on the reconstructed side was 39.3%. Preservation of function was adequate in 42 patients (81%); 10 were considered to have inadequate preservation. The most significant patient variable influencing preservation was transfusion requirement. Renovascular injury and severe concomitant injuries with shock and extensive blood loss were also associated with poor preservation of functioning renal parenchyma.

Conclusion.—Radionuclide renal scintigraphy confirmed that a high rate of adequate renal preservation (81%) can be achieved in patients undergoing reconstruction after major blunt or penetrating trauma. Renal reconstruction is, thus, an appropriate method of treating major renal trauma.

▶ The authors of this article have had extensive experience with traumatic renal injuries. This is the first quantitative documentation of the success of renal reconstruction in the trauma setting. The authors' data suggest that, when feasible, renal reconstruction should be aggressively pursued.

D.A. Goldfarb, M.D.

Method of Urinary Diversion in Nonurethral Traumatic Bladder Injuries: Retrospective Analysis of 70 Cases

Thomae KR, Kilambi NK, Poole GV (Univ of Mississippi, Jackson)
Am Surg 64:77–81, 1998   3–2

Introduction.—Traumatologists, general surgeons, and urologists continue to debate the management of penetrating or blunt traumatic bladder injuries, whether intraperitoneal or extraperitoneal. Depending on the physician's training, diversion is achieved either by a suprapubic catheter or by a simple transurethral Foley catheter. A review of patients who had penetrating or blunt nonurethral bladder injuries was conducted to determine management options and morbidity.

Methods.—There were 70 patients with bladder injuries who were reviewed to determine whether a suprapubic catheter or a transurethral Foley catheter was more effective in terms of mechanism, degree, treatment, and morbidity of injury. Forty patients (57%) were diagnosed with blunt trauma with either a cystogram (55%), a CT scan alone (15%), or by exploration (30%). A transurethral catheter was used to treat 22 patients (55%) nonoperatively for extraperitoneal extravasation or partial bladder wall laceration. There were 30 patients (43%) who had gunshot wounds, and all but 1 of these patients had a celiotomy and bladder repair. Three blunt trauma patients had suprapubic catheters placed. Seventeen patients who had sustained penetrating trauma had a suprapubic catheter placed intraoperatively. A suprapubic catheter was not used for 50 patients; 27 of these patients had repair with transurethral catheter; and 23 had transurethral catheter alone.

Results.—In the suprapubic group, all bladder or urethral morbidity occurred with 3 strictures, 2 urinary retentions, 1 suprapubic infection, and 1 urinary infection. With or without a suprapubic catheter, degree of bladder injury was the same. Patients treated with transurethral catheters alone had no urethral strictures, urinary tract infections, or retention in isolated bladder injuries. The average suprapubic catheter duration was 42 days and the average transurethral catheter duration was 13 days.

Conclusion.—For management of blunt or penetrating bladder trauma, transurethral catheters are effective, cause fewer strictures and less morbidity, and may be removed more rapidly than suprapubic catheters for any degree of bladder injury.

▶ A suprapubic tube is not required after repair of a traumatic bladder injury. Concerns about adequate bladder drainage, clot occlusion of smaller caliber catheters, and increased patient morbidity are not justified, based upon the results of this retrospective review. The bladder should be repaired in a hemostatic, watertight fashion. The first layer should be a running, inverting closure, and the second layer may be running or interrupted.

D.E. Coplen, M.D.

Burns to the Genitalia and the Perineum

Michielsen D, Van Hee R, Neetens C, et al (Academic Surgical Centre Stuivenberg, Antwerp, Belgium)

J Urol 159:418–419, 1998

3–3

Background.—Perineal or genital burns, usually part of large surface injuries, are of major concern to patients and clinicians. In the current patient review, healing and complications of such burns were assessed.

Methods.—The records of 4,216 patients treated at one burn center between 1981 and 1995 were reviewed. One hundred seventeen patients, aged 6 months to 86 years, had associated burns to the perineum or genitalia. Eighty-seven were male. The average burn size was 21% of total body surface area. Burns were caused by scalding in 55% of the patients, flame in 24%, and chemicals in 16%.

Findings.—Sixteen patients (13.6%) died. None of the deaths were caused by the perineal or genital burns. Forty-one percent of the 101 survivors needed Foley catheters. However, these catheters were indwelling only during resuscitation, required for 1 to 99 days. Topical antimicrobial agents were used to treat perineal and genital burns. Only 9.9% of the patients needed split-thickness grafts. Late complications included scar formation of the penile shaft and prepuce in 2 patients. These complications were treated with multiple Z-plasties and circumcision, respectively. One patient presented with erectile dysfunction, but the diagnostic assessment was negative.

Conclusions.—Conservative treatment with topical agents is recommended for perineal and genital burns. Surgery is rarely indicated. The most common complication is contracture, which should be treated with plastic surgery.

▶ Burns to the genitalia and perineum should be managed conservatively without radical debridement. A catheter is required only if the patient is having difficulty voiding or if it is required during resuscitation. Suprapubic tubes were not required in this series, but in situations where there is full thickness injury to the phallus it may be advantageous. When skin grafting is required, non-meshed full thickness grafts are best on the phallus and meshed grafts can be used on the scrotum.

D.E. Coplen, M.D.

4 Calculus Disease

Ureteral Stones Clinical Guidelines Panel Summary Report on the Management of Ureteral Calculi
Segura JW, Preminger GM, Assimos DG, et al
J Urol 158:1915–1921, 1997   4–1

Background.—Technological and technical advances have greatly increased the options for management of ureteral calculi in recent years. This has led to many questions regarding the best treatment choices, based on such factors as stone size, location, and composition. The Ureteral Stones Clinical Guidelines Panel of the American Urological Association was charged with the development of evidence-based recommendations for clinical practice. The panel's report was summarized.

Methods.—The panel performed a literature search to identify all studies of ureteral stones published from 1966 to 1996. Three hundred twenty-seven articles with acceptable outcomes data were found, and the outcomes data were extracted using a comprehensive form. The Confidence Profile Method was then used for meta-analysis to create outcome estimates for the various alternative treatments for ureteral calculi. The recommendations were based mainly on outcomes-based evidence and partially on the expert opinions of the panel members.

Results.—The results suggested that as many as 98% of stones measuring less than 0.5 cm in diameter will pass spontaneously. This is particularly true for stones located in the distal ureter. For stones up to 1 cm in size that are located in the proximal ureter, shock wave lithotripsy is preferred as first-line therapy. For stones of this size located in the distal ureter, either shock wave lithotripsy or ureteroscopy can be used. The evidence does not support the use of traditional blind basket extraction, without fluoroscopic control and guide wires. When other treatments fail or in certain unusual circumstances, open surgery is still an option.

Conclusion.—Most ureteral calculi will pass spontaneously; for calculi that do not, other treatment options are available. The recommendations must be interpreted in the light of varying practice patterns. Three main areas for future research include stone prevention, a uniform system for stone reporting, and predictability of stone response to shock wave lithotripsy.

▶ Management options for ureteral calculi include observation, extracorporeal shock-wave lithotripsy (ESWL), and endoscopic manipulations. Review of the literature shows that up to 98% of calculi smaller than 5 mm will pass spontaneously. Given the high success rates with ESWL and ureteroscopy, open surgery is not the first-line treatment, except in unusual cases. Extracorporeal shock-wave lithotripsy is recommended for proximal ureteral calculi, and there is no evidence that an indwelling stent increases the chance of the patient being stone-free. Ureteroscopy and ESWL are equally effective in the management of distal ureteral stones, and each has its advantages and disadvantages. Blind stone-basketing without fluoroscopy or direct stone visualization should be avoided. Cost factors, available endoscopic equipment, and patient preference influence the treatment decision regarding distal calculi.

D.E. Coplen, M.D.

Ureteroscopic Management of Ureteral Calculi: Electrohydraulic Versus Holmium:YAG Lithotripsy

Teichman JMH, Rao RD, Rogenes VJ, et al (Univ of Texas, San Antonio)
J Urol 158:1357–1361, 1997   4–2

Background.—Both electrohydraulic lithotripsy and holmium:YAG lithotripsy have been used to manage ureteral calculi. Electrohydraulic lithotripsy is generally cheaper, but it may fail to fragment all stones, cause mucosal injury, and even propel stones further into the ureter. Holmium:YAG lithotripsy fragments stones regardless of their composition and it rarely propels stones in a retrograde fashion, but it can cause thermal injury to soft tissue. With these advantages and disadvantages in mind, these authors compared the efficacy of these 2 modalities in the treatment of ureteral calculi.

Methods.—Patients with ureteral calculi too large for basketing were treated with electrohydraulic lithotripsy (n = 23) or holmium:YAG lithotripsy (n = 47). Standard techniques were used. Electrohydraulic lithotripsy involved a 1.9F fiber with an initial energy setting of 50 V, increasing to 100 V as needed. Holmium:YAG lithotripsy involved a 365 µm end-firing fiber with power output ranging between 1 and 60 W (0.6 to 1.5 J). Patients were followed for 3 months with imaging studies to ensure successful treatment.

Findings.—Patients undergoing the holmium:YAG procedure were significantly more likely than those undergoing electrohydraulic lithotripsy to be stone free both immediately after the procedure (44 of 47, or 94%, vs. 13 of 23, or 56%, respectively) and at 3 months of follow up (46 of 47, or 98%, vs. 20 of 23, or 87%, respectively). Overall operative time (105 minutes) or the mean stone size (11 or 14 cm) did not differ significantly between the 2 groups. However, when the groups were further subdivided into those with stones smaller than 15 mm and those with stones 15 mm or larger, significant differences between the 2 techniques were found (Table 3). For stones smaller than 15 mm, electrohydraulic lithotripsy had a significantly shorter operative time (72 vs. 102 minutes) and an improved

TABLE 3.—Patients With Ureteral Calculi < 15 mm and ≥ 15 mm

	Electrohydraulic Lithotripsy	Holmium: YAG Laser	p Value
	Less than 15 mm.		
No. pts.	17	32	
Mean stone size ± SD (mm.)	9 ± 3	12 ± 4	0.2
No. stones impacted (%)	3 (18)	7 (22)	0.9
Mean operative time ± SD (mins.)	72 ± 21	102 ± 38	0.004
No. pts. stone-free (%):			
At end of ureteroscopy	11 (65)	31 (97)	0.001
3 Mos. after ureteroscopy	16 (94)	31 (97)	0.3
	15 Mm. or greater		
No. pts.	6	15	
Mean stone size ± SD (mm.)	19 ± 5	19 ± 4	0.9
No. stones impacted (%)	6 (100)	15 (100)	1.0
Mean operative time ± SD (mins.)	159 ± 61	108 ± 27	0.01
No. pts. stone-free (%):			
At end of ureteroscopy	2 (33)	13 (87)	0.001
3 Mos. after ureteroscopy	4 (67)	15 (100)	0.02

(Courtesy of Teichman JMH, Rao RD, Rogenes VJ, et al: Ureteroscopic management of ureteral calculi: electrohydraulic versus holmium:YAG lithotripsy. *J Urol* 158:1357–1361, 1997.)

stone-free rate at 3 months (94% vs. 97%, nonsignificant difference). For stones 15 mm or larger, holmium:YAG lithotripsy had a significantly shorter operative time (108 vs. 158 minutes) and maintained its significant advantages in stone-free status immediately and after 3 months. Each group experienced 3 complications, consisting of a proximal ureteral calculus, gross extravasation, propulsion of a stone fragment into the lower pole, and fever.

Conclusions.—Holmium:YAG lithotripsy was substantially superior to electrohydraulic lithotripsy in most instances. However, when the stones were smaller than 15 mm, electrohydraulic lithotripsy did require a significantly shorter operative time yet provided good stone-free status at 3 months. The fact that these procedures involve different lithotripsy mechanisms (electrohydraulic lithotripsy fragments calculi via a cavitation bubble, and holmium:YAG lithotripsy vaporizes calculi) may account for the differences in results.

▶ The holmium:YAG laser vaporizes stones and does take longer to "fragment" stones. Since it is the most powerful device available and effectively treats even cystine and calcium oxalate monohydrate calculi, fragmentation occurs nearly 100% of the time and the smaller dust is more easily passed, resulting in a higher stone-free rate. This is a nonrandomized comparison of electrohydraulic lithotripsy and the holmium laser that shows safety and efficacy of the holmium laser. There is a significant capital cost associated with the laser, but it is completely portable so sharing of laser costs between multiple institutions is possible.

D.E. Coplen, M.D.

Complete Staghorn Calculi: Random Prospective Comparison Between Extracorporeal Shock Wave Lithotripsy Monotherapy and Combined With Percutaneous Nephrostolithotomy

Meretyk S, Gofrit ON, Gafni O, et al (Hadassah Med Ctr, Jerusalem, Israel)
J Urol 157:780–786, 1997

4–3

Introduction.—Four treatment modalities are available for the treatment of staghorn calculi: open surgery, percutaneous nephrostolithotomy, extracorporeal shock wave lithotripsy (ESWL), and the combination of percutaneous nephrostolithotomy and ESWL. Although ESWL is less invasive and less likely to require blood transfusions than other approaches, it does require multiple treatment sessions and has high complication and secondary unplanned procedure rates. Percutaneous nephrostolithotomy, alone or in combination with ESWL, is more invasive but offers a greater stone-free rate and is less likely to result in complications or require secondary unplanned procedures. A prospective, randomized study was conducted to compare these 2 approaches.

Methods.—Over a period of 3 years (1992–1994), 59 patients were treated for staghorn stones at the study institution. Calculi typically occupied the renal pelvis and at least 2 of 3 groups of calices. Eleven patients declined to be randomized or were ineligible, leaving 48 for analysis. Twenty-seven (group 1) were allocated to ESWL monotherapy and 23 (group 2) to initial percutaneous nephrostolithotomy with or without subsequent ESWL. The 2 groups were compared for number of required treatment sessions, narcotic doses, renal colic episodes, septic complications, unplanned ancillary procedures, length of hospitalization, total treatment duration, and stone-free rate at 6 months.

Results.—Treatment groups 1 and 2 were statistically similar in age, sex, stone dimensions, grade of collecting system dilation, and percentage with a positive urine culture at baseline. All stones treated were of large volume and complex configuration. At the conclusion of therapy, the stone-free rate was significantly higher in group 2 (74%) than in group 1 (22%). The residual stone load was also much greater in group 1. Whereas only 8% in group 2 had a residual stone load greater than 16 mm, 50% of group 1 patients had a load of this extent. There were 15 episodes of septic complications in group 1, but only 2 in group 2. Patients in the ESWL monotherapy group had a significantly higher rate of unplanned ancillary procedures and a significantly longer duration of treatment (6 months vs. 1 month). The 2 groups did not differ significantly in days of hospitalization or in number of procedures with anesthesia.

Conclusion.—For patients with staghorn calculi, a combined percutaneous nephrostolithotomy and ESWL approach offers numerous advantages over ESWL monotherapy and should be considered the preferred treatment in most cases. The combined approach best meets the goal of treatment: to remove the stone safely and expeditiously.

▶ This prospective, randomized single institution study shows percutaneous treatment of staghorn calculi is clearly better than ESWL alone. If stones are not cleared, infection persists and stone regrowth occurs. While ESWL is appealing in this situation, it ultimately is a much more expensive approach because of the very low stone-free rate (20% to 30%).

D.E. Coplen, M.D.

Holmium:Yttrium-Aluminum-Garnet Laser Cystolithotripsy of Large Bladder Calculi

Teichman JMH, Rogenes VJ, McIver BJ, et al (Univ of Texas Health Science Ctr, San Antonio)
Urology 50:44–48, 1997   4–4

Introduction.—A number of treatment modalities are available for patients with a large (4 cm or greater) bladder calculus. These calculi are hard to fragment, whether the approach is extracorporeal shock wave-lithotripsy, cystolithotripsy with electrohydraulic lithotripsy, cystolithotripsy with ultrasonic lithotripsy, or open cystolithotomy. Each of these modalities has both advantages and disadvantages. Fourteen patients underwent holmium:yttrium-aluminum-garnet (YAG) laser cystolithotripsy for bladder calculi of 4 cm or larger.

Methods.—All patients were treated endoscopically, with the understanding that open cystolithotomy would be performed if laser lithotripsy were not feasible. The procedure was performed with the patient in the dorsal lithotomy position and under spinal or general anesthesia. Laser energy was delivered using either the 365-μm end-firing fiber or the 550-μm side-firing fiber. Holmium energy settings were started at 0.6 J with a frequency of 6 Hz, then raised in increments up to a maximum of 1.4 J at a frequency of 15 Hz if needed to achieve fragmentation. Completeness of stone removal was determined by the absence of bladder calculus endoscopically and on postoperative kidney-ureter-bladder film.

Results.—The average patient age was 46; average stone size was 6 cm. Median anesthesia time was 57 minutes and median total energy required was 8.7 kJ. A single endoscopic procedure was sufficient for complete stone fragmentation and removal in all 14 patients. Stone fragmentation was achieved in 11 patients at a maximum energy setting of 1.0 J or less. Ten patients voided by the first postoperative day. Trauma to the bladder mucosa and hematuria were minimal in all cases. Twelve of 14 patients were discharged by postoperative day 1. One patient required a 4-day stay for percutaneous nephrostomy management and another, with a 15-cm stone, was hospitalized 3 days because of the lengthy duration (5.5 hours) of anesthesia.

Conclusion.—Holmium:YAG cystolithotripsy proved safe and effective for the removal of large bladder calculi. The procedure is considered technically simple and may spare patients the morbidity of open cystolithotomy. The 550-µm side-firing fiber may be more efficient than the 365-µm end-firing fiber for larger calculi.

▶ Bladder calculi are typically extremely hard and difficult to fragment. Electrohydraulic lithotripsy has low power and often results in large fragments that are difficult to "chase down" and remove. The ultrasonic lithotripsy probe is much more efficient but the probe is large and often necessitates percutaneous bladder access. The holmium:yttrium-aluminum-garnet laser causes an efficient vaporization or powdered fragmentation that is likely the result of a thermal lithotripsy mechanism. Whether this dust can be completely evacuated from an augmented bladder so that the patient is truly stone-free is doubtful. There is still a role for open cystotomy, as evidenced by the 7-hour laser session for the largest stone in this study.

D.E. Coplen, M.D.

Crystalluria and Urinary Tract Abnormalities Associated With Indinavir
Kopp JB, Miller KD, Mican JM, et al (Natl Inst of Diabetes and Digestive and Kidney Diseases, Bethesda, Md; Warren Grant Magnuson Clinical Ctr, Bethesda, Md; Natl Inst of Allergy and Infectious Diseases, Bethesda, Md)
Ann Intern Med 127:119–125, 1997   4–5

Background.—The protease inhibitor indinavir has become the most widely prescribed antiretroviral agent in the United States. It carries a 4% incidence of nephrolithiasis. The authors recently observed the appearance of distinctive urinary crystals in their patients taking indinavir, along with urinary tract symptoms. Patients receiving indinavir were studied to determine the makeup of the urinary crystals, the frequency of asymptomatic crystalluria, and the incidence of urinary tract symptoms.

Methods.—Participants included 240 adult patients who received indinavir in the course of clinical trials of HIV infection conducted at the NIH. The patients had received indinavir for a mean of 30 weeks, at a maximum dose of 2,400 mg/day in 3 or 4 divided doses. Urinalysis was performed in a subgroup of 142 patients without symptoms to determine the incidence of crystalluria. The urinary crystals and stones were evaluated by high-performance liquid chromatography (HPLC) and mass spectrometry. Patients with urologic symptoms underwent clinical evaluation.

Results.—Twenty percent of asymptomatic patients were found to have distinctive crystals on urinalysis, consisting of platelike rectangles and fan-shaped or starburst forms (Fig 4). The indinavir composition of these crystals was confirmed by mass spectrometry and HPLC. None of 40 patients who were not taking indinavir had similar crystals. The incidence of urologic symptoms in the overall study group was 8%, including a 3% incidence of nephrolithiasis. The remaining 5% of patients had crystalluria associated with dysuria or with back or flank pain. Four patients with this previously undescribed syndrome showed radiographic signs of intrarenal sludging.

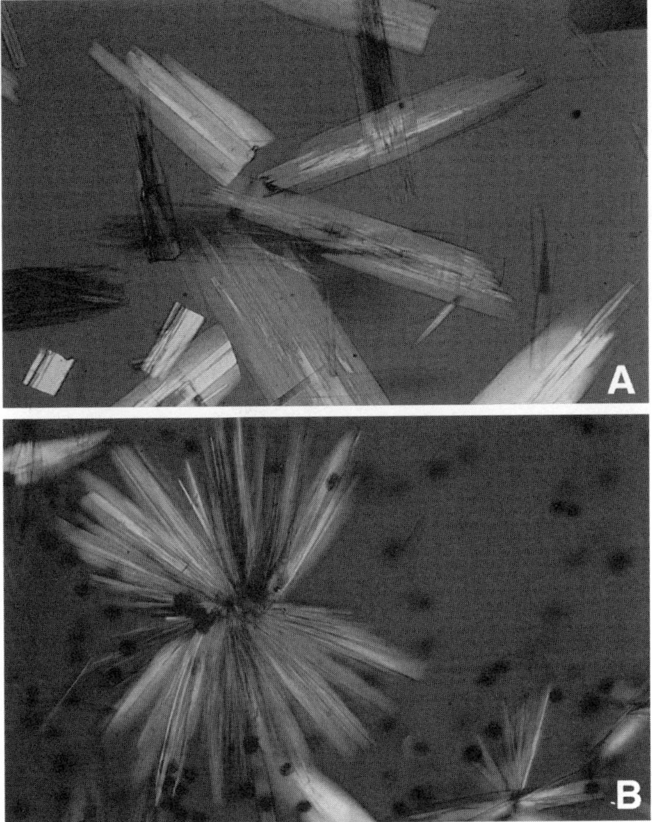

FIGURE 4.—Microscopic appearance of indinavir crystals. Crossed polarizing filters and a lambda wave plate produce variation in the color of the crystals and background as one filter is rotated. **A,** irregular plate forms (×40) in urine from an asymptomatic patient. **B,** starburst forms (×80) in urine from an asymptomatic patient. (Courtesy of Kopp JB, Miller KD, Mican JM, et al: Crystalluria and urinary tract abnormalities associated with indinavir. *Ann Intern Med* 127:119–125, 1997.)

Conclusions.—Patients taking indinavir may have characteristic crystals present in their urine. Indinavir crystalluria is linked to a spectrum of urologic findings, including dysuria and urinary frequency, dysuria with flank or back pain and intrarenal sludging, or classic renal colic. When patients taking indinavir have urologic symptoms, they can generally be treated with hydration and drug withdrawal. Later, indinavir therapy may be restarted.

▶ Indinavir is an inhibitor of the HIV protease required for cleavage of the precursor viral polypeptides into functional proteins. In treated patients, viral particles are non-infectious. Up to 20% of patients treated with the drug have crystalluria (Fig 4, A and B), and half of these have dysuria, urinary frequency, hematuria, or back or flank pain. Colic may be related to stone formation or to intrarenal sludge. Indinavir is poorly soluble in aqueous solutions and is admixed with H_2SO_4 to improve gastrointestinal absorption. Hydration and urinary acidification are recommended, although the in vitro pH of 4.5 cannot be achieved in vivo. In acute situations, the medication should be stopped for 2–3 days and the patients should be treated symptomatically.

D.E. Coplen, M.D.

5 Endourology

Endopyelotomy for Primary Ureteropelvic Junction Obstruction: Risk Factors Determine the Success Rate
Danuser H, Ackermann DK, Böhlen D, et al (Univ of Berne, Switzerland)
J Urol 159:56–61, 1998   5–1

Introduction.—The classic surgical treatment for primary ureteropelvic junction obstruction has been open pyeloplasty. Endopyelotomy was the next logical step for minimally invasive treatment of ureteropelvic junction obstruction after the successful introduction of percutaneous stone surgery. For primary ureteropelvic junction obstruction, the feasibility, complications, and short-term and long-term results of endopyelotomy were prospectively assessed.

Methods.—Excretory urogram or nephrostomogram, retrograde pyelography, diuresis renography, and Whitaker test were used to diagnose primary ureteropelvic junction obstruction in 80 consecutive patients. A cold knife was used to perform antegrade endopyelotomy in all patients, and for 6 weeks an indwelling stent was left. An excretory urogram and/or diuretic renography, questionnaire, and ultrasound were used to assess the results at 6 and 24 months postoperatively.

Results.—After the first endopyelotomy, the primary success rate was 89%, and increased to 91% after 2 patients had a second endopyelotomy. Six of the 73 initially successfully treated patients had relapse after a median follow-up of 26 months. There was then an overall success rate of 81% after 2 were successfully retreated by a second endopyelotomy, and the rate increased to 86% after a second endopyelotomy was performed in 4 patients. Six months after endopyelotomy, mean preoperative pyelocaliceal volume decreased from 64 to 41 mL, and remained unchanged during the following 18 months. In patients with a preoperative pyelocaliceal volume of less than 50 mL (87%), the probability of successful endopyelotomy was better. In patients with a volume greater than 50 mL, the probability of successful endopyelotomy was worse (76%). In 6 of 10 patients retreated by open pyeloplasty or nephrectomy, a crossing vessel to the lower pole of the kidney causing persistent functional obstruction of the ureteropelvic junction was found. In patients with failed nephrotomy, preoperative mean renal function as determined by diuretic renography was significantly lower than in successfully treated patients. There was no

27

change in renal function 6 and 24 months postoperatively in successfully treated patients.

Conclusions.—Having a high primary success rate and a low relapse rate, endopyelotomy in primary ureteropelvic junction obstruction is a safe, minimally invasive procedure. In 86% of patients, open pyeloplasty could be avoided. Pyeloplasty is more invasive and has more functional and aesthetic sequelae than endopyelotomy, which does not compromise open surgery if that becomes necessary. As a first-line treatment for patients with primary ureteropelvic junction obstruction, endopyelotomy is recommended.

▶ Endopyelotomy is a successful treatment of ureteropelvic junction (UPJ) obstruction in 80% to 90% of patients. Risk factors for failure are felt to be a redundant pyelocaliceal system that precludes a postoperative-dependent funneled UPJ, poor preoperative renal function (decreased urine flow influences healing and scarring?), and a lower-pole crossing vessel. In this series, endoscopy of failed endopyelotomies with crossing vessels revealed no intrinsic narrowing but persistent extrinsic compression. However, Nakada and associates show that endopyelotomy is successful in the presence of a crossing vessel in 40% of cases, and conclude that preoperative evaluation for the vessel (angiography, spiral CT, or endoluminal ultrasound) is not required.[1] Should endopyelotomy be applied indiscriminately in all adults with UPJ obstruction? This is an unanswered question. Open pyeloplasty after endopyelotomy is reportedly not more difficult, and the endopyelotomy with a crossing vessel is not associated with a higher risk of bleeding and transfusion.

D.E. Coplen, M.D.

Reference

1. Nakada SY, Wolf JS, Brink JA, et al: Retrospective analysis of the effect of crossing vessels on successful retrograde endopyelotomy outcomes using spiral computerized tomography angiography. *J Urol* 159:62–65, 1998.

Open Surgical Exploration After Failed Endopyelotomy: A 12-Year Perspective

Gupta M, Tuncay OL, Smith AD (Long Island Jewish Med Ctr, New Hyde Park, NY)
J Urol 157:1613–1619, 1997

5–2

Introduction.—Endopyelotomy failure is fairly common, but the factors leading to failure of this procedure have not been evaluated fully. A retrospective analysis of 401 percutaneous antegrade endopyelotomies was conducted to determine the importance of renal function, hydronephrosis, ureteral stents, surgeon experience, and crossing vessels on patient outcome.

TABLE 1.—Type of Stent, Degree of Hydronephrosis and Preoperative Renal Function in Relation to Outcome of Endopyelotomy

	No. Pts. (%)		
	Success	Failure	% Success Rate
Stent type:			
Universal (Smith)	66 (19)	8 (13)	89
Repeat nephrostomy tube	7 (2)	3 (5)	70
Endopyelotomy	268 (79)	49 (82)	85
Totals	341	60	85
Preop. hydronephrosis grade:			
4 (massive)	11 (4)	11 (20)	50
3 (severe)	151 (50)	37 (69)	80
2 (moderate)	138 (46)	6 (11)	96
1 (mild)	0 (0)	0	—
0 (none)	0 (0)	0	—
Insufficient information	41	6	—
Totals	341	60	85
% Renal function:			
More than 40 (good)	145 (58)	13 (28)	92
25–40 (moderate)	99 (39)	25 (58)	80
Less than 25 (poor)	7 (3)	6 (14)	54
Insufficient information	90	16	—
Totals	341	60	85

(Courtesy of Gupta M, Tuncay OL, Smith AD: Open surgical exploration after failed endopyelotomy: a 12-year perspective. *J Urol* 157:1613–1619, 1997.)

Methods.—The procedures were performed on 393 patients with uteropelvic junction obstruction. Percutaneous endopyelotomy failed in 60 patients, for an overall success rate of 85.0%. Outcome was considered successful if the patient was completely asymptomatic after at least 6 months of follow-up and exhibited significant improvement in the flow of contrast medium from the renal pelvis through the ureter on excretory urography. Those whose surgery failed were considered for open exploration and underwent nuclear scintigraphy to assess renal failure.

Results.—The average patient age at endopyelotomy was 41. Success rates were similar for male and female patients, but patients with primary ureteropelvic junction obstruction had a lower success rate (82%) than those with secondary obstruction (89%). There was a highly statistically significant correlation between degree of hydronephrosis and likelihood of failure. Success rates were 96% for patients with grade 20 (moderate) hydronephrosis, but only 50% for those with grade 40 (massive). Poor preoperative renal function had a similar influence (Table 1) on the success rate of endopyelotomy. The most common findings at exploration in 54 patients with endopyelotomy failure were extrinsic fibrosis (37%), intrinsic fibrosis (31%), and an obstructive crossing vessel (24%). Surgeon experience did not appear to affect the rate of success.

Conclusion.—Endopyelotomy is more likely to fail in patients with high grade nephrosis and poor preoperative renal function. The role of crossing vessels on outcome is less than previously thought.

▶ Endopyelotomy is now the initial procedure of choice in adult ureteropelvic junction (UPJ) obstruction. However, the success rate remains approximately 10% less than that reported in most series of dismembered pyeloplasties and has not changed appreciably as surgeons get more experience with the procedure. Seventy-five percent of failures occurred in the first 3 months. Fibrosis was the cause of failure in nearly 70% of cases and a crossing vessel was the cause of failure in only 25% of cases. Open exploration and UPJ repair after failed endopyelotomy is not associated with increased morbidity and has a 92% success rate.

D.E. Coplen, M.D.

Long-term Results of Endoureterotomy for Benign Ureteral and Ureteroenteric Strictures

Wolf JS Jr, Elashry OM, Clayman RV (Univ of Michigan, Ann Arbor; Tanta Univ, Egypt; Washington Univ, St Louis)
J Urol 158:759–764, 1997

5–3

Introduction.—Benign ureteral strictures and ureteroenteric strictures can be treated through endoscopic ureteral incisions, or endoureterotomy. However, there have been few studies of the long-term results or prognostic factors after endoureterotomy. The results of endoureterotomy for benign ureteral and ureteroenteric strictures were reviewed, including prognostic and treatment factors associated with a good outcome.

Methods.—The retrospective study included 77 endoureterotomies performed in 69 patients. All procedures were performed to treat benign intrinsic ureteral obstruction, excluding those located at the ureteropelvic junction. The success of the procedures was judged according to symptomatic improvement and radiographic resolution of the obstruction. Survival curves were constructed according to the Kaplan-Meier method, and prognostic factors were evaluated with a Cox proportional hazards model.

Results.—In 9 cases, the ipsilateral kidney accounted for <25% of total renal function; none of these procedures was successful. This left 38 benign ureteral strictures in 36 patients and 30 ureteroenteric strictures in 25 patients. Median follow-up in successful cases was 28 and 13 months, respectively. In the benign ureteral strictures, the 3-year success rate was 80% (Fig 1). There were no treatment failures after 11 months, with 25 patients at risk beyond this point. For the patients with ureteroenteric strictures, success rate was 73% at 1 year, 51% at 2 years, and 32% at 3 years (Fig 2). There were no treatment failures after 3 years, with 5 patients at risk beyond this point. Treatment was generally less successful for complete or tight strictures. In strictures longer than 1 cm, factors associated with a better outcome included nonischemic cause, stent size

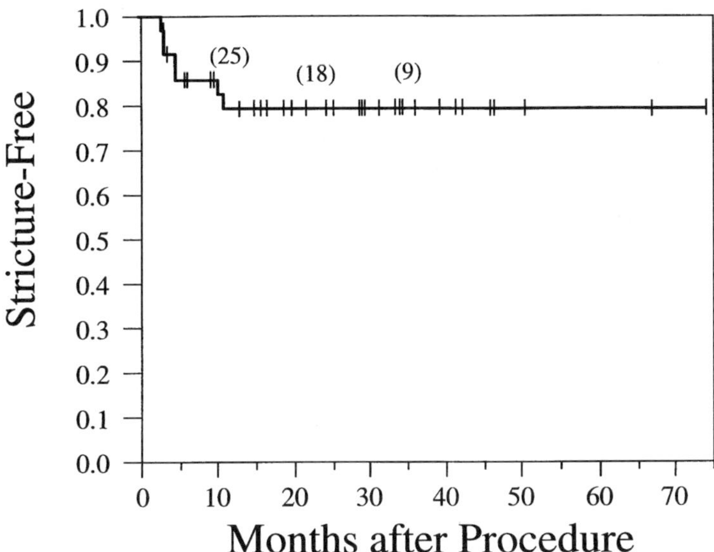

FIGURE 1.—Kaplan-Meier curve illustrates success rate of endoureterotomy for benign ureteral strictures. *Crosshatches* indicate censored procedures (obstruction not present at last follow-up). Figures in parentheses indicate number of patients at risk at 1, 2, and 3 years. (Courtesy of Wolf JS Jr, Elashry OM, Clayman RV: Long-term results of endoureterotomy for benign ureteral and ureteroenteric strictures. *J Urol* 158:759–764, 1997.)

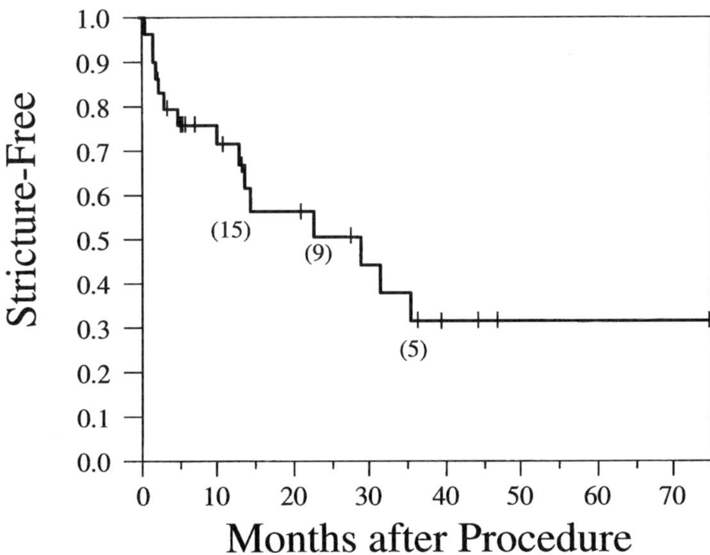

FIGURE 2.—Kaplan-Meier curve illustrates success rate of endoureterotomy for ureteroenteric strictures. *Crosshatches* indicate censored procedures (obstruction not present at last follow-up). Figures in parentheses indicate number of patients at risk at 1, 2, and 3 years. (Courtesy of Wolf JS Jr, Elashry OM, Clayman RV: Long-term results of endoureterotomy for benign ureteral and ureteroenteric strictures. *J Urol* 158:759–764, 1997.)

12F or larger, and triamcinolone injection into the bed of the incised stricture.

Conclusions.—Endoureterotomy offers excellent results in benign ureteral strictures. The results are not so good for ureteroenteric strictures, though the procedure is still a reasonable first step. Endoureterotomy is unlikely to give good results if renal function on the affected side is poor. Use of a stent 12F or larger and injecting triamcinolone appear to be associated with better results in strictures longer than 1 cm.

▶ Endoscopic management of short ureteral strictures has the same success rate (80%) as endopyelotomy for ureteropelvic junction obstruction. Whether the injection of steroids in the stricture bed is important cannot be determined from the paper, although it would appear that in longer strictures (more fibrosis?) it may be beneficial. Long-term success in ureteroenteric strictures is only 32%, probably because of the ischemic nature of all these strictures. In the younger patient with a long ureteroenteric stricture, open reconstruction should be utilized, while an older or poor-risk patient should probably have an indwelling stent after opening the narrowing.

D.E. Coplen, M.D.

Ureterorenoscopic Approach to the Symptomatic Caliceal Diverticulum

Batter SJ, Dretler SP (Massachusetts Gen Hosp, Boston)
J Urol 158:709–713, 1997   5–4

Background.—Methods that have been used to treat symptomatic caliceal diverticula include open surgery, a percutaneous approach, shock wave lithotripsy, and ureterorenoscopy. These authors report their experience over a 6-year period with ureterorenoscopy.

Methods.—Ureterorenoscopy was used to treat symptomatic caliceal diverticula in 26 patients (20 women, 6 men) 20 to 60 years old (mean 40 years). Symptoms included flank pain (81%), recurrent urinary tract infection (54%), pyelonephritis (12%), and urosepsis (8%). The abnormality included an upper caliceal diverticulum in 14 patients, a middle one in 5 patients, and a lower one in 7 patients. The procedure involved a retrograde approach in which the flexible ureteroscope was advanced into the diverticular cavity to dilate the neck of the diverticulum and to deliver pulsed-dye laser or electrohydraulic lithotripsy when needed.

Findings.—Operative time ranged from 1.25 to 4 hours. Success rates were better for upper and middle caliceal diverticuli (16 of 19 patients, or 84%) and worse for lower caliceal diverticuli (2 of 7 patients, or 29%). Of the 18 diverticuli that were successfully entered (70% of total), stones were completely removed in 15 patients (83%), while additional shock wave lithotripsy was needed for removal of stones in the other 3 patients. The procedure was performed on an outpatient basis in 13 of 26 patients (50%); 10 patients (38%) required a 1-night hospital stay, and the other 3 needed 3, 7, and 10 days in the hospital because of bleeding, pain, or sepsis. At an average of 45 months of follow up (range 15 to 84 months), all 18 patients with a successful retrograde treatment were symptom free, and only 1 showed a residual fragment (embedded in the diverticular wall) that required further treatment (endoscopy).

Conclusions.—The ureterorenoscopic approach provided very good short- and long-term results with very limited morbidity, particularly for upper and middle caliceal diverticuli. In the 3 upper caliceal diverticuli that were not successfully treated, the main reason was that the calix came off the infundibulum at an angle that was too acute or the infundibulum was too narrow to allow the ureteroscope to flex. Lower caliceal diverticuli were more difficult to locate, and inserting a dilating balloon into the diverticular neck in this area was more difficult. This less invasive method, then, should be considered for patients with symptomatic upper or middle caliceal diverticuli.

▶ The treatment of caliceal diverticuli with calculi and/or recurrent infections no longer requires open surgery. A retrograde ureteroscopic approach can be used in upper and middle pole diverticuli. Lower pole diverticuli are harder to access in retrograde fashion and are best approached percutaneously.

D.E. Coplen, M.D.

Conservative Management of Colon Injury Following Percutaneous Renal Surgery
Gerspach JM, Bellman GC, Stoller ML, et al (Kaiser Permanente Med Ctr, Los Angeles; Good Samaritan Hosp, Los Angeles; Univ of California, San Francisco)
Urology 49:831–836, 1997   5–5

Objective.—Colon injury is a rare complication of renal surgery. However, when it occurs, it can be difficult to diagnose and can cause serious morbidity. This retrospective study sought to identify risk factors for colon injury during percutaneous renal surgery, to identify effective preventive measures, and to optimize the treatment approach to such injuries.

Methods.—The 5-year review included more than 1,000 percutaneous renal surgeries performed at 3 California kidney stone centers. Five cases associated with kidney injury were identified. These were analyzed, together with 13 additional reports from the literature.

Results.—The patients were 4 men and 1 woman with a mean age of 31 years. All were injured during percutaneous nephrolithotomy, and all of the injuries were extraperitoneal in nature. Body habitus was judged to be lean in 3 patients in average in the other 2. There were 3 left-sided and 2 right-sided kidney injuries. The colon injury was unrecognized until after

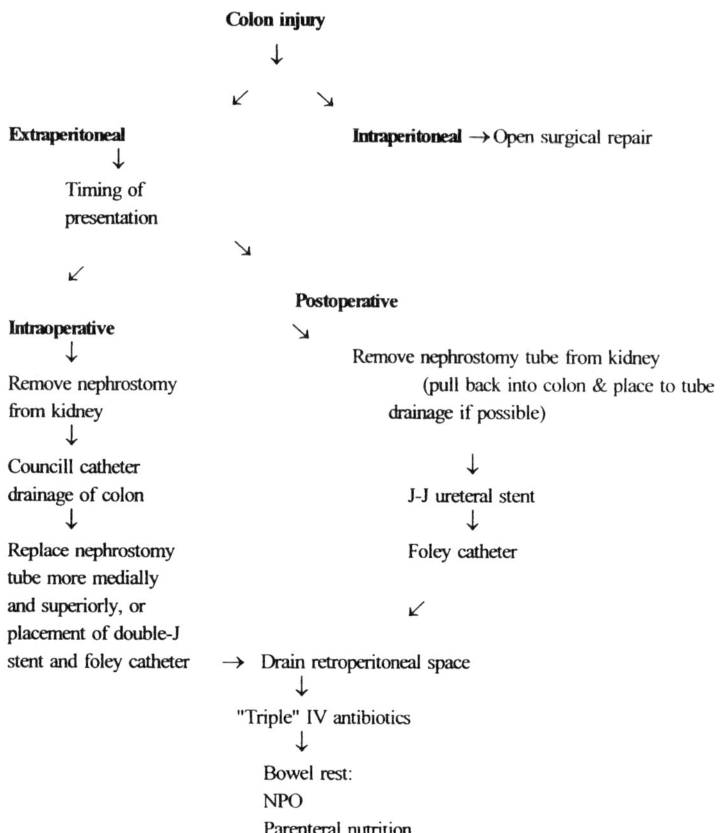

FIGURE 4.—Colon injuries related to percutaneous nephrostomy injuries. Algorithm for treatment. (Reprinted by permission of the publisher from Gerspach JM, Bellman GC, Stoller ML, et al: Conservative management of colon injury following percutaneous renal surgery. *Urology* 49:831–836, copyright 1997 by Elsevier Science, Inc.)

surgery in 4 patients. Clinical findings associated with the injuries included fever, fecaluria, abdominal pain, and leukocytosis. With prompt management, all patients recovered without adverse sequelae.

Conclusion.—Patients who appear to be at high risk of colon injuries during percutaneous renal surgery are young men of lean body habitus and with minimal retroperitoneal fat who are more likely to have colon located behind the kidney. The puncture should be made more superiorly and medially in such patients. With early recognition and drainage of the intestinal urinary and intestinal tracts, these injuries are easily managed. Based on their cases and reports from the literature, the authors presented an algorithm for the management of colon injuries related to percutaneous nephrostomy (Fig 4).

▶ The majority of colonic injuries will be retroperitoneal and, if identified early, can be managed nonoperatively. The symptoms may be nonspecific.

The incidence is very small (0.5% in this series) and can be decreased by avoiding a percutaneous approach lateral to the posterior axillary line and by using an upper pole approach when technically feasible.

D.E. Coplen, M.D.

Diagnosis and Management of Ureteroiliac Artery Fistula: Value of Provocative Arteriography Followed by Common Iliac Artery Embolization and Extraanatomic Arterial Bypass Grafting

Vandersteen DR, Saxon RR, Fuchs E, et al (Oregon Health Sciences Univ, Portland)

J Urol 158:754–758, 1997

5–6

Introduction.—Diagnosis of ureteroarterial fistula is difficult in the absence of active bleeding, and the reported mortality rate is high. A multidisciplinary approach resulted in salvage of all affected renal units and no deaths in 4 patients.

Patients and Methods.—The patients were 4 women aged 24–68 years. Three were referred for evaluation of gross hematuria, and 1 came to the emergency room with clot retention. All had previously been treated for intrapelvic cancer (osteosarcoma of the sacrum, endometrial carcinoma, or squamous cell carcinoma of the cervix) and had received pelvic irradiation. One patient had a second fistula 1 year after the first episode. The precipitating incident in 4 of the 5 fistulas was ureteral stent exchange. Diagnosis was established using standard and provocative arteriography (arteriography combined with ureteral manipulation). Lesions were then treated with percutaneous embolic occlusion of the common iliac artery followed by extra-anatomical arterial bypass grafting.

Results.—Provocative arteriography was required to obtain a diagnosis of ureteroarterial fistula in all 4 patients. Embolization of the common iliac artery and extra-anatomical arterial bypass grafting were successful in managing the fistulas. No patient required laparotomy, and ipsilateral renal function was preserved. At follow-up ranging from 6 to 27 months, no further interventions were necessary.

Discussion.—Risk factors for ureteroarterial fistulas include pelvic surgery, pelvic radiation, pelvic vascular disease, and chronic ureteral intubation. The number of reported cases of ureteroarterial fistulas has increased in recent years. Although mortality rates have declined since 1980, laparotomy rates have remained high. In approximately one third of published cases, function was lost in the ipsilateral renal unit. Diagnosis with provocative arteriography avoids the risks associated with surgical exploration.

▶ This group reports an innovative way to manage a very complex and life threatening circumstance. Ureteroiliac artery fistulas typically occur in the setting of prior pelvic malignancy, surgery, radiation, or chronic ureteral stenting. Historically, this pathology has been associated with high morbidity and mortality rates. The authors reported several cases of successful management using endovascular iliac artery embolization and extra-anatomical arterial bypass grafting. This approach was successful in preserving the affected renal unit and avoided the morbidity of an intra-abdominal surgical procedure.

D.A. Goldfarb, M.D.

Liquid Sterilization Versus High Level Disinfection in the Urologic Office
Fuselier HA Jr, Mason C (Ochsner Clinic, New Orleans, La)
Urology 50:337–340, 1997   5–7

Background.—Outpatient flexible cystoscopy is increasingly performed in the office setting. Instruments must be sterilized between patients. In this study, liquid sterilization (LS) with the Steris System 1 Processor (SSP1) was compared with high-level disinfectant (HLD) processing using the Voluntary Hospital Association Plus Glutaraldehyde system.

Methods.—The LS system was used at the Ochsner Clinic Department of Urology from June 1993 to June 1994, and the HLD system was used from June 1994 to July 1995. The cost of purchase, cost of operation, and processing time are reported.

Results.—The SSP1 system cost $16,200, plus $8,645 for accessories, service contract and training; and $5,800 for installation. Two gallons of glutaraldehyde plus container cost $15.60. Some facilities may need to install a ventilation system to maintain glutaraldehyde levels <0.2 ppm. There were no clinical differences between these 2 systems. The yearly operating expenses for the SSP1 were $6,037 and for HLD were $445. The average processing time was 35 minutes for SSP1, and 20 minutes for HLD. Seven cystoscopes required repair during the SSP1 period, and none required repair during the HLD period.

Conclusions.—Both an LS and an HLD system were used to sterilize flexible cystoscopes at a single urological institution. The results demonstrate that HLD is as effective as LS, and is significantly less costly.

▶ Glutaraldehyde (Cidex) is a good choice for office-based endoscopy instrument cleaning, because more than one instrument can be cleaned at a time, the cleaning time is short, and operating costs are minimal. However, glutaraldehyde may be noxious to those with chronic exposure. Watery eyes, rhinitis, and throat irritation may occur. Some type of ventilation system is usually required to get the ambient air concentration <0.2 ppm. Glutaraldehyde only disinfects and does not sterilize, but is not associated with a higher infection rate, and is not less safe under usual clinical situations.

D.E. Coplen, M.D.

6 Laparoscopy

The Role of Computerized Tomography in the Evaluation of Complications After Laparoscopic Urological Surgery
Cadeddu JA, Regan F, Kavoussi LR, et al (Johns Hopkins Med Institutions, Baltimore, Md)
J Urol 158:1349–1352, 1997   6–1

Background.—Although laparoscopic surgery for urologic procedures is becoming more widespread, many urologists remain unfamiliar with its possible postoperative complications. Various methods can be used to assess these complications, and these authors evaluated the usefulness of computed tomography (CT) in this regard.

Methods.—Over a 3-year period, 20 patients (8 men, 12 women, mean age 46 years) who underwent laparoscopic urologic surgery had postoperative symptoms that were not explained by routine tests (physical examination, blood and urine culture, chest or abdominal radiography). Symptoms included pain (n = 12), fever and leukocytosis (n = 5), and a falling hematocrit (n = 3). Each patient received an abdominal CT scan from 1 day to 4 months after surgery to help determine the cause of his or her symptoms.

Findings.—CT identified significant procedure-related complications in 13 of the 20 patients. CT also revealed pathology that was unrelated to the surgery in 2 patients. Thus in 15 of 20 patients (75%), CT revealed a symptom-related diagnosis. For patients with a falling hematocrit, fever, or leukocytosis, CT correctly identified the cause in all patients (including hematoma, pneumonia, urine leak, perforated duodenal ulcer, or ileus). For the 12 patients with pain, CT identified a cause that was directly related to laparoscopic surgery in 5 patients. CT in another 2 patients with pain revealed pathologic conditions unrelated to the surgery (enlarged gallbladder and ovarian cyst). Thus, CT revealed a symptom-related diagnosis in 7 of 12 (57%) patients with pain. In 4 of 20 patients, additional procedures were necessary (including CT-guided percutaneous hematoma aspiration, nephrostomy placement, transfusion, or laparoscopic drainage of a pelvic abscess). In 4 of 8 patients who received a CT scan by postoperative day 6, intraperitoneal or retroperitoneal gas was found.

Conclusions.—CT has a role in the diagnosis of significant unexplained postoperative symptoms after laparoscopic surgery. CT was particularly accurate in revealing the sites of hemorrhage, obstruction, or leakage.

Furthermore, CT can help in the planning of further therapeutic interventions, such as CT-guided aspiration. Pneumoperitoneum may be a common complication after urologic laparoscopic surgery (found in 50% of evaluated patients).

▶ Symptoms after any surgical procedure can often not be explained by physical examination or routine diagnostic studies. Computerized tomography is a useful adjunct in these situations, revealing an etiology in the majority of cases with unexplained pain, fever, and leukocytosis. Although there were no hernias in this series, CT helps to localize which port site has broken and directs laparoscopic reduction of the herniated bowel. CT also helps direct percutaneous approaches to hematomas, lymphoceles, or abscesses as clinically indicated.

D.E. Coplen, M.D.

Role and Long-term Results of Laparoscopic Decortication in Solitary Cystic and Autosomal Dominant Polycystic Kidney Disease

Lifson BJ, Teichman JMH, Hulbert JC (Univ of Minnesota; Univ of Texas, San Antonio)
J Urol 159:702–706, 1998   6–2

Background.—The use of the laparoscope for access to the retroperitoneal structures is minimally invasive and has distinct advantages over conventional surgery. One experience with laparoscopic cyst decortication for kidney diseases was presented.

Patients and Findings.—Seventeen patients underwent a total of 20 procedures. Nine procedures were for nonpolycystic kidney disease, and 11 were for polycystic disease. Three of the 8 patients with polycystic kidney disease had repeat procedures. The patients were followed up for 3 to 63 months (mean, 26). All patients with simple cysts treated for pain were free of pain at their most recent follow-up. Nine of the 10 procedures done for pain relief in patients with polycystic kidney disease successfully alleviated pain. Pain-free status declined over time: 87.5% were pain free after 6 months, 71.4% at 1 year, 66.7% at 2 years, and 25% at 3 years. In 2 of 3 patients, repeat operation successfully relieved recurrent pain. Currently, 71% of the 7 patients with polycystic kidney disease who had surgery for pain relief are free of pain.

Conclusions.—Laparoscopic renal cyst decortication is effective in patients with painful simple cysts. In patients with polycystic kidney disease, the procedure effectively alleviates pain in the short and intermediate term. In the long term, a repeat procedure may be needed to maintain adequate control of symptoms in these patients.

▶ Symptomatic, single, peripherally located cysts are best managed with percutaneous drainage and sclerosis. The peripelvic cyst is rare, but percutaneous management is difficult and contraindicated because of proximity to the great vessels and renal pelvis. Cyst decortication in polycystic disease is time consuming and technically demanding. Longer follow-up is required to determine the role of this procedure with respect to pain relief and potential improvements in both renal function and hypertension.

D.E. Coplen, M.D.

7 Adrenal

The Natural History and Treatment of Adrenal Myelolipoma
Han M, Burnett AL, Fishman EK, et al (Johns Hopkins Med Institutions, Baltimore, Md)
J Urol 157:1213–1216, 1997   7–1

Objective.—Adrenal myelolipomas are rare, benign, usually asymptomatic tumors. Whether these tumors may progress is not known. Records of a large series of patients with adrenal myelolipoma treated operatively and nonoperatively were reviewed to identify a treatment strategy and an improved understanding of the natural course and clinical features of the tumor.

Methods.—From 1982 to the present, 20 patients (8 men) aged 26–82 years received diagnoses of 21 adrenal myelolipomas on the basis of CT and MRI results.

Results.—Four patients had abdominal pain and 1 had Cushing's syndrome. The average tumor size was 5.1 cm. Twelve patients had hypertension, 10 had cancer, 12 were obese, and 5 had diabetes mellitus. Four patients had surgery: 2 for abdominal pain, 1 with Cushing's syndrome, and 1 for a large (10.3 cm) tumor. Fifteen patients were followed up for an average of 3.2 years. Of 12 patients with 13 tumors, serial radiographs showed that mean tumor size increased from 5.1 cm to 5.6 cm. Two patients continued to have pain. The tumor is thought to be an adrenocortical cell metaplasia of the reticuloendothelial cells of blood capillaries. Differential diagnoses include retroperitoneal lipoma or liposarcoma, exophytic renal angiomyolipoma, adrenal adenoma, adrenal metastasis, and primary adrenal malignancy.

Conclusion.—Adrenal myelolipomas should be treated conservatively. Surgery is necessary only for symptomatic patients. Although tumors may grow, they are not life-threatening and do not necessarily become symptomatic.

▶ Adrenal myelolipomas are rare, benign tumors of the adrenal gland that contain adipose tissue and hematopoietic elements. Often this tumor is asymptomatic unless it enlarges, and most patients with this condition can be monitored expectantly. The clinical diagnosis of adrenal myelolipoma relies upon radiographic evaluation. Computed tomography scanning will usually demonstrate that the tumor does not arise from the kidney, it is seemingly well encapsulated, and it contains areas of fat with negative Hounsfield units, calcification, and soft-tissue density regions. The differential diagnosis may include retroperitoneal tumors (lipoma or liposarcoma), renal angiomyolipoma, or other primary adrenal masses such as adenoma, metastases, or adrenal corticocarcinoma. This tumor is usually hormonally inactive and only rarely do these tumors spontaneously hemorrhage. On the basis of these considerations, biopsy is usually not necessary to make the diagnosis, and all that is required is occasional repeat imaging unless the patient becomes symptomatic.

G.L. Andriole, Jr., M.D.

Adrenocortical Oncocytoma: Two Case Reports and Review of Literature

Waters PR, Haselhuhn GD, Gunning WT III, et al (Med College of Ohio, Toledo)
Urology 49:624–628, 1997   7–2

Background.—Oncocytomas—rare, often benign tumors composed chiefly of oncocytes (large, eosinophilic, granular cells with numerous mitochondria)—are found in varied locations.

Case 1.—White man, 47, had a right adrenal mass found in an evaluation for microhematuria. He reported no headaches, palpitations, or diaphoresis. Physical and cystourethroscopic examinations were unrevealing. Renal US showed a large right adrenal mass, confirmed by CT and removed uneventfully by right adrenalectomy. The capsule was complete, uniform, fairly thick, and fibrous, without vascular invasion. Polygonal cells had abundant granular, eosinophilic cytoplasm and, rarely, bizarre, multiple nuclei. Ultrastructural morphological features consistent with oncocytoma showed many mitochondria, often with electron-dense inclusions; some lysosomal granules; a few crystalline inclusions; and few other organelles. Patient 1 is doing well without recurrence at 30 months.

Case 2.—White woman, 41, had a renal mass found during evaluation of flank pain and emesis. She reported no hematuria, headaches, palpitations, or diaphoresis. Physical examination showed mild left flank tenderness without palpable mass or other findings. Abdominal CT showed a partially necrotic mass. This thinly encapsulated mass, without vascular invasion, was carefully and uneventfully removed by left radical nephrectomy. It was spherical, grayish, and soft, with a cut surface characteristic of hemorrhage and necrosis. Large, abundantly eosinophilic and granular cells with pleomorphic nuclei were seen in solid sheets, with occasional macronucleoli and multinucleated cells as in case 1. Ultrastructural morphological features consistent with oncocytoma showed many round mitochondria, but without inclusions as in case 1. Patient 2 is doing well without recurrence at 9 months.

Discussion.—Postoperative analysis in both cases yielded the rare diagnosis of adrenal oncocytoma for masses found incidental to evaluation for other conditions. The tumor in case 1 was removed because of its size. In case 2, the tumor was removed because of presumed renal origin. Increased CT allows more frequent detection of nonfunctional adrenal masses; those larger than 6 cm must be surgically removed.

▶ This manuscript reviews an uncommon entity, oncocytomas arising in the adrenal glands. Adrenocortical oncocytomas are different from renal oncocytomas in that they may be associated with internal hemorrhage, and the typical central scar that is observed in patients with renal oncocytomas is generally not present within those that originate from the adrenal gland. However, like their renal counterpart, the cells comprising this tumor are strongly eosinophilic and contain numerous mitochondria. These tumors are usually benign but may behave in a malignant manner and should be treated by surgical excision.

G.L. Andriole, Jr., M.D.

8 Renal Tumors

Lymphatogenous Spread of Renal Cell Carcinoma: An Autopsy Study
Johnsen JA, Hellsten S (County Hosp, Karlskrona, Sweden; Univ Hosp of Malmö, Sweden)
J Urol 157:450–453, 1997   8–1

Objective.—About one third of patients with renal cell carcinoma have metastatic spread at the time of diagnosis, most commonly to the lungs, lymph nodes, bone, and liver. Reported rates of lymph node spread range from 6% to 45%. This extreme variation may only reflect the extent of lymph node dissection performed. There are questions regarding the incidence, extent, and clinical significance of lymphatogenous spread of renal cell carcinoma. The metastasis of clinically unrecognized renal cell carcinoma was analyzed, emphasizing its relationship to primary tumor stage.

Methods.—The 24-year review included 1,063 cases of renal cell carcinoma detected in 1 Swedish city. Of these, 554 were recognized only at autopsy. The findings of the clinically and autopsy-recognized cases were reviewed. Analysis of lymph node metastases included histologic examination of the retroperitoneal, mediastinal, supraclavicular, axillary, and inguinal lymph nodes.

Findings.—The rate of distant metastases in the autopsy cases was 21.5%, including single metastases in 5.6%. Eighty-eight percent of autopsy subjects died of renal cancer. Sixty-seven percent of cases of metastases showed lymphatogenous dissemination; most of these showed additional, mostly multifocal, metastatic spread. There was only 1 case of metastases in which the primary tumor did not show aggressive growth and only 5 cases of lymph node metastases of only the paracaval and/or para-aortic lymph nodes.

Conclusion.—In cases of clinically unrecognized renal cell carcinoma with lymphatic spread, additional distant metastatic sites are almost always present. Thus, patients with renal cell carcinoma are unlikely to derive substantial benefit from extensive lymphadenectomy. However, limited unilateral lymph node dissection may still have a useful role as a staging procedure.

▶ This manuscript addresses the presence of lymph node and distant metastases in patients who were found only on autopsy to have renal cell carcinoma. One noteworthy finding is that among 80 patients with lymphatic metastases, 75 had additional, usually multifocal, metastatic disease. Therefore, this calls into question the necessity of performing a paracaval or paraortic lymph node dissection as a therapeutic maneuver during a radical nephrectomy.

The second interesting point is that 3.5% of tumors that were smaller than 3 cm had documented metastases, and about half of these small tumors showed other local histologic findings (such as pericapsular or vascular invasion) that indicated the propensity for aggressive behavior. These data call into question historical series suggesting that small cortical tumors (less than 3 cm) be considered benign.

G.L. Andriole, Jr., M.D.

Prognostic Factors and Surgical Treatment of Osseous Metastases Secondary to Renal Cell Carcinoma

Althausen P, Althausen A, Jennings LC, et al (Harvard Med School, Boston)
Cancer 80:1103–1109, 1997   8–2

Objective.—Renal cell carcinoma commonly metastasizes to bone. Prognostic factors for such patients have not been well defined. Data from an analysis of the survival of 38 patients with metastatic renal cell carcinoma treated at Massachusetts General Hospital were used to identify prognostic factors.

Methods.—Survival was analyzed in 38 patients (14 women) aged 36–88 years treated between 1977 and 1996 for metastases to bone secondary to renal cell carcinoma. At last follow-up, 17 had died of their disease and 3 had died of other causes. In 21 patients, the metastasis-free interval was as long as 22.4 years, and averaged 3.0 years. Renal cell carcinoma was discovered concurrently with metastatic disease in 17 patients. Age, sex, site of primary tumor, presence of pathologic fracture, disease-free interval, initial presentation with metastasis, solitary vs. multiple metastases, and axilla vs. appendicular metastases and their effect on survival were analyzed.

Results.—The maximum time from diagnosis to death was 23 years. The average time was 6.0 years. The maximum time from first appearance of bone metastases to death was 14.7 years. The average time was 3.0 years. Survival was 90% at 6 months, 84% at 1 year, 55% at 5 years, and 39% at 10 years (Table 4). No metastases at presentation, a longer time to metastasis, metastases to the axial skeleton, and solitary metastases were significant factors predicting survival. Aggressive surgical resection may improve survival. Only 2.5% of these patients have solitary metastases.

Conclusion.—No metastases at presentation, a longer time to metastasis, metastases to the axial skeleton, and solitary metastases were significant factors predicting survival. Aggressive surgery involving wide marginal excision, particularly of appendicular lesions, in patients with late-onset metastases may increase survival time.

TABLE 4.—Survival of Patients With Metastatic Renal Cell Carcinoma:
A Survey of the Literature

		% surviving	
Study	1 yr	5 yrs	10 yrs
Tobisu et al.*	77	45	0
Montie et al.*	36	7	0
Smith et al.*	53.8	7.7	0
Maldazys and Dekernion	48	9	—
Thompson et al.	21.5	0	0
Dekernion et al.	42	13	—
Skinner et al.	—	8	7
Middleton et al.	10	0	0
Tolia et al.†	—	35.8	7.7
Patel et al.	26	0	0
Giuliani et al.	—	7	0
Current study	84	55	39

*Data from patients with only metastases to bone was used.
†Solitary metastases only.
(Courtesy of Althausen P, Althausen A, Jennings LC, et al: Prognostic factors and surgical treatment of osseous metastases secondary to renal cell carcinoma. *Cancer* 80:1103–1109, Copyright 1997 American Cancer Society. Reprinted by permission of Wiley-Liss, Inc., a subsidiary of John Wiley & Sons, Inc.)

▶ This manuscript presents results of 54 patients with renal cell carcinoma metastatic to the bone. These patients generally underwent aggressive excision of the bone metastasis and nephrectomy. This aggressive approach was associated with an astonishing 55% 5-year survival (as shown in Table 4 that compares the current study to several others in the literature). These results are extremely encouraging for the approximately 2.5% of all patients with renal cell cancer who have a solitary bone metastasis. Among this group of patients, this study confirms that metastases to the extremities generally are associated with a better survival than metastases to the axial skeleton.

This study confirms that an aggressive approach to acceptable surgical candidates with solitary osseous metastasis from renal cell carcinoma may be associated with prolonged survival.

G.L. Andriole, Jr., M.D.

Natural History and Therapy of Metastatic Renal Cell Carcinoma: The Role of Interleukin-2

Bukowski RM (Cleveland Clinic Cancer Ctr, Ohio)
Cancer 80:1198–1220, 1997   8–3

Objective.—Renal cell carcinoma (RCC) affects twice as many males as females, commonly occurs in the fifth through seventh decade of life, and accounts for 3% of adult malignancies. Familial patterns of RCC have been identified. Metastatic RCC is almost always fatal. Immunotherapeutic agents such as recombinant human interleukin-2 (rIL-2) and interferon-α (IFN-α) have shown promise in the treatment of RCC.

Methods.—The role of rIL-2 with or without IFN-α was reviewed.

Results.—Results of IFN-α and rIL-2 therapies, alone or in combination, were reviewed. Overall response rates in patients with RCC given rIL-2 alone or in combination with IFN-α ranged from 15% to 21%. Patients given rIL-2 alone had a higher frequency of complete response and a longer duration of response compared with patients given IFN-α alone. Patients receiving subcutaneous therapy had less toxicity that did patients receiving IV therapy. Patient performance status is the most significant predictor of outcome in individuals with metastatic RCC.

Conclusion.—Whereas the optimal treatment for RCC remains to be discovered, there is a role for cytokines such as rIL-2 alone or in combination with other immunotherapeutic or chemotherapeutic agents.

▶ This excellent review article summarizes studies using rIL-2 alone or in combination with interferon or lymphokine activated killer cells. This is a very evenhanded presentation of the data, and it underscores the fact that whereas there has been considerable progress in the last 10 years in developing immunotherapy for urologic cancer, more work needs to be done. The authors suggest that this treatment is only appropriate for patients with the best overall performance status and, point out that they would generally recommend use of the least toxic regimen (i.e., a regimen that can be administered on an outpatient basis as opposed to intensive high-dose therapies that require admission to the hospital). This is a nice article that may be helpful to patients and their families if immunotherapy is being considered.

G.L. Andriole, Jr., M.D.

Cytoreductive Surgery Before High Dose Interleukin-2 Based Therapy in Patients With Metastatic Renal Cell Carcinoma

Walther MM, Yang JC, Pass HI, et al (Natl Cancer Inst, Bethesda, Md)
J Urol 158:1675–1678, 1997   8–4

Objective.—In patients with metastatic renal cell carcinoma, performing nephrectomy before immunotherapy with interleukin-2 (IL-2) may have some important advantages, including reducing the number of cancer cells present, removing a trap for trafficking lymphocytes, preventing complications of IL-2 treatment, and reducing a potentially immunosuppressive tumor burden. However, the uses of such cytoreductive surgery remain to be clarified. The authors report a total of 11 years' experience with preimmunotherapy cytoreductive surgery for metastatic renal cell carcinoma.

Methods.—One hundred ninety-five patients had cytoreductive nephrectomy in preparation for high-dose IL-2-based adoptive immunotherapy. There were 134 men and 61 women, mean age 49 years. At surgery, any primary and locoregional disease that could be safely resected was removed. Eight weeks after recovery, the patients were re-staged. Various immunotherapy-based regimens were used during the experience. One to 2 months after the end of treatment, evaluation of disease for complete or partial response was performed.

Results.—Ninety percent of patients required transabdominal incision for large primary renal tumors. Twenty-three percent required significant additional resection after nephrectomy, most commonly extraction of vena caval thrombus requiring cavotomy and regional lymph node dissection. The unresectability rate was 2.6%, and the perioperative death rate was 1%. Sixty-two percent of patients were eligible for immunotherapy after cytoreductive surgery, and 55% received it. The objective response rate to immunotherapy was 18%, including 4 complete and 15 partial responses.

Conclusions.—In selected patients with advanced renal cell carcinoma, cytoreductive surgery before immunotherapy appears to be feasible. The efficacy of this approach can only be determined by randomized trials. However, in some patients, primary debulking followed by systemic IL-2 therapy can produce complete and lasting tumor regression.

▶ The authors of this article demonstrate that in specialized centers of excellence, cytoreductive surgery can be safely performed in select patients who have metastatic renal cell carcinoma. However, just because it can be done does not necessarily mean that it should be done, particularly at centers without the excellence and expertise of the National Cancer Institute. The precise contribution of cytoreductive surgery in preparing a patient for immunotherapy is undefined, and despite the aggressive resections, only 62% of patients remained eligible for immunotherapy after surgery and only 55% were eventually treated. This must be balanced against the approximate 25% of patients who had disease progression after surgery before immunotherapy could even be started. Another important consideration is that the authors observed only an 18% objective response rate and only 4 complete responses.

To me these data indicate that extensive cytoreductive surgery is not to be widely recommended except in the context of an organized program investigating immunotherapy for renal cell carcinoma.

G.L. Andriole, Jr., M.D.

Low-grade Collecting Duct Carcinoma of the Kidney: Report of 13 Cases of Low-grade Mucinous Tubulocystic Renal Carcinoma of Possible Collecting Duct Origin
MacLennan GT, Farrow GM, Bostwick DG (Case Western Reserve Univ, Cleveland, Ohio; Mayo Clinic, Rochester, Minn)
Urology 50:679–684, 1997   8–5

Objective.—There is little information about outcome, and there are no convincing reports of rare low-grade collecting duct carcinoma. Thirteen cases of low-grade mucinous tubulocystic renal cancer, likely to be of collecting duct origin, were reviewed.

Methods.—Clinical, pathologic, and radiologic findings of 13 patients (5 women) with unusual low-grade renal carcinomas evaluated between 1985 and 1995 were reviewed.

Results.—Eight patients had no symptoms, and 4 had pain and hematuria. Radiologic studies revealed 8 solid tumors, 2 apparently cystic tumors, and 1 solid/cystic mass. One radiologically undetected renal tumor was found at autopsy. Renal angiography showed avascularity in 2 patients and slightly enhanced avascularity in a third. Tumors averaged 6 cm in their greatest dimension and ranged from 2 to 17 cm. Pathologic findings revealed circumscribed tumors that were cystic, nodular, or both, minimal hemorrhage, little extension beyond the kidney, and little necrosis. Tumors expressed keratin AE1/AE3, keratin Cam, keratin 34β-E12, and UEA-1. No metastatic disease was detected in 12 patients. One patient died of metastatic disease morphologically identical to his primary renal tumor. Patients were followed for an average of 62 months. Nine patients were alive at last follow-up, and 5 had survived longer than 70 months.

Conclusion.—These tumors are believed to be low-grade cancers arising in collecting duct epithelium.

▶ Collecting duct carcinoma is a rare form of renal cancer whose clinical course has generally been considered aggressive. In this report, the authors describe 13 low-grade renal tumors that shared many of the histopathologic and immunophenotypic characteristics of collecting duct carcinoma but which permitted prolonged, metastasis-free survival (a range of 112 to 114 months with a mean of 62 months). The characteristic finding in these tumors were their tubulocystic architecture and the presence of mucin. Additional immunohistochemical findings were consistent with a collecting duct origin. Although the histopathologic features were distinctive, there were no characteristic radiologic findings. This is an interesting report of a newly recognized entity.

G.L. Andriole, Jr., M.D.

9 Transplantation

The Current Level of Involvement of Urological Trainees and Faculty in Clinical Kidney Transplantation in the United States and Canada
Flechner SM, Novick AC (Cleveland Clinic Found, Ohio)
J Urol 157:1223–1225, 1997   9–1

Background.—What types of exposure do urology trainees and faculty have to renal transplantation? This study surveyed all the urology training programs in the United States and Canada regarding aspects of their renal transplantation program.

Methods.—In 1995, surveys were sent to every urology training program in the United States (n = 123) and Canada (n = 13) regarding the involvement of residents and faculty in renal transplantation. The response rate was 100%. Institutional data were also examined as to how many urologists were directors of the renal transplant program.

Findings.—In the United States, 116 of 123 programs (94%) were associated with renal transplantation, and 100 (81%) exposed residents to the procedure. All programs in Canada were associated with renal transplantation and all exposed residents to the procedure. More U.S. postgraduates gain this exposure in the earlier years of residency, whereas in Canada the exposure occurs more often in senior years of training. Another difference between the countries is the number of renal transplant programs directed or codirected by urologists (21.9% in the United States and 83.7% in Canada). Most residents in both countries (almost 80% in the United States and more than 90% in Canada) gain exposure in all aspects of transplant surgery, and about half of residents in each country are trained in immunosuppression. Faculty in the United States perform fewer of the kidney transplant operations (25% of programs) than faculty in Canada (92% of programs), but more faculty in the United States are responsible for operative complications and immunosuppression (23% in the United States vs. 15% in Canada).

Conclusion.—The number of renal transplant programs in the United States directed or codirected by urologists remains strong and has not changed since an earlier study reported in 1988. Residents must continue to be exposed to this important aspect of urologic medicine.

▶ Despite the explosion of transplantation programs across North America in the past 10 years, urologic involvement has remained stable. Approximately 25% of United States programs have urology faculty involved in transplantation surgery and immunosuppression. In Canada, there is a higher proportion of urology faculty involved in transplantation surgery (somewhat under 90%); however, they are less involved in immunosuppressive treatment (15%). It is important for urologists (the primary specialty involved with kidney surgery) to maintain their visibility and strength in renal transplantation. Furthermore, renal transplantation represents an important exposure to open renal reconstructive surgery for urology trainees.

D.A. Goldfarb, M.D.

Complications and Risks of Living Donor Nephrectomy

Johnson EM, Remucal MJ, Gillingham KJ, et al (Univ of Minnesota, Minneapolis)
Transplantation 64:1124–1128, 1997

9–2

Introduction.—The number of donor kidneys has failed to keep pace with the growing number of potential recipients, and the median waiting period for a kidney increased from 400 days in 1988 to 842 days in 1994. Although living donor organs are associated with improved patient and graft survival and would increase the number of available organs, donor nephrectomy does carry a risk of morbidity and mortality. To determine the incidence of perioperative morbidity, investigators reviewed donor nephrectomies performed over a 10-year period.

Methods.—The nephrectomies took place at a single institution from 1985 through 1995. Records of 871 donors (491 women and 380 men) were available for review. Donor data collected included age, gender, race, weight, body mass index, and smoking history. Operative and postoperative data were also recorded. All but 2 donor nephrectomies involved the standard subcostal flank incision. Graft ischemia time was minimized by beginning the donor and recipient operations simultaneously.

Results.—Donors had a mean age of 38.2 years, a mean weight of 76.3 kg, a mean body mass index of 26.3 kg/m^2, and a mean operative duration of 4 hours 9 minutes. The mean postoperative stay was 4.9 days. Most donors (93.2%) were white and more than half had never smoked (56.7%) or had not smoked for at least 6 months (11.2%). One or more ribs were excised in 644 cases. The peritoneum was entered inadvertently in 109 donors. There were 2 major and 86 minor complications, for an overall complication rate of 8.2%. One patient required reoperation for a retained sponge but had no ill effects; another experienced left lower extremity weakness attributed to femoral nerve compression and had residual effects at 6-month follow-up. No donor died or required ventilation or intensive care. Three significant risk factors for perioperative complications were identified as follows: male gender, pleural entry, and weight of 100 kg or greater. Significant risk factors for a postoperative stay of more than 5 days were operative duration of 4 hours or more, and age 50 years or older.

Conclusion.—A statistical risk of mortality is associated with all major surgery, but kidney donation can be performed with little major morbidity and a reported mortality rate of only 0.03%. There may be a slightly increased risk for certain potential donors.

▶ This is a large, single-center contemporary review of the live donor nephrectomy operation. Nearly all operations were done through the flank. The finding of no mortality and an extremely low major complication rate of 0.2% confirms the safety of live donor nephrectomy. The authors also identified risk factors for perioperative complications that included male gender, pleural entry, and weight 100 kg or greater. These are certainly reassuring statistics to discuss with patients who are contemplating live donor nephrectomy.

D.A. Goldfarb, M.D.

Pregnancy After Donor Nephrectomy

Wrenshall LE, McHugh L, Felton P, et al (Univ of Minnesota, Minneapolis)
Transplantation 62:1934–1945, 1996   9–3

Background.—Women considering donating a kidney often ask whether unilateral nephrectomy will impair their ability to have children in the future. One group of kidney donors was surveyed to investigate this question.

Methods and Findings.—Two hundred twenty women donating a kidney between 1985 and 1992 were included. The response rate was 65%. Thirty-three of the 144 responders became pregnant after donation. The total number of pregnancies was 45. Three fourths of the pregnancies went to term with no difficulties. Miscarriage occurred in 13.3%, pre-eclampsia in 4.4%, gestational hypertension in 4.4%, proteinuria in 4.4%, and tubal pregnancy in 2.2%. Difficulties occurring in another 4 pregnancies necessitated preterm hospitalization. The overall morbidity was 8.8%. There were no pregnancy-related deaths and no fetal abnormalities. There were no cases of persistent hypertension, proteinuria, or changes in renal function. None of these findings differed significantly from outcomes in the general population. Infertility was a problem in 8.3% of the survey respondents, compared to 16.7% worldwide.

Conclusions.—Donor nephrectomy does not appear to be detrimental to the prenatal course or outcome of pregnancies after donation. The incidence of perinatal complications in this series was comparable to that in the general population.

▶ This article addresses a very important concern for women of reproductive age who are considering renal donation, that is, the issue of pregnancy after donor nephrectomy. Based upon the results of the authors' survey, it would appear that donor nephrectomy is not detrimental to the conception, prenatal course, or outcome of pregnancy. This is reassuring information for women of reproductive age interested in donating to a relative or spouse.

D.A. Goldfarb, M.D.

Helical CT Angiography for Examination of Living Renal Donors

Cochran ST, Krasny RM, Danovitch GM, et al (Univ of California, Los Angeles)
AJR 168:1569–1573, 1997

9–4

Introduction.—Subjects being investigated as potential living related kidney donors usually undergo excretory urography and renal arteriography. With helical CT, it is now possible to image the entire renal region in a single breath-hold and to image the renal arteries. The combination of helical CT arteriography and conventional radiography was investigated as a possible alternative to excretory urography and conventional renal arteriography for the investigation of living related renal donors.

Methods.—Helical CT arteriography was prospectively performed in 57 consecutive potential renal donors. During the pyelographic phase, conventional radiographs were performed to assess the urothelium. The findings were compared with those of conventional arteriography in 46 patients. The surgical findings of 40 patients were analyzed as well. The accuracy and cost of helical CT arteriography plus conventional radiography were compared with those of excretory urography and conventional arteriography.

Results.—The results of CT and conventional arteriography agreed in 89% of kidneys. The results of surgery agreed with those of CT arteriography in 90% of kidneys and with those of conventional arteriography in 87%. In 11% of patients, the findings of CT arteriography precluded kidney donation.

Conclusion.—Helical CT arteriography appears to be as accurate as conventional arteriography in demonstrating the number of vessels perfusing and draining the kidneys. For patients being considered as potential living related renal donors, CT arteriography can be used instead of conventional arteriography. Helical CT angiography plus conventional radiography can significantly reduce the cost of imaging studies, compared with the conventional approach of excretory urography and conventional renal arteriography.

▶ This paper documents the accuracy of helical CT angiography for assessment of living renal donors. The accuracy in depicting renal arterial anatomy was approximately 90% and was comparable to conventional angiography. The advantages of helical CT include accurate assessment of renal vessels and simultaneous assessment of the renal parenchyma and urinary drainage system. If other centers confirm the excellent results of this paper, this technique will emerge as a radiographic assessment of choice for living donors.

D.A. Goldfarb, M.D.

Immunologic and Patient Selection Strategies for Successful Utilization of Less Than 15 Kg Pediatric Donor Kidneys: Long Term Experiences With 40 Transplants
Bretan PN Jr, Friese C, Goldstein RB, et al (Univ of California at San Francisco)
Transplantation 63:233–237, 1997
9–5

Background.—Kidneys from donors under 5 years of age are rarely used because they are associated with very poor graft survival. Using strict donor, recipient, immunologic, and surgical strategies, these authors investigated whether graft survival with young and/or low-weight donor kidneys could be improved.

Methods.—Forty adult recipients were identified who were at low risk. Low risk was defined as age between 25 and 55 years, no diabetes, no coronary artery disease or angina, no congestive heart failure, no lupus, no previous transplantation, panel reactive antibodies less than 15%, and a normal urinary tract. Recipients received 10 days of postoperative therapy with OKT3, after which they received prednisone with either azathioprine or CellCept. FK506, Sandimmune, or Neoral were also used to maintain immunosuppression. Pulse steroids or OKT3 were used to manage rejection crises.

Findings.—The mean donor age was 23.6 ± 18.4 months, and the mean donor weight was 14.4 ± 4.5 kg. Donor kidneys were kept in cold storage for a minimal time, and revascularization times were minimal. Grafts survived in 35 of 40 patients (88%). Graft losses were caused by noncompliance, life-threatening pneumonitis, cardiac dysfunction, lymphoma, and thrombosis (1 each). Twelve rejections occurred (30%), but appropriate therapy led to recovery in all patients. Serum creatinine levels decreased steadily over the course of the study, and single kidney volumes increased rapidly, roughly doubling, tripling, and quadrupling at 1, 3, and 6 months, respectively, after transplantation.

Conclusion.—These results of 88% success with small donor kidneys are in striking contrast with other reports of an 80% failure rate with donors 24 months of age or younger. Factors that maximized graft survival included carefully selecting the recipients, en bloc grafting of donor kidneys, preventing early rejection, matching smaller recipients with smaller kidneys, and using quadruple immunosuppression. The success reported here can dramatically increase the pool of donors for kidney transplant procedures.

▶ The national shortage of organs for transplantation has led to the use of organs from older donors or very young donors. Historically, the outcomes when using pediatric kidneys of donors less than 2 years of age have been poor. Furthermore, there is the theoretical concern that with transplantation of a smaller renal mass, there is a risk for hyperfiltration-induced injury. This paper describes excellent results obtained by transplanting 2 kidneys en-bloc from very young donors (less than 2 years of age) or very small (less than 15 kilogram) renal donors. The authors' success is based upon stringent criteria for patient selection (low-risk recipients), as well as the use of OKT3 induction therapy to prevent early rejection.

D.A. Goldfarb, M.D.

When Should Expanded Criteria Donor Kidneys Be Used for Single Versus Dual Kidney Transplants?

Alfrey EJ, Lee CM, Scandling JD, et al (Stanford Univ, Calif)
Transplantation 64:1142–1146, 1997   9–6

Introduction.—The liberalized criteria for kidney transplantation have led to an increase in the number of patients on the waiting list for a donor organ. Some centers have also expanded their acceptance criteria for kidney donors, particularly older donors with a history of hypertension. In such cases, both donor kidneys may be transplanted into a single recipient. A retrospective review of 52 recipients of expanded criteria donor (ECD) kidneys was undertaken to define when these kidneys should be used as a single, vs. a dual, kidney transplant.

Methods.—Between January 1, 1995 and November 15, 1996, 52 of 263 adult cadaveric renal transplants performed at the study institution involved ECD kidneys that all other local transplant centers had declined. Recipients of single vs. dual ECD kidneys were compared for 7 donor variables and 16 recipient variables. Fifteen patients received dual transplants and 37 received single kidneys. In the dual-recipient group, most of the donors were aged 59 years or older (14 of 15), hypertensive (10 of 15), or both (9 of 15). In the single-recipient group, 11 of 37 ECD donors were aged 59 years or older, 11 of 37 were hypertensive, and 7 of 37 were both. The single and dual transplants were subgrouped by donor admission creatinine clearance of less than 90 mL/min, donor age of 59 years or older, and cold storage time (under or over 24 hours).

Results.—Delayed graft function occurred at a significantly higher incidence in single compared with dual recipients when the donor admission creatinine clearance was less than 90 mL/min (45% vs. 9%). When donor age was 59 years or older, recipients of single kidneys had significantly higher mean serum creatinine clearance at 1, 4, and 12 weeks, compared with recipients of dual kidneys. Cold storage time also had an effect on delayed graft function and early outcome. The incidence of delayed graft function was significantly lower among recipients of dual kidneys stored for less than 24 hours than among recipients of single kidneys stored for more than 24 hours. Early graft function at 1, 4, and 12 weeks, as measured by mean serum creatinine clearance, was also better for those receiving dual kidneys stored for less than 24 hours. Overall 1-year patient and graft survivals, however, did not differ significantly between recipients of single vs. dual ECD kidneys (96% and 81% vs. 93% and 87%, respectively).

Conclusion.—Kidney transplant recipients can have an excellent outcome after receiving ECD kidneys, both as single and dual grafts. When used for dual grafts, donors 59 years of age or older with creatinine clearance of less than 90 mL/min are acceptable for size- and age-matched adult recipients. Single ECD grafts may be less successful when the donor has a long history of hypertension.

▶ In an effort to increase the total number of available cadaver organs, the criteria for what is an acceptable organ has recently been expanded. One way this has been accomplished is by raising the age limitations. Still, lower graft survival with the use of single kidneys over the age of 60 years has been a problem. In an effort to reconcile this issue, many centers adopted a policy of using both kidneys from older donors in an attempt to increase the amount of nephron mass delivered at the time of transplantation. This study presents the Stanford criteria for determining when kidneys should be used as single or as dual transplants. Most of the experience to date has relatively short follow-up. It will be interesting to see whether a policy of dual transplantation yields improved long-term results.

D.A. Goldfarb, M.D.

The Use of Kidneys From Living Donors With Renal Vascular Disease: Expanding the Donor Pool
Serrano DP, Flechner SM, Modlin CS, et al (Cleveland Clinic Found, Ohio)
J Urol 157:1587–1591, 1997   9–7

Introduction.—The shortage of kidneys available for donation has led many transplant centers to use organs from donors categorized as "marginal." Such donors are younger than 5 years, older than 55 years, or with a history of certain medical conditions. Although most of these considerations relate to cadaveric donors, success was reported in the transplantation of kidneys from living donors with renovascular disease.

Methods.—During routine preoperative evaluation, 5 living donors aged 30–56 years were found to have unilateral renovascular abnormalities. All were asymptomatic and normotensive, with otherwise normal renal function. Conditions identified by abdominal aortograms and selective renal angiograms included saccular renal artery aneurysms, an arteriovenous malformation, localized atherosclerosis, and fibromuscular renal artery stenosis. The kidney lesions were repaired after donor nephrectomy and before transplantation into the recipient.

Results.—All recipients were related to their donors: 2 recipients were brothers; 1 was a sister; 1, a daughter; and 1, a father. Each kidney showed prompt diuresis, and blood flow was excellent at the initial postoperative renal scans. There were no cases of posttransplant delayed graft function. Recipients were immunosuppressed with cyclosporine, azathioprine, and steroids. One patient had a reversible acute rejection episode at 5 months. At follow-up ranging from 17 to 32 months, all patients had serum creatinine levels less than 2 mg/dL, and no donor had hypertension or renal deterioration.

Discussion.—Because ideal kidney donors, young adult trauma victims, make up a small percentage of the available donor pool, marginal cadaveric donor organs are used more often. For living potential donors, the presence of bilateral renal abnormalities makes donation impossible. Kidneys from living donors with unilateral renovascular disease can be transplanted successfully, however, if precautions are carefully followed, informed consent obtained, and the donor confirmed to have a normal remaining kidney.

▶ There is a tremendous disparity between the number of patients awaiting kidney transplantation and the number of organs available for transplantation. United Network of Organ Sharing (UNOS) data suggest that there are approximately 30,000 patients awaiting kidney transplantation in the United States. On an annual basis there are approximately 10,000 transplantations performed, and this number has not changed significantly during the past several years. The criteria for what is an acceptable donor kidney has been expanded in recent years. One source has been the use of kidneys with either urologic or renal vascular abnormalities. This study very nicely supports the use of kidneys with repairable renal vascular abnormalities, provided there is satisfactory renal parenchyma, the donor is left with the normal kidney, and there are no other comorbid medical conditions to preclude donation.

D.A. Goldfarb, M.D.

The Asystolic, or Non-Heartbeating, Donor
Kootstra G (Univ Hosp Maastricht, The Netherlands)
Transplantation 63:917–921, 1997   9–8

Introduction.—Kidney transplantation results in a markedly improved quality of life, particularly when compared with dialysis, and nearly all patients who had a first graft fail are willing to go through transplantation again. Other sources for kidneys are being sought because of the discrepancy between demand and supply. The asystolic, or non-heartbeating, donor is being considered. To be defined as an asystolic donor, there must be no circulation to the organs for a certain period.

Methods.—Cooling helps delay the decay of organs after cardiac arrest, and in situ cooling involves the double-balloon, triple-lumen catheter. The cold preservation solution of 4°C flows through a catheter into the kidneys and the other visceral organs. The preservation solution can be histidine-tryptophan-ketoglutarate, which is cheaper than the University of Wisconsin solution, which is the best solution available, but also very expensive. Waiting 10 minutes without perfusion of the brain before inserting the cooling catheter in the body is suggested.

Results.—The short- and long-term outcomes of transplantation of kidneys from non-heartbeating donors were good. The outcome of 57 kidneys from non-heartbeating donors were compared with those from matched heartbeating controls. There was a higher delayed function rate among the non-heartbeating donor kidneys than the heartbeating donor kidneys (60% vs. 35%). The long-term outcome of the heartbeating donor kidneys was equal to that of the non-heartbeating donor kidneys. Kidney function did not differ between both groups at 3, 6, and 12 months.

Conclusion.—The primary hurdle to overcome in worldwide acceptance of this technique is determining the point of death—when the cooling device can be introduced—and developing a viability test for kidneys from non-heartbeating donors. Machine preservation should be a prerequisite.

▶ There is a well-recognized shortage of organs for renal transplantation. This discrepancy between demand and supply has led to the use of transplantation of donor organs at the extremes of age as well as from living, unrelated donors. Another potential source of organs is the non-heartbeating donor, which represents up to 10% of cadaver donors at some institutions. Recently, this approach has received adverse media criticism because of ethical concerns. This article is an excellent contemporary review of issues and results related to the non-heartbeating donor.

D.A. Goldfarb, M.D.

Clinical Xenotransplantation of Solid Organs
Dorling A, Riesbeck K, Warrens A, et al (Hammersmith Hosp, London)
Lancet 349:867–871, 1997   9–9

Background.—The current supply of cadaveric organs cannot meet the present demands for transplantation. As an alternative to human donors, animal donors (xenografts) are being investigated. This article examines the current status of xenotransplantation and discusses the existing barriers to xenograft survival.

Xenograft Donor Selection.—Although primates would seem the most suitable donors for human transplantation because of their similar immunologic makeup, for many ethical and practical reasons (e.g., slow breeding, endangered species status for chimpanzees) they are not the most likely candidates. Pigs have emerged as a more likely xenograft model, although infections and hyperacute rejection are serious concerns.

Short-term Barriers to Xenograft Survival.—Hyperacute rejection occurs with all discordant species transplants (i.e., rejection is similar to that of primed allograft recipients). In hyperacute rejection, preformed IgM xenoreactive natural antibodies bind to carbohydrate epitopes on the endothelium of the graft and cause complement activation. This severe rejection could be overcome by preventing the binding of xenoreactive natural antibodies to the endothelium or by preventing complement activation. Preliminary studies suggest that both these approaches may have clinical applications. Ideally, the goal of xenograft transplantation is to provide grafts that last at least as long as allografts.

Long-term Barriers to Xenograft Survival.—Examination of grafts with delayed xenograft rejection reveal a prominent infiltration of natural killer cells, among others. Natural killer cells are cytotoxic to xenogenic tissues. The IgG xenotropic natural antibodies may encourage the transmigration of natural killer cells into the graft, thereby activating production of tumor necrosis factor-α. T-cell–mediated xenograft rejection also is a serious concern. Strategies to prevent delayed xenograft rejection are thus focusing on both IgG (and its associated xenotropic natural antibodies) and natural killer cells. Such immunosuppressive strategies hold promise in that the very nature of the xenograft model offers opportunities to develop graft-specific approaches to immunosuppression that are not available in the allograft model.

Other Barriers to Xenograft Survival.—Not all of the barriers to be overcome are immunologic. For example, how long would a xenograft last in a human? Is transplanting organs from other animals into humans ethically justified? These other issues may not be resolved until the immunologic barriers have been addressed. In the meantime, research continues to exploit the opportunities of xenotransplantation in providing organs to an increasingly large pool of human recipients.

▶ This is an excellent overview of a very important developing field in transplantation. A consistent problem across the board in solid organ transplantation is a shortage of organs. Significant research efforts are ongoing to develop the field of xenotransplantation (solid organs of other species transplanted into humans). The major hurdle to be overcome for xenotransplantation is that of hyperacute rejection. This is an excellent and well-illustrated introductory article that explains basic concepts related to this field.

D.A. Goldfarb, M.D.

Morphology of hDAF (CD55) Transgenic Pig Kidneys Following Ex-Vivo Hemoperfusion With Human Blood
Storck M, Abendroth D, Prestel R, et al (Ludwig-Maximilian Univ of Munich; Univ of Ulm, Germany; Univ of Cambridge, England)
Transplantation 63:304–310, 1997

9–10

Background.—Complement activation is one of the current pitfalls in the discordant xenotransplantation of pig kidneys into human recipients. Other studies have used a human decay accelerating factor (hDAF [CD55]) to control complement activation in vivo. In this ex vivo experiment, transgenic pig kidneys were perfused with human blood to examine the activity of hDAF.

TABLE 2.—Histologic and Immunocytochemical Evaluation of Transgenic and Control Kidneys Following 1 Hour of Ex Vivo Hemoperfusion With Unmodified, Unpooled Heparinized Human Blood*

Feature	Transgenic	Control	P
Glomerular edema	1.62 (0.91)	4 (0)	<0.01
Glomerular rupture	0.75 (0.88)	4 (0)	<0.01
Glomerular hemorrhage	0.25 (0.46)	3.25 (0.83)	<0.01
Vascular thrombosis	1.25 (0.71)	3.87 (0.33)	<0.01
Platelet thrombi	2.38 (0.51)	4 (0)	<0.05
Tubular hemorrhage	0.5 (0.53)	3.5 (0.5)	<0.01
Tubular necrosis	0.13 (0.35)	4 (0)	<0.01
hDAF on glomerula	3.38 (0.91)	0	<0.001
hDAF on endothelium	2 (0.93)	0	<0.001
C3	1.3 (0.51)	3.75 (0.46)	<0.01
C4	4 (0)	3.8 (0.35)	N.S.
C9	2.1 (1.24)	3.3 (0.51)	<0.05
P-selectin	2.6 (0.51)	3.6 (0.51)	<0.05
IgG	3 (0.53)	3 (0)	N.S.

*Values are expressed as mean (SD) of a severity score ranging from 0 to 4 (Student's t test).

(Courtesy of Storck M, Abendroth D, Prestel R, et al: Morphology of hDAF [CD55] transgenic pig kidneys following ex-vivo hemoperfusion with human blood. *Transplantation* 63:304–310, 1997.)

Methods.—After cold ischemia for 1–4 hours, kidneys from transgenic pigs with adequate endothelial CD55 (n = 8) and nontransgenic control pigs (n = 9) underwent ex vivo hemoperfusion with fresh single-donor human blood. The blood was heparinized, reduced to a hematocrit of 25%, and adjusted within the perfusion circuit until blood gas and electrolyte levels were physiologic for the pig. This hemoperfusion system has been shown not to activate leukocytes or complement. Blood samples from the venous effluate were drawn regularly, and levels of blood chemistries, soluble inflammatory mediators, and soluble adhesion molecules were measured. At 60 minutes of reperfusion, the specimen was shock frozen and immunohistologic and electron microscopic studies were performed.

Findings.—Although the transgenic kidneys had significantly lowered resistance values, compared with controls, this decrease was not to the level of resistance found in autologous reperfusion. Also, as the resistance increased, urine output decreased. Except for IL-10, all cytokine levels were significantly higher in the control kidneys than they were in the transgenic kidneys. In particular, transgenic kidneys had almost no human tumor necrosis factor-α. Staining (Table 2) revealed hDAF on the glomerular capillary and vascular endothelium of all transgenic kidneys, but no control kidneys. C4 staining was similar in both groups, but staining of C3 and C9 was significantly less in the glomerular capillary and vascular endothelium of the transgenic mice. Control kidneys did show a higher expression of P-selectin and neutrophil extravasation.

Conclusions.—Human decay accelerating factor was found on all transgenic kidneys but on no controls, and C3 and C9 staining was significantly less in the transgenic kidneys. Thus, despite xenoantibody deposition after hemoperfusion with human blood, hDAF inhibited complement activation beyond C3. This approach shows promise in avoiding the hyperacute rejection that occurs after xenotransplantation.

▶ A major impediment to xenotransplantation is hyperacute rejection. In the discordant combination of pig to human transplantation, this is caused by naturally occurring antibody to galactose α (1-3) galactose, and complement activation. The strategy for inhibiting complement activation in this study is the use of transgenic pig kidneys for CD55, which is a human complement regulatory protein (hDAF). There was less evidence of rejection damage in the transgenic kidneys (expressing hDAF) than in control kidneys. Research such as this will pave the way for successful xenotransplantation for humans.

D.A. Goldfarb, M.D.

Senior Citizens Pool for Aged Kidneys

Gjertson DW, Terasaki PI, Cecka JM, et al (Univ of California, Los Angeles)
Transplant Proc 29:129, 1997   9–11

Objective.—Several approaches have been considered for expanding the availability of cadaveric kidneys. These include the use of kidneys from more marginal donors, for example, from older donors. Cadaveric kidneys from older donors are relatively abundant. The possibility of using a separate "senior citizens' pool" of waiting patients to receive these older kidneys was investigated.

Methods and Results.—Data from the United Network for Organ Sharing Renal Transplant Registry were used to analyze the effects of donor age on the results of transplantation. One-year graft survival decreased from 86% for kidneys from donors aged 21 to 30 years to 73% for kidneys from patients older than 60 years. Beyond 1 year, graft half-lives were 10 and 5 years, respectively. However, kidneys from older donors had better survival in older than in younger recipients. The half-life of kidneys older than 60 years was 5 years in recipients aged 21 to 30 years vs. nearly 7 years in recipients older than 60 years. The immunologic failure rate was 36% for older recipients of aged kidneys, compared with 61% for younger recipients of aged kidneys.

Conclusion.—Although they may be inadequate for use in younger patients, cadaveric kidneys from older donors may be appropriate for use in older, less active recipients. Kidneys from donors aged 60 years or older might be best designated for older recipients, in whom the renal outcomes are relatively good. This approach could make use of the more abundant kidneys from older donors while shifting the use of younger donor kidneys to younger recipients.

▶ The shortage of available organs for transplantation has led to the use of expanded criteria for donor organs, such as those from older donors. Still, long-term survival of grafts from donors over 60 years of age is less than what can be obtained with younger donors. This paper demonstrates that the older donor kidneys give better results when they are transplanted into older recipients. The authors suggest a "senior citizens pool" for the older donor kidneys. This would make the younger donor kidneys available to younger recipients.

D.A. Goldfarb, M.D.

Risks of Transplanting Kidneys From Hepatitis B Surface Antigen-Negative, Hepatitis B Core Antibody-Positive Donors
Satterthwaite R, Ozgu I, Shidban H, et al (Natl Inst of Transplantation, Los Angeles)
Transplantation 64:432–435, 1997   9–12

Introduction.—The chronic shortage of donor organs for kidney transplantation has led investigators to examine the possibility of transplanting organs previously considered marginal or undesirable. Kidneys from donors with positive hepatitis B serology results were thought to have an adverse effect on recipient and graft outcome. The risks of using kidneys from hepatitis B (HB) surface-antigen (sAg)–negative (−) but HB core-antibody (cAb)–positive (+) donors were examined.

Methods.—Between 1990 and 1994, 1,067 cadaveric kidneys were transplanted at the study institution. Thirty-eight kidneys were from HBsAg(−)/HBcAb(+) donors. Twenty-seven recipients (group 1) were HBcAb(−) and 11 (group 2) were HBcAb(+). Both groups received no hepatitis immunoglobulin therapy after transplantation, and all recipients were given the same immunosuppression and rejection therapies as patients who received kidneys from HBcAb(−) donors. Primary study endpoints were recipient hepatitis B seroconversion, graft failure, and recipient death.

Results.—Among the group 1 patients, none of whom were HBcAg(+) or HBsAb(+) before transplantation, 3 (11%) became HBsAb(+) and 2 (7%) became HBcAb (+). No patient became HBsAg(+) or both HBsAb (+) and HBcAb (+). One group 1 patient had elevated transaminase levels 4 years after transplantation, but this finding resolved after 5 months and the patient did not have jaundice. No patient exhibited signs or symptoms of acute or chronic HB. Eight of the 11 group 2 patients were HBsAb(+) and 1 was HBsAg(+) before transplantation. None became newly HBsAg(+) or HBsAb(+), and none had signs or symptoms of acute or chronic HB during follow-up. Three patients died during follow-up, all with a functioning graft. The 2 groups had similar graft and patient survival rates, and these rates were similar to those of kidney recipients whose donors were HBcAb(−).

Conclusion.—Kidneys from HBsAg(−)/HBcAb(+) donors present a small risk of HB seroconversion, but none of the recipients in this series had clinical signs or symptoms of acute or chronic HB. Short-term graft and patient survival were not adversely affected by the use of these donors.

▶ Although the transplant community would like to increase the total number of donors available for transplantation, one must also minimize the risk of transmission of infectious agents. Donors who are HBsAg(+) cannot be used because of the high risk of viral transmission. There are little data regarding the outcome of the use of HBsAg(−)/HBcAB(+) donors. This article demonstrates the relative safety of using these kidneys for transplantation. At the present time, many centers are using HBsAg(−)/HBcAB(+) donors providing that the HBcAb is an IgG. If the antibody is an IgM, the infectious risk is considered significant and these organs are not used.

D.A. Goldfarb, M.D.

Urological Complications of Pancreatic Transplantation

Hickey DP, Bakthavatsalam R, Bannon CA, et al (Beaumont Hosp, Dublin)
J Urol 157:2042–2048, 1997   9–13

Objective.—Pancreatic transplantation is an increasingly accepted treatment option for patients with insulin-dependent diabetes and end-stage renal disease. The exocrine pancreatic secretions are usually drained via the bladder; thus, urologic complications are common. As the use of pancreatic transplantation increases, so will the need to manage the postoperative urologic complications. Complications occur because of the unphysiologic nature of pancreatico-urinary fistula created by duodenocystostomy. The literature on urologic complications of pancreatic transplantation was reviewed.

Duodenocystostomy Fistula.—Duodenocystostomy fistula develops after pancreatic transplantation in 7% to 14% of recipients. Fistulas are most common in the early posttransplant period because of duodenal ischemia, but they may also occur later. The main clinical findings are abdominal pain and tenderness, hyperamylasemia, leukocytosis, and increased serum creatinine. Bladder catheterization is indicated for patients with these symptoms; if a leak is present, treatment depends on the size and timing of the leak.

Hematuria.—The reported incidence of posttransplant hematuria is 9% to 28%. Although early, microscopic hematuria requires no treatment, gross, persistent hematuria is clinically significant. Pancreatic exocrine secretions are probably the major cause. The bleeding usually responds to hydration and bed rest, with identification and treatment of such conditions as pancreatitis, rejection, and cytomegalovirus infection. Cystoscopy is necessary if conservative treatment fails. For patients with late, chronic hematuria, cystoscopic fulguration is not always successful.

Urinary Tract Infections.—Many factors can contribute to the occurrence of lower urinary tract infections after pancreatic transplantation. The causative organisms may be changing in response to immunosuppression, but also because of breakdown of the normal bladder and duodenal mucosal barriers. Antibiotic therapy is usually successful; if infections recur, cystoscopy and other investigations are necessary.

Reflux Pancreatitis.—Reflux pancreatitis develops in 11% to 17% of transplant recipients and can occur immediately or after a period of several years. It probably results from urine reflux into the pancreatic duct during the high-pressure phase of micturition. Treatment is urinary catheterization and continuous drainage, repeated in case of recurrences.

Bladder and Urethral Complications.—Irritative bladder and urethral complications occur in 8% to 14% of pancreatic transplant recipients. The most serious of these is urethral disruption. Most patients with such complications will respond to catheter drainage and antibiotic therapy. For the rest, enteric conversion almost always leads to the resolution of complications.

Cancer Risk.—As the results of pancreatic transplantation improve, there is growing concern regarding the possibility of long-term malignancy risk. Experimental and clinical studies have shown that tumors can occur after bladder augmentation, with many of the predisposing factors similar to those encountered in patients with bladder-drained pancreatic transplants. Chronic immunosuppression may play a role as well. Although no cases of tumor in a bladder-drained pancreas transplant have been reported, long-term cystoscopic follow-up seems prudent.

Summary.—Urologic complications are common in recipients of bladder-drained pancreatic transplants, affecting 50% to 60% of patients. As the number of pancreas transplants increases, the urologist will play an increasingly important role in posttransplant management.

▶ This is a timely review for urologists who work in centers with an active pancreas transplant program.

D.A. Goldfarb, M.D.

Peripheral Vascular Disease After Kidney-Pancreas Transplantation in Diabetic Patients With End-stage Renal Disease

Morrissey PE, Shaffer D, Monaco AP, et al (Beth Israel-Deaconess Med Ctr, Boston; Harvard Med School, Boston)
Arch Surg 132:358–362, 1997   9–14

Background.—Peripheral vascular complications (PVCs) are greatly increased in diabetic patients. Theoretically, replacement of the malfunctioning pancreas with a functioning one should reduce these complications by achieving euglycemia. This study evaluated the rate of PVCs after either kidney transplantation alone or kidney plus pancreas transplantation in patients with diabetes.

Methods.—The study group included 39 diabetic patients with a kidney plus pancreas transplant. The control group included 65 diabetic patients with a kidney transplant only. Both groups received long-term immunosuppressive therapy. Peripheral vascular complications were defined as any midfoot or limb amputation caused by arterial occlusive disease (amputations resulting from an ulcer were not included), an ischemic ulceration that required treatment, lower-extremity bypass surgery, or angioplasty.

Findings.—Allograft function after 6 months was slightly better in the group that received a kidney transplant alone. Of patients undergoing kidney plus pancreas transplantation, 35 of 39 patients (90%) were no longer taking insulin at the end of the study, indicating euglycemia. The group that received a kidney transplant alone had more atherosclerotic risk factors, yet the pretransplantation incidence of PVCs was similar in both groups. After transplantation, however, the patients receiving a dual transplant experienced significantly more PVCs than the patients receiving a kidney-only transplant (46% vs. 31%).

Conclusion.—Diabetic patients receiving a kidney plus pancreas transplant enjoyed drastic improvement in their dependence on insulin. However, this group actually had more PVCs after transplantation than the group that received a kidney transplant alone. These contradictory findings indicate that, whereas pancreas transplantation can improve some measures of diabetic function, it has no effects—or perhaps even detrimental ones—on other complications of diabetes, such as peripheral vascular disease.

▶ This paper evaluates PVCs in diabetic patients after either kidney-only transplant or combined kidney/pancreas transplantation. Despite more risk factors for atherosclerotic disease in the kidney-only group (hypertension, hypercholesterolemia, hypertriglyceridemia, coronary artery disease), patients who received a combined kidney/pancreas transplant more frequently experienced a PVC. In other words, the euglycemic state offered no protection from the development of PVCs.

This is somewhat unexpected; however, a recent Office of Health Technology Assessment report revealed that although patients' quality of life improved after successful pancreas engraftment, improvement in the end-organ complications of diabetes were minimal. The reasons for this observation are unclear. Some have attributed this to systemically drained pancreas allografts that bypass the normal portal metabolism and may result in hyperinsulinemia. This may contribute to progressive atherosclerosis by stimulating vascular smooth-muscle growth and arterial wall lipid deposition.

D.A. Goldfarb, M.D.

Cellular and Molecular Predictors of Chronic Renal Dysfunction After Initial Ischemia/Reperfusion Injury of a Single Kidney

Azuma H, Nadeau K, Takada M, et al (Harvard Med School, Boston; Brigham and Women's Hosp, Boston)
Transplantation 64:190–197, 1997   9–15

Introduction.—Among the factors contributing to late renal allograft failure are initial ischemia/reperfusion injury and synergy between the initial injury and acute rejection. Nephron loss may also influence allograft failure. Potential causes of permanent nephron deficit include the early acute ischemia/reperfusion episode and replacement of 2 native kidneys with a single graft. These possibilities were investigated.

Methods.—Male Lewis and Fischer rats were divided into 4 groups. Group 1 animals had the left kidney subjected to unilateral ischemic injury and the right kidney removed; the right kidney was retained in group 2 to assess the influence of additional functioning renal mass during follow-up. Controls were age-matched, uninephrectomized (group 3) and nonoperated (group 4) rats. To examine the early effects of injury, ischemic kidneys were excised at periods ranging from 4 hours to 7 days after operation. Cellular and molecular changes and indices of renal injury thought to develop secondary to the initial ischemic insult were examined in kidneys collected at 12 periods from 2 to 52 weeks after operation.

Results.—Acute polyuria and transient mild proteinuria developed in group 1, peaking at 7 days and then returning to baseline. Progressive proteinuria developed again at approximately 12 weeks later. The remaining 3 groups showed no changes in rate of protein excretion during 52 weeks of follow-up. Group 1 kidneys were found to have small numbers of infiltrating cells, tubular atrophy, and moderate numbers of sclerotic glomeruli by 16 weeks; glomerulosclerosis was widespread at 32 weeks. Although immunohistology showed acute early changes in both groups 1 and 2, later changes occurred almost exclusively in kidneys from group 1. Cytokine activity in kidneys from groups 3 and 4 remained at baseline, in contrast to those from groups 1 and 2, and changes were diminished in group 2 compared with group 1.

Discussion.—Ischemia/reperfusion injury and uninephrectomy appear to interact, producing progressive fibrotic changes and a reduction in total nephron number. Chronic injury may occur after significant ischemia and reperfusion together with a 50% reduction in renal mass, as in a recipient with a single transplanted kidney.

▶ The authors of this article provide insight into the molecular basis for long-term renal dysfunction in a solitary kidney after an ischemic insult. They identified a number of proinflammatory mediators (chemokines/cytokines) that were generated in the setting of a solitary ischemic kidney but remained at baseline when a normal contralateral kidney was in place. With a better knowledge of the molecular events that produce chronic renal dysfunction after ischemic injury, it may be possible to develop an interventive strategy to ameliorate this process.

D.A. Goldfarb, M.D.

Evaluation of Injury Preservation in Pig Kidney Cold Storage by Proton Nuclear Magnetic Resonance Spectroscopy of Urine

Hauet T, Mothes D, Goujon JM, et al (Hôpital Saint Louis, Paris)
J Urol 157:1155–1160, 1997

9–16

Background.—Determining the amount of tubular damage in cold-stored cadaver kidneys would help determine which specimens are most suited for transplant. This study evaluated the utility of nuclear magnetic resonance (NMR) spectroscopy in identifying urinary markers of tubular injury after transplantation of cold-stored cadaver kidneys.

Methods.—Isolated, perfused pig kidneys were flushed in situ with cold (4°C) Euro-Collins solution and then reperfused with heparinized saline either immediately (group 1, controls), after 24 hours of cold storage (group 2), or after 48 hours of cold storage (group 3). Biochemical markers in urine samples (glucose, alanine, etc.) were evaluated during reperfusion with a commercial kit and with NMR spectroscopy at 400 MHz. Amino acid excretion and renal glucose excretion rates were determined. After reperfusion, kidneys underwent histopathologic examination, and lesion extent was rated on a 5-point scale.

Findings.—After prolonged perfusion (group 3), glucose excretion, the fractional reabsorption of sodium and creatinine clearance were significantly worse than in the other groups. Lactate dehydrogenase, N-acetyl-βD-glucosaminidase, trimethylamine-N-oxide, and lactate levels were also significantly greater in group 3. Glomerular filtration and the perfusate flow rate were significantly worse after prolonged cold storage. Nuclear magnetic resonance spectroscopy identified another peak in group 3 between the peaks of alanine and threonine plus lactate. Histologic analysis revealed progressive damage of kidney ultrastructures with increased cold storage.

Conclusion.—These results confirm the fact that prolonged cold storage results in greater tubular necrosis. An advantage of NMR spectroscopy was its ability to detect multiple markers (amino acids, trimethylamine-N-oxide, etc.) in the same experiment. Furthermore, NMR spectroscopy identified a new peak in group 3. This new peak may be useful as a marker of prolonged ischemia after cold storage. Thus, the use of NMR spectroscopy of urine should be pursued not only for its use in identifying current markers of cadaver kidney damage, but also in screening future preservation solutions and methods.

▶ This study correlated the level of renal injury markers in urine (lactate, N-acetyl-βD-glucosaminidase, and trimethylamine-N-oxide) as measured by NMR spectroscopy with renal functional outcome in an isolated perfused pig kidney model. With greater ischemic time, there were higher levels of these markers. Additionally, at the most prolonged ischemic time (48 hours), a new unidentified NMR peak was noted.

Delayed graft function still remains an important issue within the field of transplantation. It increases cost and morbidity of the transplantation process, and the renal injury itself may predispose kidneys to rejection. There is still no good way to predict which kidneys will experience delayed graft function. If markers like these can be identified rapidly in the urine of prospective donors, one may implement preservation using pulsatile perfusion or ensure short ischemic times. Also, these markers may be used as end points to study new methods to help preserve kidney function before kidney donation.

D.A. Goldfarb, M.D.

Nitric Oxide Synthase Activity in Renal Ischemia-Reperfusion Injury in the Rat: Implications for Renal Transplantation

Shoskes DA, Xie Y, Gonzalez-Cadavid NF (Harbor-UCLA Med Ctr, Torrance, Calif)
Transplantation 63:495–500, 1997

9–17

Background.—The delayed graft function that can occur after ischemia-reperfusion injury in cadaveric renal transplants is associated with decreased allograft survival. Attenuating the ischemia-reperfusion injury might lessen the effects of delayed graft function and thus improve graft survival. One substance known to improve recovery from ischemia is nitric oxide, which is produced by nitric oxide synthase (NOS). Whether NOS activity is increased in a rat model of acute tubular necrosis (ATN) was examined.

Methods.—In male rats, the left renal pedicle was clamped for 60 minutes to produce ischemic ATN. Also, in some rats the right kidney was removed to assess serum creatinine levels with a solitary kidney. Some rats were given an NOS substrate (L-arginine, at 2 dose levels) and a corticosteroid (dexamethasone) before surgery, and U74389G (which prevents lipid peroxidation) was given before clamping and after release. An additional dose of U74389G was given to rats studied for longer than 6 hours. Rats were killed at various times (2 hours to 14 days) after the ischemia-reperfusion injury to evaluate the short- and long-term effects of ATN. An enzymatic method was used to determine NOS activity.

Findings.—In the unnephrectomized right kidney NOS activity did not change significantly after ATN. However, NOS activity was significantly greater in the ischemic left kidney by 2 hours after the induction of ATN (79.8 pmol/min/mg) compared with baseline (33.7 pmol/min/mg). By 24 hours, NOS activity in the ischemic kidneys had decreased (57 pmol/min/mg) to a level similar to that of control kidneys. By day 3, NOS levels in the ischemic kidney were significantly lower than at baseline (15.8 pmol/min/mg). NOS levels did not return to baseline until day 21. Changes in the serum creatinine level in animals whose right kidney was removed at ATN induction showed an opposite pattern. The serum creatinine level peaked on day 3 (5.6 mg/dL) and returned to near baseline by day 21 (1.4 mg/dL). The 5 g/L dose of L-arginine caused a significant reduction in the serum creatinine level at 7 days (2.1 mg/dL). U74389G administration significantly blocked the initial increase in NOS activity, and it significantly lowered serum creatinine levels at days 7 (2.0 mg/dL) and 14 (1.3 mg/dL).

Conclusions.—The reduced levels of NOS immediately after ischemia-reperfusion injury reflect poor blood flow. Therefore, improving renal function by increasing NOS activity, in this case by administering L-arginine, may keep blood flow from worsening. Also, U74389G helped normalize the responses to ATN, which indicates that this substance may also be useful in improving graft function and survival.

▶ This paper examines the role of nitric oxide in an ischemic renal injury model. Although nitric oxide synthase is initially up-regulated early after reperfusion, its levels were ultimately significantly depressed. Recovery of nitric oxide synthase activity paralleled the improvement in creatinine. Supplementing substrate (L-arginine) or a lazaroid compound, which reduces lipid peroxidation, hastens the recovery of the kidney. Better understanding of the molecular mechanisms involved with ischemic renal injury will ultimately lead to improvement and possible prevention of delayed graft function in transplantation. Furthermore, there may be some implications of this research in other urologic cases, such as preventing ischemic renal dysfunction after partial nephrectomy.

D.A. Goldfarb, M.D.

Antilymphocyte Induction Therapy in Cadaver Renal Transplantation: A Retrospective, Multicenter United Network for Organ Sharing Study

Shield CF, Edwards EB, Davies DB, et al (Via Christi Regional Med Ctr, Wichita, Kan; United Network for Organ Sharing, Richmond, Va)
Transplantation 63:1257–1263, 1997   9–18

Introduction.—There is an ongoing debate over the use of antilymphocyte induction therapy in cadaver renal transplantation, particularly with regard to the indications for its use. Some authors question the effectiveness of antilymphocyte induction therapy when cyclosporine and tacrolimus immunosuppressive therapy are available. Data from the United Network for Organ Sharing (UNOS) Center-Specific Outcomes Analysis were used to assess the length of treatment and efficacy of antilymphocyte preparations in cadaver renal transplantation.

Methods.—The analysis included data on 24,191 cadaver renal transplants performed between 1987 and 1991. Participating centers were asked to provide information on whether they were using antilymphocyte preparations, whether treatment began within 24 hours after transplantation, and the duration of administration. The effects of antilymphocyte treatment on graft outcome were analyzed, with adjustment for other variables.

Results.—Sixty percent of transplant recipients received an antilymphocyte preparation. Graft outcomes were better for patients who received at least 5 days of therapy with Minnesota antilymphocyte globulin or at least 7 days of treatment with OKT3. Relative risks were 0.82 and 0.86, respectively. There was no evidence to suggest that a longer duration of therapy might benefit certain patient subgroups. In a semiparametric model, antilymphocyte treatment improved outcome in patients with a 3-or-more-antigen mismatch and those with a 0-antigen mismatch.

Conclusion.—Early use of antilymphocyte preparations after cadaver renal transplantation improves graft outcomes, even with the availability of cyclosporine immunosuppression. This study demonstrates the effectiveness of antilymphocyte therapy across all covariates. The study did not include sufficient data on the effectiveness of antithymocyte globulin. Further data on the duration of treatment with currently available antilymphocyte preparations are being collected by the UNOS Scientific Registry.

▶ The effectiveness of antilymphocyte preparations in an era of cyclosporine and tacrolimus use has been questioned. Furthermore, in an era of cost containment, the use of expensive antilymphocyte products should be validated. To date, there has been conflicting evidence regarding the value of induction antilymphocyte therapy after cadaveric renal transplantation. This article shows a clear-cut benefit for the use of antilymphocyte products based upon their duration of treatment. Readers should note that the Minnesota antilymphocyte globulin product is no longer available and that the outcomes quoted in this article are for UNOS data collected between 1987 and 1991. Outcomes should be validated now with antithymocyte globulin.

D.A. Goldfarb, M.D.

Steroid Withdrawal in Mycophenolate Mofetil-Treated Renal Allograft Recipients
Grinyo JM, Gil-Vernet S, Serón D, et al (Univ of Barcelona; F Hoffman-La Roche Ltd, Basel, Switzerland)
Transplantation 63:1688–1690, 1997   9–19

Background.—Discontinuing steroid use may improve quality of life for transplant recipients, but it carries a risk of acute rejection. The new immunosuppressive agent mycophenolate mofetil (MMF), given in combinations with cyclosporine (CsA) and steroids, greatly reduces the incidence of acute rejection. It may also improve the chances of steroid withdrawal without increasing the risk of rejection. This open study examined the results of steroid withdrawal in renal transplant recipients treated with MMF and CsA.

Methods.—The study included 26 consecutive patients with their first adult cadaveric kidney transplant. All were receiving CsA, prednisone at 0.1 mg/kg/day, and MMF. The MMF was given at 3 g/day to 19 patients and 2/g/day to 7 patients. Steroid withdrawal was attempted after the patients had had stable renal function for at least 2 months. It was initiated at a mean of 17 months after transplantation. The patients were followed for a mean of 10 months after steroid withdrawal. The metabolic changes and incidence of acute rejection after steroid withdrawal were investigated.

Results.—The mean CsA dose decreased from 4.2 mg/kg/day at the time of steroid withdrawal to 3.0 mg/kg/day at last follow-up. Cyclosporine blood levels at these times were 170 and 113 ng/mL, respectively. There was no significant change in serum creatinine: 133 µM/L at the time of steroid withdrawal and 130 µM/L at follow-up. None of the patients had any episodes of rejection, and all allografts were still functioning at follow-up.

Conclusion.—Although more study is needed, MMF appears to prevent graft damage after steroid withdrawal. There is no decline in renal function after steroid withdrawal, even though the CsA dose is significantly reduced.

▶ This is one of the first papers to examine steroid withdrawal in the setting of treatment with MMF as opposed to azathioprine. The favorable results indicating stable renal function in the absence of rejection are provocative. Larger prospective studies of steroid withdrawal are needed in this era of Neoral, tacrolimus, and MMF.

D.A. Goldfarb, M.D.

Tacrolimus Rescue Therapy for Renal Allograft Rejection: Five-Year Experience

Jordan ML, Naraghi R, Shapiro R, et al (Univ of Pittsburgh, Pa)
Transplantation 63:223–228, 1997   9–20

Background.—The immunosuppressive agent tacrolimus has shown promise in attenuating renal allograft rejection after cyclosporine therapy. This study built on previous experience with a large patient group.

Methods.—One hundred sixty-nine patients (mean age, 36.2 years; range, 2 to 75 years) with biopsy-proven renal allograft rejection who had been taking cyclosporine were converted to tacrolimus. All patients had received antirejection therapy with high-dose steroids before conversion to tacrolimus, and 85% had also received a monoclonal or polyclonal antilymphocyte preparation. Tacrolimus conversion occurred at a mean of 4.3 months (range, 2 days to 55 months) after transplantation. Conversion was considered successful if the serum creatinine level improved, if follow-up renal biopsy showed improvement, or (for those patients who had been dependent on dialysis, $N = 28$) if dialysis was no longer necessary.

TABLE 1.—Outcome of Tacrolimus Conversion in Renal Transplant Recipients Failing Primary Cyclosporine Therapy

Preconversion biopsy	Number of Pts. (%)	Success	(%)*
Acute cellular rejection	91 (54%)	70	(77%)
Vascular rejection	62 (37%)	47	(75%)
Acute cellular rejection with primary nonfunction	16 (9%)	8	(50%)
Total	169	125	(74%)

*$P = 0.1$.

(Courtesy of Jordan ML, Naraghi R, Shapiro R, et al. Tacrolimus rescue therapy for renal allograft rejection: Five-year experience. *Transplantation* 63(2):223–228, 1997.)

Findings.—Over a mean follow-up of 30.0 months (range, 12 to 62 months) after tacrolimus conversion, 159 of 169 patients (94%) survived and 125 (74%) had a salvaged renal graft. Table 1 shows the success of tacrolimus conversion based on preconversion biopsy results. Thirteen (46%) of the 28 patients who were dialysis dependent before tacrolimus had functioning grafts after conversion. One hundred seventeen (81%) of the patients who had been treated with antilymphocyte antibody responded to tacrolimus therapy. Prednisone doses were lowered from 28.0 ± 9.0 mg/day during cyclosporine therapy to 6.6 ± 5.1 mg/day during tacrolimus; in fact, 28 patients (22%) were no longer using prednisone by the end of the study. Earlier conversion to tacrolimus (within 6 months of transplantation) was significantly more likely to be successful than later conversion. In the 44 patients in whom tacrolimus conversion failed, 22 had ongoing allograft rejection, 11 had rejection after initial successful rescue, 8 patients were not saved, 2 were noncompliant and lost their graft, and 1 died with a functioning graft.

Conclusion.—Tacrolimus rescue therapy after renal allograft rejection with cyclosporine therapy had significant effects on long-term survival. Tacrolimus should be considered an effective alternative to the conventional drugs used in managing renal allograft rejection.

▶ Cyclosporine is the core of immunosuppression at most transplant centers. A small percentage of patients may experience refractory rejection, despite adequate cyclosporine treatment. On the basis of a large experience over an extended period, Dr. Jordan and his group from the University of Pittsburgh have now established the use of tacrolimus rescue therapy for refractory rejection. Tacrolimus is most effective when the preconversion biopsy specimen demonstrates acute rejection. The finding of chronic rejection will decrease the success rates. Outcomes in patients receiving dialysis at conversion, with vascular rejection, or with a serum creatinine greater than 3 are also not as favorable. This paper attests to the long-term efficacy of tacrolimus conversion for refractory rejection and it is the current method by which this problem is managed now at our center in this setting.

D.A. Goldfarb, M.D.

A Comparison of Tacrolimus (FK506) and Cyclosporine for Immunosuppression After Cadaveric Renal Transplantation

Pirsch JD, Miller J, Deierhoi MH, et al (Univ of Wisconsin, Madison; Univ of Miami, Fla; Univ of Alabama, Birmingham; et al)

Transplantation 63:977–983, 1997

9–21

Background.—Tacrolimus (FK506) is a potent inhibitor of interleukin-2 expression T lymphocytes. In an open-label, randomized study, tacrolimus was compared with cyclosporine for cadaveric kidney transplantation (CRT).

Methods.—In sum, 412 patients were randomly assigned to receive tacrolimus (n = 205) or cyclosporine (n = 207) after CRT. They were monitored for 1 year for patient and graft survivals and other clinical data.

Results.—During the study, 16 patients (9 in the tacrolimus group and 7 in the cyclosporine group) died, most commonly of infection (overall infection rates were comparable). The tacrolimus group had nonsignificantly fewer graft failures ($P = 0.098$). Survival at 1 year for the tacrolimus group was 95.6% and for the cyclosporine group was 96.6% ($P = 0.576$). The tacrolimus group had significantly lower rates of biopsy-confirmed acute rejection (30.7% vs. 46.4%, $P = 0.001$) and of use of antilymphocyte therapy (10.7% vs. 25.1%, $P < 0.001$). In both treatment groups, impaired renal function, gastrointestinal disorders, and neurologic complications were common, although tremor and paresthesia not requiring treatment or dosage change were more frequent in the tacrolimus group. Post-CRT diabetes mellitus, which occurred in 19.9% of the tacrolimus group and in 4% of the cyclosporine group ($P < 0.001$), was reversible in some cases. Hyperlipidemia and hypercholesterolemia were substantially decreased in the tacrolimus group. Although such well documented side-effects of cyclosporine as hirsutism, gingivitis, and gum hyperplasia were rarely seen with tacrolimus, alopecia and pruritus were more frequent.

Conclusions.—The dramatic reduction in biopsy-proved acute rejection, significantly reducing the need for antilymphocyte antibody treatment, has great clinical significance. Neurologic events were increased but were rarely treatment limiting, and post-CRT diabetes mellitus was increased but was reversible in some cases. Increasing clinical experience should foster better management. Tacrolimus is safe, effective, and superior to cyclosporine in CRT.

▶ This important study is the first direct comparison of FK506 and cyclosporine in renal transplantation. Although patient and graft survivals were comparable, there was less rejection in the FK506 group. Nephrotoxicity was similar; however, there was a higher incidence of posttransplant diabetes in the tacrolimus group. In interpreting this article, it is very important to understand that the cyclosporine group was treated with Sandimmune. This preparation of cyclosporine is not as reliably absorbed as the newer product Neoral. Although these findings are certainly notable, the results will ultimately have to be updated with the use of Neoral because it is the most common preparation of cyclosporine offered to new transplant recipients over the past several years.

D.A. Goldfarb, M.D.

Clinical Significance of Renal Allograft Biopsies With "Borderline Changes," as Defined in the Banff Schema
Saad R, Gritsch HA, Shapiro R, et al (Univ of Pittsburgh, Pa)
Transplantation 64:992–995, 1997   9–22

Introduction.—Biopsies with changes insufficient for a diagnosis of mild acute rejection are classified as having "borderline changes" under the Banff Schema. While some suggest that patients under this classification should receive no treatment, others believe these patients would benefit from increased immunosuppression. There was a study of patients with borderline changes who were compared to patients with mild acute rejection to further clarify the clinical course of and response to antirejection therapy.

Methods.—There were 14 patients with mild acute rejection who received antirejection therapy, and who were compared to 24 patients with borderline changes who also received antirejection therapy. Patients were classified as showing complete response if the posttreatment fall in serum creatinine was more than 70%, a partial response if the serum creatinine was 30%–70%, and no response if the serum creatinine fell to less than 30%. In accordance with the Banff Schema, renal allograft biopsies were systematically evaluated.

Results.—In 15 of 24 patients (63%), complete response to antirejection therapy was seen. In 3 patients (13%), there was a partial response, and 6 patients (25%) had no response with borderline change. Nonresponse was associated with higher scores of acute tubular necrosis and chronic allograft nephropathy, when nonresponding patients were compared with patients showing complete response. Compared with patients with borderline change, 12 of 14 (86%) patients with mild acute rejection showed complete response to antirejection therapy. A higher score for chronic allograft nephropathy was associated with a lack of response.

Conclusion.—Borderline changes frequently require increased immunosuppression when biopsies are done in the context of renal allograft dysfunction. This therapeutic response, however, is limited by intercurrent conditions, such as acute tubular necrosis or chronic allograft nephropathy. These findings should not be extrapolated to protocol biopsies performed in the setting of stable graft function.

▶ According to the Banff Schema for renal transplant histopathology, "borderline changes" refer to those changes insufficient for diagnosis of mild acute rejection. Still, little is known regarding the outcome of these patients. This article demonstrates that in the setting of renal allograft dysfunction, a majority of the patients respond to intervention aimed at treatment of rejection. In general, the patients who did not respond had other biopsy parameters (glomerulosclerosis, interstitial fibrosis) as a reason for nonresponse.

D.A. Goldfarb, M.D.

Critical Evaluation of the Association of Acute With Chronic Graft Rejection in Kidney and Heart Transplant Recipients
Opelz G, for the Collaborative Transplant Study (Univ of Heidelberg, Germany)
Transplant Proc 29:73–76, 1997   9–23

Introduction.—Acute transplant rejection occurs less frequently with the use of current immunosuppressive methods, but chronic rejection is a growing concern. Because most cases of chronic rejection occur in patients who have experienced episodes of acute rejection, more aggressive immunosuppressive induction treatment might prevent the development of chronic rejection. An analysis of heart and kidney transplant recipients examined the relationship between acute and chronic graft rejection.

Methods.—Transplants included in the analysis were performed from 1983 to 1994 and reported to the Collaborative Transplant Study by 305 kidney and 104 heart transplant centers. Clinical follow-up data were reported at 3, 6, and 12 months, then yearly.

Results.—Patients treated for acute rejection of kidney grafts were separated into those whose serum creatinine values returned to a level considered "normal" for transplant patients and those who did not have a return to normal values. The former had only a slightly lower long-term graft survival compared with patients who experienced no rejection during the first posttransplant year. In contrast, those who continued to have higher creatinine values after treatment for acute rejection had an inferior long-term outcome. Even severe rejection had no adverse effect on long-term outcome as long as it was completely reversible. Outcome was not influenced by the use of aggressive induction treatment with monoclonal or polyclonal antibodies. The analysis of heart transplants showed very little evidence that acute rejection episodes were predictive of chronic rejection.

Discussion.—The incidence of chronic kidney graft rejection may be reduced by successful treatment of episodes of acute rejection. Aggressive induction treatment with monoclonal or polyclonal antibodies does not appear, however, to reduce the rate of chronic kidney graft rejection. Treatment for acute rejection had no effect on long-term outcome after heart transplantation.

▶ This is confirmation that not all rejections are equal. There was little difference in long-term graft survival with or without rejection if the creatinine value was low at 1 year. In contrast, for patients with higher creatinine values, the presence or absence of rejection had a significant impact on long-term graft survival. This substantiates the concept that the ultimate level of renal function at 1 year is a major predictor of long-term graft success.

D.A. Goldfarb, M.D.

Impact of Acute Rejection and Early Allograft Function on Renal Allograft Survival

Cosio FG, Pelletier RP, Falkenhain ME, et al (Ohio State Univ, Columbus)
Transplantation 63:1611–1615, 1997   9–24

Introduction.—Understanding the relationship between acute rejection (AR), graft function, and graft survival can enhance understanding of chronic transplant nephropathy and its prevention. The relationship between AR and graft function was assessed in 843 adult recipients of first cadaveric renal grafts to determine the impact of these factors alone or in combination.

Findings.—Follow-up was a minimum of 3.5 years. During follow-up, 23% of patients died and 15% lost their allograft. Patients were placed in 1 of 4 groups, depending on history of AR and concentration of serum creatinine during the first 6 months after transplantation (SCr_{6mo}). There were no significant between-group differences in death censored allografts in 376 patients without AR and with low SCr_{6mo} (group 1); in 117 patients without AR but with an elevated SCr_{6mo} (group 2); or in 185 patients with AR but with low SCr_{6mo} (group 3). Compared with these 3 groups, the 165 patients in group 4 with AR and elevated SCr_{6mo} had a significantly worse graft survival. In group 4, 32% of patients had an elevated SCr at 10 days after transplantation (SCr_{10d}), before onset of AR, that was higher than or equal to SCr_{6mo}. Using these observations, the implications of SCr_{10d} concentration on graft prognosis were evaluated. There was a weak correlation between SCr_{10d} and graft survival. An elevated SCr_{10d} was significantly correlated with other potential risk factors for graft survival: male recipient, older donors, heavier recipients, and the posttransplant factors of increasing numbers of AR, high posttransplant blood pressure, and lower doses of cyclosporine.

Conclusions.—When correlated with AR, graft dysfunction predicts poor graft survival. Acute rejection predicts poor allograft survival only when correlated with graft dysfunction. The SCr_{10d} may be considered an indicator of risk factors from the donor and recipient and predicts a higher risk of acquiring additional risk factors in the early transplantation period.

▶ This article deals with an old subject and clarifies issues pertaining to it. For some time it has been recognized that any episode of AR is associated with a poorer long-term prognosis. This article clearly demonstrates that only those patients who have renal dysfunction as a consequence of AR are at risk for a long-term poor prognosis. Furthermore, early allograft dysfunction in the absence of AR does not impart a serious long-term adverse risk.

D.A. Goldfarb, M.D.

Long-term Renal Allograft Survival: Prognostic Implication of the Timing of Acute Rejection Episodes
Leggat JE Jr, Ojo AO, Leichtman AB, et al (Univ of Michigan, Ann Arbor)
Transplantation 63:1268–1272, 1997   9–25

Introduction.—Despite improvements in short-term survival of renal allografts, there has been relatively little change in long-term survival. The pathogenesis of chronic rejection, the major cause of late allograft loss, is unclear; however, acute transplant rejection (ATR) is a known risk factor for chronic rejection. The effects of the timing of ATR on long-term allograft survival were analyzed,

Methods.—The study used United States Renal Data System data on adult transplant patients whose initial renal allografts were still functioning at 1 year. The analysis included 31,600 patients operated on from 1984 through 1992 at 217 centers. Based on time to their first ATR, the patients were divided into 4 groups: 21% of patients had no episodes of ATR in the first year (group I), 17% had an episode of ATR before discharge (group II), 17% had their first episode of ATR between discharge and 6 months later (group III), and 4% had their first ATR between 7 months and 1 year after discharge (group IV). A Cox proportional hazard model, with adjustment for 19 cofactors, was used to examine 5-year allograft survival among the various groups.

Results.—Estimated 5-year graft survival decreased progressively with increasing time to first ATR: 78% in group I, 72% in group II, 69% in group III, and 54% in group IV. Graft survival was significantly better in group I than in all other groups; it was significantly worse in group IV than in all other groups. The half-life of allograft loss after 1 year of allograft survival was 9.5 years for group I, 8.3 years for groups II and III, and 5.0 years for group IV. Compared with group I, relative risks of graft loss were 1.24 in group II, 1.50 in group III, and 5.0 in group IV. For patients with episodes of ATR in more than 1 time period, later episodes were linked to worse long-term graft survival. This relationship was unrelated to previous episodes of ATR.

Conclusion.—In renal allograft recipients whose grafts survive for 1 year, a later initial episode of ATR is associated with a worse prognosis for long-term graft survival. Survival may also be worse for later rejections in combination with previous rejections. Later episodes of ATR may be related to inadequate immunosuppression from noncompliance or disruption of immune tolerance to the graft. These behavioral and immunologic factors must be considered in any attempt to reduce late transplant loss.

▶ Not all rejections are similar in their impact upon long-term allograft survival. In a large review of U.S. Renal Data System data, the authors demonstrate the more serious consequences of rejection that occurs after the first 6 months.

D.A. Goldfarb, M.D.

Risk Factors for Vascular Thrombosis in Pediatric Renal Transplantation: A Special Report of the North American Pediatric Renal Transplant Cooperative Study

Singh A, Stablein D, Tejani A (State Univ of New York, Brooklyn; EMMES Corp, Potomac, Md; New York Med College, Valhalla)
Transplantation 63:1263–1267, 1997   9–26

Purpose.—Vascular thrombosis is responsible for graft failure in 12% of initial and 19% of repeat pediatric renal transplants. The events leading to thrombosis are unclear, but several factors are thought to play a role. Risk factors for vascular thrombosis after renal transplantation in children were investigated.

Methods.—The study used data from the North American Pediatric Renal Transplant Cooperative Study. Of the 4,394 transplants considered, 2,060 were living donor (LD) transplants and 2,334 were cadaver donor (CAD) transplants. Vascular thrombosis occurred in 1.8% of the LD transplants and 4.2% of the CAD transplants. Univariate and multivariate analyses were performed to identify risk factors for vascular thrombosis.

Results.—On univariate analysis, thrombosis was a more frequent cause of graft loss in recipients aged less than 2 years, compared with older recipients. For children under 2 years, the rate of graft loss caused by thrombosis was 9.0% for CAD transplant recipients and 3.5% for LD transplant recipients; for children older than 12 years, these rates were 3.5% and 1.9%, respectively. The thrombosis rate was 8.3% for recipients of kidneys from donors less than 5 years of age, compared to 4.5% with organs from 5- to 10-year-old donors and 3.2% for organs from donors over 10 years of age. The thrombosis rate was 5.6% when the cold ischemia time was greater than 24 hours vs. 3.2% with shorter cold ischemia times. Risk of graft loss to thrombosis was reduced for recipients who received antilymphocyte therapy on the day of, or the day after, transplantation (2.2% vs. 4.1%). These patterns were similar for the LD and CAD groups. Among LD recipients, those who had received previous transplants had a higher thrombosis rate than those receiving their first transplant (4.6% vs. 1.6%). Regardless of the source of the organ, acute tubular necrosis significantly increased the risk of thrombosis.

On regression analysis, previous transplantation was associated with an increased risk of thrombosis in the LD group. Risk decreased in linear fashion with increasing recipient age, and with use of antilymphocyte antibody or cyclosporine on day 0 or 1. In the CAD group, thrombosis risk increased with cold ischemia time of greater than 24 hours and decreased with antibody induction therapy, donor age older than 5 years, and increased recipient age.

Conclusion.—For pediatric LD kidney recipients, previous transplantation and young recipient age are significant risk factors. For pediatric CAD kidney recipients, risk factors include younger recipient and donor age and prolonged cold ischemia time. Immediate prophylactic antibody therapy does not increase thrombosis risk for either group.

▶ Graft thrombosis remains a significant cause of graft loss in the pediatric population. This is the largest study to date examining risk factors for vascular thrombosis in pediatric transplantation. One of the most significant findings of this paper was that antilymphocyte therapy diminished graft loss from thrombosis. Furthermore, there was no difference between antithymocyte globulin/antilymphocyte globulin and OKT3. Previously, OKT3 had been associated with a higher incidence of graft thrombosis in pediatric patients.

D.A. Goldfarb, M.D.

Patterns of Graft Infiltration and Cytokine Gene Expression During the First 10 Days of Kidney Transplantation
McLean AG, Hughes D, Welsh KI, et al (Oxford Univ, England)
Transplantation 63:374–380, 1997   9–27

Background.—Although the histologic and immunohistologic evidence of acute transplant rejection is beginning to unfold, the role of T-cell–mediated damage is less well studied. A theory holds that the immune response to an allograft is determined by the balance between circuits involving T-helper (Th) 1 cells (producing interleukin 2 [IL-2] and γ-interferon [γ-IFN]) and Th2 cells (producing interleukins 4 and 10 [IL-4 and IL-10]). Also, previous research has shown that interleukin 2 (IL-2) gene expression correlates closely with acute rejection. These authors looked for evidence of these mechanisms during the acute period after kidney transplantation.

Methods.—Twenty patients received kidney transplants and were monitored for 10 days. All received postoperative triple-drug immunosuppressive therapy, and any episodes of rejection were treated with methylprednisolone. Each graft provided paired fine-needle aspiration samples for cytologic and immunocytologic analysis of morphological cytology and for reverse transcriptase–polymerase chain reaction analysis of cytokine gene expression.

Findings.—Interleukin 10 gene expression was measurable in all 20 grafts, but its presence bore no relationship to the development of rejection. Only 2 samples (of 84 data points) contained IL-6, and no IL-4 was detected in any grafts. A low-grade, monocyte-rich mononuclear cell infiltrate was evident in all grafts during the first 3 days after transplantation, after which the infiltrates became more lymphocytic. Of 20 grafts, 13 had dense infiltrates. Acute cellular rejection and graft dysfunction developed in 7 of these, whereas in 6, no rejection was seen. All 13 grafts with dense infiltrates showed a biphasic pattern of gene expression for IL-2 and γ-IFN. However, no IL-2 or γ-IFN was seen in the 7 grafts without dense infiltrates, nor did these grafts experience rejection. Donor recipient mismatching at one or both loci was largely responsible for the episodes of rejection.

Conclusions.—Rejecting and nonrejecting infiltrates cannot be distinguished based on their pattern of gene expression for Th1 cells in the first 10 postoperative days. Although IL-2 and γ-IFN had to be present before acute rejection developed, their presence was not sufficient to cause rejection. No evidence was found that Th2 (IL-4 and IL-10) cells play a significant role in acute cellular rejection.

▶ Great strides have been made regarding control of rejection for renal transplant recipients in the past 10–15 years. Still, within 6 months of transplantation, between 20% and 50% of patients may experience an episode of acute cellular rejection. Any episode of rejection has been associated with a poor long-term prognosis. Rejection is usually manifest as renal dysfunction. At this point, renal damage has occurred. This article examines cytokine expression in that period which leads to rejection. Although a reliable predictor was not identified, it is the approach adopted by this group that may lead to better prediction of rejection. In this way, graft dysfunction may be prevented at a stage before loss of nephrons occurs.

D.A. Goldfarb, M.D.

Molecular Executors of Cell Death: Differential Intrarenal Expression of Fas Ligand, Fas, Granzyme B, and Perforin During Acute and/or Chronic Rejection of Human Renal Allografts
Sharma VK, Bologa RM, Li B, et al (New York Hosp-Cornell Med Ctr; Hennepin County Med Ctr, Minneapolis)
Transplantation 62:1860–1866, 1996   9–28

Background.—Two distinct cytolytic pathways have been described. In one, the interaction between the Fas antigen and its ligand results in apoptosis. In the other, the pore-forming protein perforin and the serine protease granzyme B contribute to DNA fragmentation and cell death. The intrarenal expression of these molecular executors of cell death was studied in light of the potential participation of cytolytically active cellular elements in the antiallograft repertory.

Methods.—Eighty human renal allograft biopsies were studied. Intrarenal expression of Fas antigen, Fas ligand, granzyme B, and perforin was identified using reverse transcriptase-polymerase chain reaction. Display of messenger RNA (mRNA) was correlated with the Banff histologic diagnosis of renal allografts.

Findings.—Intrarenal expression of Fas ligand mRNA and of granzyme B mRNA was found to be a correlate of acute but not chronic rejection. In the absence of rejection, Fas ligand mRNA was not detectable. The intrarenal coexpression of members of each lytic pathway and that of both pathways were associated with acute rejection. In addition, there was a direct correlation between the histologic severity of acute rejection and intrarenal coexpression of mRNA encoding Fas ligand, Fas, granzyme B, and perforin.

Conclusions.—These data demonstrate the differential expression of the 2 major lytic pathways in acute and chronic allograft rejection. Specific treatment aimed at the cytotoxic attack molecules may be effective in preventing and/or treating acute rejection.

▶ Acute rejection remains an important cause for early renal allograft dysfunction and is now well recognized to have adverse effects on long-term renal function. Still, the precise mechanism by which acute rejection mediates renal damage is unclear. This article analyzes the differential intrarenal expression of several molecular executors of cell death that work through a variety of mechanisms. With a more precise knowledge of the molecular events associated with acute rejection, better strategies for prevention and treatment may be developed.

D.A. Goldfarb, M.D.

Nephron Mass Modulates the Hemodynamic, Cellular, and Molecular Response of the Rat Renal Allograft
Azuma H, Nadeau K, Mackenzie HS, et al (Harvard Med School, Boston; Brigham and Women's Hosp, Boston)
Transplantation 63:519–528, 1997   9–29

Background.—Some have suggested that the number of nephrons at transplantation (i.e., renal mass) can affect renal allograft function over the long term. These investigators examined the hemodynamic, cellular, and molecular responses to the effects of varying renal mass as a factor in chronic renal allograft rejection.

Methods.—Fisher 344 rats were divided into 4 groups. In group 1, functioning renal mass was reduced to one sixth via nephrectomy or ligation of blood supply. In group 2, rats were bilaterally nephrectomized and received a single allograft or isograft. Rats in group 3 were either bilaterally or unilaterally nephrectomized, then received either 2 allografts or 1 allograft, respectively, for a total of 2 functioning kidneys. In group 4, rats were unilaterally nephrectomized, received an allograft, and then either retained their native kidney (group 4A) or had it removed after 8 weeks (delayed single-kidney state, group 4B). At various intervals, kidneys were weighed and sectioned for immunohistologic analysis and polymerase chain reaction analysis.

Findings.—Proteinuria was progressive and significantly worse in group 1, with group 2 showing proteinuria after 12 weeks. Groups 3 and 4A experienced no proteinuria; proteinuria in group 4B paralleled that in group 2. By 24 weeks, the weight of single allografts in group 2 was similar to total renal weight in groups 3 and 4A. By the end of the study (40 weeks), rats with only 1 kidney (groups 2 and 4B) had significantly more glomerulosclerosis than groups 3 and 4A. Arteriosclerosis at 40 weeks was significantly more common in group 2 than in groups 3, 4A, and 4B. Antigen expression in group 1 peaked early (between 6 and 9 weeks). Antigen expression in group 2 peaked at 16 weeks and declined thereafter; it peaked at 32 weeks in group 4B, and it was delayed with a significantly lower peak at 40 weeks in groups 3 and 4B. Findings from polymerase chain reaction analysis bolstered the results from immunohistologic study.

Conclusion.—The patterns of proteinuria, glomerulosclerosis, and arteriosclerosis support the idea that total renal mass at transplantation has significant effects on when and to what extent graft injury develops. Furthermore, given the changes in macrophages and their associated cytokines, renal mass at transplantation also influences the long-term immunologic mechanisms of injury.

▶ In a well-established experimental model of chronic renal allograft rejection, the authors, once again, demonstrate that modulation of the total renal mass supplied at transplantation can induce hyperfiltration-related injury such as proteinuria, glomerulosclerosis, and arterial hyalinization. These changes occur earlier and more profoundly with a greater reduction in overall renal mass.

In this paper, the authors identify a predictable pattern of sequential expression of macrophage chemoattractants (regulated upon activation, normal T cell expressed and secreted chemokine), monocyte chemotactic protein, adhesion molecules (intercellular adhesion molecules), endothelin, HLA class II molecules, and cytokines (transforming growth factor–β, tumor necrosis factor–α). The sequential changes in these chemical mediators occurs in an accelerated manner in reduced-mass kidneys. Therefore, any renal injury in a transplanted kidney that reduces mass below some critical level has the ability to set off a cascade of molecular events that culminates in graft sclerosis. This may have implications with regard to nephron dosing in clinical transplantation. With further understanding of these mechanisms of injury, it will be interesting to see whether strategies are developed to ameliorate the effects of hyperfiltration.

D.A. Goldfarb, M.D.

Should Obese Patients Lose Weight Before Receiving a Kidney Transplant?

Modlin CS, Flechner SM, Goormastic M, et al (Cleveland Clinic Found, Ohio)
Transplantation 64:599–604, 1997   9–30

Introduction.—Some studies have found that obese recipients of kidney transplants have increased mortality, reduced long- and short-term graft survival, and more surgical and medical complications than nonobese recipients. Other reports, however, do not support the idea that obesity is associated with a worse outcome after renal transplantation. A study of obese and nonobese patients sought to determine whether those with excess body weight should undergo transplantation.

Methods.—The study population included 127 obese patients transplanted between 1970 and 1994. Controls were 127 nonobese patients who received their renal transplant within approximately 5 years of the study group. The 2 groups were comparable in cause of renal failure, sex, donor source, and immunosuppression. Pretransplant and posttransplant clinical data were collected and compared for the obese and nonobese patients.

Results.—Obese patients were significantly older than nonobese patients at the time of transplant (mean, 43.8 years vs. 39.8 years). Although generally comparable in pretransplant data, significantly more obese patients had a history of angina or myocardial infarction (11.2% vs. 3.2% and 5.6% vs. 0.8%, respectively). The 2 groups were similar in need for dialysis for the first 7 days after transplant, length of hospital stay, and operative blood loss. Obese patients experienced significantly more complications per patient, required significantly increased operative and renal revascularization, and had a significantly higher incidence of posttransplant diabetes. At an average follow-up of 58.9 months, patient survival was greater in nonobese patients (89% vs. 67%). The most common causes of death were a cardiac event in the obese group (39.1%) and infectious complications in the nonobese group (28%). When death with graft function was censored, the 2 groups did not differ significantly in graft survival. Obese patients were receiving less cyclosporine than nonobese patients, but their cyclosporine trough blood levels were similar.

Conclusion.—Although the 5-year mortality rate was increased in obese vs. nonobese kidney transplant recipients, cardiac events in the obese patients accounted for most of this difference. Weight reduction is recommended for the high-risk cohort of obese patients with coronary artery disease.

▶ Some have questioned the wisdom of transplanting normal-sized adult kidneys into overweight patients. The concern is over the disparity between transplanted nephron mass and excessive metabolic demand from an overweight patient. The findings of this paper suggest that there is no increase in graft loss from immunologic causes or chronic rejection in an obese population. The significant differences in 5-year graft loss related purely to an increase in the risk of death with a functioning graft. Significantly over-weight patients need to understand this issue before their transplants.

D.A. Goldfarb, M.D.

Results of Renal Transplantation in Patients With Renal Cell Carcinoma and Von Hippel-Lindau Disease

Goldfarb DA, Neumann HPH, Penn I, et al (Cleveland Clinic Found, Ohio; Albert-Ludwigs Univ, Freiburg Germany; Univ of Cincinnati, Ohio)
Transplantation 64:1726–1729, 1997   9–31

Introduction.—Renal cell carcinoma is reported to occur in up to 45% of patients with von Hippel-Lindau disease (VHL) and is a leading cause of death for those with this autosomal dominant syndrome. Compared with sporadic cases, renal cell carcinoma associated with VHL occurs at a younger age and is more frequently bilateral and multicentric. A review of 32 patients with VHL who underwent renal transplantation for localized renal cell carcinoma was conducted to determine outcome of the proce-dure.

Methods.—The study group consisted of 23 men and 9 women (mean age, 36 years) who received transplants between 1974 and 1996. Their mean duration of dialysis before transplantation was 26 months. Donor sources were cadaveric in 62.5% of cases, living-related in 28.1%, and living-unrelated in 9.4%. Patients were followed for a mean of 48 months and compared for outcome with a cohort of 32 renal transplant recipients without VHL disease. The 2 groups were matched for age, gender, primary or regraft transplant, and date of transplantation.

Results.—The 32 study patients received 33 kidney transplants; 1 pa-tient had a nonfunctioning graft and received a successful transplant 24 months later. Graft survival in patients with VHL disease was 100% at 1 year and 62.6% at 5 years. The control group had graft survival rates of 87.5% and 76.1%, respectively, at 1 and 5 years. Neither graft survival nor renal function, as assessed by mean serum creatinine value, differed between the 2 groups. There were 5 deaths in each group; 3 patients with VHL disease died with metastatic disease and all 5 in the control group died of cardiovascular disease.

Conclusion.—End-stage renal failure is common in patients with renal cell carcinoma and VHL, and the preferred treatment in such cases is renal transplantation. Although there is concern that immunosuppression may predispose to tumor recurrence, a review of outcomes supports the value of renal transplantation in this population.

▶ Patients with VHL have germ-line mutation in chromosome 3p. They are prone to the development of renal carcinoma. Although a nephron-sparing approach provides effective initial management, many patients with VHL ultimately go on to require removal of all renal tissue. This study summarizes the excellent results that can be obtained with renal transplantation in this population, with an acceptable rate of tumor recurrence. Overall, patients with VHL act much more like patients with acquired renal cystic disease, as opposed to patients with sporadic renal cell carcinoma, in terms of propensity for recurrence to develop after transplantation.

D.A. Goldfarb, M.D.

Nephrotic-Range Proteinuria in Renal Atheroembolic Disease: Report of Four Cases
Haqqie SS, Urizar RE, Singh J (Stratton Veterans Affairs Med Ctr, Albany, NY; Albany Med College, NY)
Am J Kidney Dis 28:493–501, 1996   9–32

Background.—Renal atheroembolic disease (AED) occurs as cholesterol-containing plaques in blood vessels that ulcerate. The movement of these cholesterol crystals into the kidney can lead to acute or chronic renal failure. However, patients with AED rarely have nephrotic proteinuria, which can thwart the diagnosis of renal failure. These investigators report on 4 patients with histologically proven AED who developed nephrotic-range proteinuria.

Methods.—Various symptoms were seen in these patients, but all 4 were elderly (60–81 years old), all 4 had hypertension, 3 were smokers, and 3 had undergone cardiac surgery. Nephrotic range proteinuria was seen in all 4 patients. All patients underwent percutaneous needle biopsy to determine the cause of the nephrotic syndrome. Samples were examined by light and electron microscopy and immunofluorescence.

Findings.—Renal biopsy sampling retrieved 102 glomeruli. Hyalinization was seen in 27% of glomeruli examined by light microscopy. Cholesterol emboli were seen in vessels. Glomerular basement membrane wrinkling also was seen with all 3 examination methods. Based on the histologic findings, no diagnoses other than AED were supported.

Conclusions.—Vascular surgery has been shown to be associated with an increased risk of AED, because the surgical or radiologic procedures cause cholesterol-containing plaques to ulcerate. Furthermore, elderly men with hypertension are more likely to have AED. Thus, AED should be part of the differential diagnosis for elderly patients with hypertension and atherosclerotic vascular disease who develop nephrotic syndrome.

▶ Atheroembolic renal disease can be seen in the setting of renal artery stenosis or generalized atherosclerosis. Manifestations of renal insufficiency usually occur after an inciting event such as vascular surgery or an interventive radiologic procedure. Historically, there has not been an association with proteinuria. This paper very nicely documents 4 cases of nephrotic-range proteinuria in patients with atheroembolic renal disease. Certainly this diagnosis should now be entertained for elderly patients with hypertension, widespread atherosclerotic vascular disease, and nephrotic-range pro-teinuria.

D.A. Goldfarb, M.D.

Epidermal Growth Factor Suppresses Renal Tubular Apoptosis Following Ureteral Obstruction

Kennedy WA II, Buttyan R, Garcia-Montes E, et al (Columbia Univ, New York; Maimonides Med Ctr, Brooklyn, New York)
Urology 49:973–980, 1997   9–33

Background.—Obstruction of the ureter can lead to the degenerative condition of hydronephrosis. This degeneration has been related to apoptosis, and apoptosis is known to result from certain growth factor deficiencies (among other causes). Could supplementation of epidermal growth factor (EGF) attenuate or prevent the cell death that occurs in obstructive nephropathy? These investigators sought to answer this question.

Methods.—Acute unilateral ureteral obstruction was surgically induced in male rats by left proximal complete ureteral ligation. An additional 2 rats were used as sham-operated controls. Animals with obstruction were then divided into 2 groups, those that received EGF supplementation at 10, 20, or 40 µg/day (test group) and those that did not receive EGF (control group). At 24, 48, and 72 hours, 2 animals at each EGF dose and 2 controls were killed, and their kidneys were snap frozen for molecular and histologic analyses. DNA was extracted to determine the laddering pattern on agarose gel electrophoresis and to determine fragmented DNA in apoptotic cells by in situ gap labeling. Also, mRNA levels of a genetic marker of apoptosis, sulfated glycoprotein-2 (SGP-2), were determined by in situ hybridization.

Findings.—The administration of EGF significantly increased renal cortex mitotic activity in the test group, with greater effects at higher doses. DNA laddering also was less in the test group, as was DNA fragmentation, and these effects were again more pronounced at higher EGF doses. In fact, at the 40 µg/day EGF dose, DNA fragmentation in the test kidneys was similar to that in the sham-operated controls. The architecture of in situ gap-labeled nuclei was most disrupted in the control rats, least disrupted in the sham-operated controls, and intermediate in the EGF-supplemented rats (closer to that of the sham-operated controls). Finally, SGP-2 as a marker of apoptosis was less pronounced in the test group than it was in the control group.

Conclusions.—EGF administration stimulated the proliferation of tubular epithelial cells. Apoptosis was less pronounced in the EGF-treated kidneys, as determined by DNA fragmentation and by the gene product SGP-2. The preservation of renal tubular epithelial cells by EGF indicates a role for EGF as adjunctive therapy in hydronephrosis and other obstructive nephropathies.

▶ Improved understanding of basic urologic pathophysiology at the molecular level will be the key to more successful treatments in the future. This paper (authored by a scholar of the American Foundation for Urological Diseases) is an excellent demonstration of how supplemental growth factors may be helpful in preventing programmed cell death in hydronephrotic kidneys. If this can be associated with a distinctive functional benefit for recovery in follow-up experiments, this concept may translate into a useful adjunct in the treatment of hydronephrosis.

D.A. Goldfarb, M.D.

10 Incontinence

A Followup on Transurethral Collagen Injection Therapy for Urinary Incontinence
Cross CA, English SF, Cespedes RD, et al (Univ of Texas, Houston; Wilford Hall Med Ctr, Lackland Air Force Base, Tex)
J Urol 159:106–108, 1998

Background.—Urinary incontinence due to intrinsic sphincter deficiency can be treated with sling procedures, artificial sphincters, and injectable agents. Since 1993, injection of glutaraldehyde cross-linked bovine collagen has been used to treat intrinsic sphincter deficiency in women. This report describes the results of 139 patients treated with transurethral collagen therapy from 1994 to 1997.

Methods.—Abdominal leak point pressure was determined using video urodynamics in patients with urinary incontinence complaints. An abdominal leak point pressure of less than 60 cm water was used to identify patients with intrinsic sphincter deficiency. These patients underwent collagen skin testing. Collagen injections were performed with local anesthesia at an outpatient clinic for 139 patients. The median patient age was 72, and the average duration of incontinence was 3.5 years. The median follow-up period was 18 months. Postprocedure evaluation included chart review and telephone questionnaire.

Results.—Of the 139 patients in this study group, 74% were substantially improved (72% after 2 or fewer procedures), and 20% were improved. Treatment failed in 7 patients who underwent successful surgical

TABLE 2.—Post-procedural Evaluation

	No. Pts.	No. De Novo Detrusor Instability (%)	No. Continued Urge Incontinence (%)	No. Repeat Collagen or Other Procedure
Substantially improved	103	23 (22)	17 (16)	10
Improved	29	12 (41)	9 (31)	6
Failed	7	4 (57)	3 (43)	4 slings, 3 myectomies

(Courtesy of Cross CA, English SF, Cespedes RD, et al: A followup on transurethral collagen injection therapy for urinary incontinence. *J Urol* 159:106–108, 1998.)

procedures. In 11.6% of the successfully treated patients, additional collagen injections were required 6 months later as efficacy decreased (Table 2). No complications developed from transurethral collagen injection.

Conclusions.—Women with stress incontinence caused by intrinsic sphincter deficiency can be treated successfully with transurethral collagen injection therapy. This procedure is minimally invasive and is associated with few side effects.

▶ Collagen injection is clearly a safe, low morbidity procedure that improves urinary incontinence, but we need to have some quality-of-life assessments in the follow-up evaluation of collagen injection patients. The cure rate in most studies is around 20% to 25%,[1] and we don't know how many patients are cured in this study though it is probably small because the authors don't list this group. However, the real issue is whether or not the women in the substantially improved group are satisfied with the results or if they will eventually require additional therapy such as a pubovaginal sling.

D.E. Coplen, M.D.

Reference

1. Swami S, Batista JE, and Abrams P: Collagen for female genuine stress incontinence after a minimum 2-year follow-up. *Br J Urol* 80:757–761, 1997.

Collagen Injection Therapy for Postradical Retropubic Prostatectomy Incontinence: Role of Valsalva Leak Point Pressure
Sánchez-Ortiz RF, Broderick GA, Chaikin DC, et al (Univ of Pennsylvania, Philadelphia)
J Urol 158:2132–2136, 1997   10–2

Introduction.—In men with a localized adenoma and a life expectancy of at least 10 years, radical prostatectomy is the standard treatment. Following this procedure, incontinence is not uncommon. Transurethral injection of glutaraldehyde cross-linked collagen has been successfully used to treat incontinence in women but has been less successful in men. To identify the subset of patients with post-radical prostatectomy urinary incontinence who might benefit from collagen injection, the relationship between urodynamics, Valsalva leak point, and outcome was retrospectively assessed in 31 men.

Methods.—The study group consisted of 31 men, aged 43 to 79, who received transurethral collagen injection therapy for postradical retropubic prostatectomy incontinence. Prior to treatment, all patients had a complete medical history, physical examination, and urodynamic evaluation and completed the American Urology Association (AUA) quality-of-life index. Each patient was skin tested for collagen hypersensitivity. Collagen injection was considered a successful treatment if follow-up AUA quality-of-life index was 3 or less or if there was a 50% reduction in the daily use of pads and the patient would recommend this treatment to others.

Results.—Of the 31 men in the study group, 11 had a successful result from collagen injection therapy. Of these 11, 2 were completely dry and 9 were improved. The successfully treated patients had an average Valsalva leak point pressure of at least 64.0 cm water, compared to an average of 42.2 cm water in patients in whom the treatment was not successful. Among patients with a Valsalva leak point pressure of at least 60 cm water, 70% had a successful result, whereas 81% of those with a lower Valsalva leak point pressure did not. There was no other significant difference between these 2 groups.

Conclusions.—This retrospective study of men who received collagen injection therapy for postradical prostatectomy incontinence demonstrates that this therapy can be effective in a minority of patients, although few will be completely dry. Patients with a pretreatment Valsalva leak point pressure of less than 60 cm water have a significantly lower chance of a successful treatment with collagen injection than those with a higher Valsalva leak point pressure. Valsalva leak point pressure may be useful to screen men with postradical prostatectomy incontinence to determine who would benefit from collagen injection therapy.

▶ Postradical prostatectomy incontinence is difficult to treat. The artificial sphincter gives the best cure rate but is associated with increased patient morbidity and complications. Collagen injection has a low cure rate (less than 10% in this series) but pre-injection Valsalva leak point pressure (VLPP) may help select appropriate patients. Seventy percent of men with leak point pressures greater than 60 cm water had improvement whereas only a minority were cured. Men with a low VLPP are probably best treated with other modalities given the cost of the collagen and the need for repeated injections in this subset. Valsalva leak point pressure is a useful measure that may help direct therapeutic interventions for postprostatectomy incontinence.

D.E. Coplen, M.D.

Morbidity and Mortality of Incontinence Surgery in Elderly Women: An Analysis of Medicare Data

Sultana CJ, Campbell JW, Pisanelli WS, et al (Case Western Reserve Univ, Cleveland, Ohio; MetroHealth Med Ctr, Cleveland, Ohio)
Am J Obstet Gynecol 176:344–348, 1997   10–3

Introduction.—In the last few decades, the proportion of surgery performed among the elderly has grown from 19% of all operative procedures in 1980 to 29% in 1989. Little data are available on surgery for urinary incontinence for older women. In women 65 years or older, surgical mortality rates and causes of mortality for needle urethropexies, retropubic suspensions, and anterior vaginal repairs were determined, as well as specific complications and causes of postoperative morbidity.

Methods.—A review was conducted of surgical procedures done for incontinence from data obtained from Medicare billing forms in the Medicare Provider Analysis and Review Record database. The procedures were performed from 1984 to 1991 for 66,478 women, with a mean and median age of 71 years, and the population was overwhelmingly white. A review of secondary diagnosis codes helped reveal comorbidities and reasons for readmission.

Results.—There was a 0.33% 30-day surgical mortality. Age affected length of stay and an increase in mortality. Death was associated with the acute events of cerebrovascular accident (stroke) (14.6%); myocardial infarction (14.2%); pulmonary embolism or deep vein thrombosis (9.7%); and pneumonia (2.7%). Higher rates of diabetes and heart failure were seen with patients who died, but they did not have higher rates of hypertension. Patients older than 80 years had higher rates of 30-day readmission than their younger counterparts who had a 4.8% rate of readmission. The most frequent diagnoses on readmission were urinary tract infection (12.2%), hypertension (16%), and unspecific complications (9%). In only 1% of the population, there was myocardial infarction, pulmonary embolism, cerebrovascular accident, deep vein thrombosis, and pneumonia. One admission for surgery for incontinence was seen with 97.7% of patients, 2.2% had 2 visits, and 0.12% had 3 or more procedures.

Conclusion.—In the "young elderly" or those younger than 80 years, incontinence surgery is safe. Increased risk is apparent with those older than 80 years and those with certain chronic illnesses.

▶ This review of Medicare data clearly shows that incontinence surgery can be safely performed in elderly women, but there is increased morbidity and mortality in women older than 85 years. Up to 16% of this group are readmitted to the hospital and 2.5% die within 90 days of surgery. This group of women should be counseled concerning increased risks.

D.E. Coplen, M.D.

Clinical and Urodynamic Characteristics of Women With Recurrent Urinary Incontinence After Burch Colposuspension

Kjølhede P, Rydén G (Univ Hosp, Linköping, Sweden)
Acta Obstet Gynecol Scand 76:461–467, 1997   10–4

Introduction.—Short-term follow-up after a Burch colposuspension (B.c.) suggests a high cure rate, but recent reports of long-term follow-up indicate a steadily decreasing cure rate over time. Women with recurrent urinary incontinence (RUI) after B.c. were evaluated to determine their clinical and urodynamic characteristics.

Methods.—Fifty women with complaints of RUI at a median of 6 years after B.c. (group 1) and 52 women with primary stress urinary incontinence with no surgical intervention (group 2) underwent medical examination, urogynecologic examination, and a urodynamic investigation conforming to the standardization recommended by the International Continence Society.

Results.—Group 1 women had significantly greater body mass index than group 2 women. Group 1 women had significantly higher incidence of concomitant diseases, recurrent lower urinary tract infections, rectocele, enterocele, and lumbago and sciatica than group 2 women. Ten percent of group 1 women and 23% of group 2 women were receiving local or systemic estrogen replacement therapy. Significantly more group 2 women had hypermobility of the bladder neck and urethra and palpable contraction of the levator ani muscles. Group 2 women had significantly more pronounced leakage, compared to group 1 women. Detrusor instability was observed significantly more often in group 1 than group 2 women. Five group 1 women had low urethra pressure.

Conclusion.—Women with RUI after B.c. appeared to have a more pronounced weakness of the pelvic floor than women with primary stress urinary incontinence. The lack of voluntary pelvic floor muscle contraction in women with RUI suggests neuromuscular damage to the pelvic floor muscles.

▶ In this series, almost half of the patients with recurrent incontinence had detrusor instability. It is not known if this was de novo or a preexisting condition. Only 40% of the women had hypermobility of the bladder neck postoperatively. This implies that some may have had intrinsic sphincteric deficiency, although leak point pressures were not determined. Both of these are significant risk factors for failure and this points out the need for complete patient evaluation before primary repair (bladder neck suspension) of stress incontinence.

D.E. Coplen, M.D.

Use of a Pedicled Rectus Abdominis Muscle Flap Sling in the Treatment of Complicated Stress Urinary Incontinence

Wall LL, Copas P, Galloway NTM (Emory Univ, Altanta, Ga)
Am J Obstet Gynecol 175:1460–1466, 1996   10–5

Introduction.—In patients with stress incontinence resulting from failure of the intrinsic sphincteric mechanism itself, surgical treatment usually requires the use of a sling beneath the bladder neck to restore normal closure. The natural and synthetic materials used to create the sling have had varying degrees of success. In the patients reported here, a pedicled muscle flap developed from the rectus abdominis muscle was used to create a suburethral sling.

Methods.—The rectus muscle sling operation was performed for 32 patients with complex urinary incontinence. These women had undergone a variety of previous operations, including 33 procedures for stress incontinence and 31 hysterectomies. Fourteen had an open vesical neck on fluoroscopy and 16 had had massive vaginal prolapse. Many additional procedures were performed at the time of the rectus muscle sling operation. Two surgeons perform the procedure which involves transecting 1 rectus abdominis muscle just above its first tendinous intersection and isolating the muscle as a flap on its inferior vascular pedicle. The flap is then swung beneath the urethra and bladder neck, pulled into the retropubic space on the contralateral side, and sewn to the obturator internus fascia or to Cooper's ligament. Follow-up averaged 6 months.

Results.—Twenty-eight patients (87.5%) reported improved bladder function and were satisfied with the results of surgery. There were 4 surgical failures; 2 women reported their bladder function was unchanged and 2 considered it worse. One woman was cured of stress incontinence but continued to have significant urinary leakage because of detrusor overactivity. Hesitancy in starting the urinary stream was present in 7 patients before surgery and resolved postoperatively in 6. An additional 6 women reported that hesitancy appeared after the sling operation.

Conclusion.—These preliminary results suggest that the pedicled rectus abdominis muscle flap offers a promising treatment for complicated stress incontinence. The soft, broad-based support created by the muscle-flap sling appears to reduce the incidence of postoperative voiding dysfunction.

▶ This is an involved operation applied in women with persistent urinary incontinence after multiple prior procedures. The broad based vascular flap is felt to compress structures with its bulk. Unlike many successful sling operations, none of the patients required post-op clean intermittent catheterization and only 3 developed symptoms of urgency after surgery. These are excellent results, but follow-up averages only 6 months.

D.E. Coplen, M.D.

The Value of Intraoperative Cystoscopy in Urogynecologic and Reconstructive Pelvic Surgery

Harris RL, Cundiff GW, Theofrastous JP, et al (Duke Univ, Durham, NC; Mountain Area Health Education Ctr, Asheville, NC)
Am J Obstet Gynecol 177:1367–1371, 1997   10–6

Background.—Though the value of intraoperative cystoscopy in the recognition and management of lower urinary tract injury during surgery has been established, it has not been widely used in a routine manner. The role of cystoscopy during surgery for pelvic organ prolapse and urinary incontinence was investigated.

Methods and Findings.—The records of 224 consecutive patients undergoing intraoperative cystoscopy after urogynecologic surgery were reviewed. Nine injuries unsuspected before cystoscopy were identified, for an incidence of 4%. Six ureteral ligations were noted, 4 occurring after Burch cystourethropexy and 2 after vaginal culdoplasty. Intravesical sutures were found after Burch procedures in 2 patients. Another injury occurred during the passing of fascia lata through the bladder in a pubovaginal sling procedure. Management of 8 injuries consisted of removal and replacement of the suture or sling. Only 1 required ureteroneocystotomy. Demographic and surgical parameters did not differ between patients with and patients without injuries.

Conclusions.—Complex urogynecologic surgery is associated with significant potential for damage to the lower urinary tract. Intraoperative surveillance cystoscopy should be included in all such procedures.

▶ Unsuspected ureteral injury or transvesical placement of sutures occurred in 4% of patients in this series. Intraoperative cystoscopy combined with or without the administration of indigo carmine dye is easily performed and should be part of any urogynecologic procedure after sutures have been tied. In suspension procedures, the ureter is usually kinked, so removal and replacement of the sutures corrects the problem. While not described in this paper, cystoscopy should also be performed in conjunction with vaginal hysterectomy.

D.E. Coplen, M.D.

Transvaginal Electrical Stimulation for Female Urinary Incontinence
Brubaker L, Benson JT, Bent A, et al (Rush Med College, Chicago; Indiana Univ, Indianapolis; Greater Baltimore Med Ctr, Md; et al)
Am J Obstet Gynecol 177:536–540, 1997   10–7

Introduction.—The efficacy of transvaginal electrical stimulation as a treatment for female urinary incontinence was investigated in this multicenter, randomized, placebo-controlled clinical study.

Methods.—The study group consisted of 121 women with urinary incontinence. Intake evaluation included a comprehensive urogynecologic history and physical, multi-channel urodynamic testing, urinary diary, and quality-of-life assessment. Participants were stratified by urodynamic diagnosis into 3 groups: genuine stress incontinence, detrusor instability, and mixed incontinence. Within these 3 groups, participants were randomized to either transvaginal electrical stimulation with the InCare Microgyn II or a sham device. After a 1 week baseline period, treatment began with use of the device for 20 minutes twice daily for 8 weeks. A posttreatment evaluation was performed at the end of the 8-week treatment period and again 2 weeks later.

Results.—Of the 33 women in the stimulation group with detrusor overactivity, half no longer had detrusor overactivity at the end of the treatment period. This decrease was highly significant and did not occur in the sham treatment group. However, there was no significant decrease in urinary incontinence or improvement in quality of life in any group in this study.

Conclusions.—Transvaginal electrical stimulation appears to be useful in the treatment of detrusor overactivity in women with urinary incontinence.

▶ In this prospective, randomized, double-blinded study, transvaginal electrical stimulation had a significant effect on detrusor instability. In 50% of treated patients detrusor, instability was eliminated. We do not know if this is a durable response. Unfortunately, even though instability was eliminated, there was no change in urinary incontinence or other quality-of-life measures. This will probably limit the utility of this device because the patients presented for management of urinary incontinence.

D.E. Coplen, M.D.

A New Intraurethral Sphincter Prosthesis With a Self Contained Urinary Pump

Nativ O, Moskowitz B, Issaq E, et al (Bnai Zion Med Ctr, Haifa, Israel)
ASAIO J 43:197–203, 1997   10–8

Introduction.—A number of treatments are available to achieve urine evacuation in patients with atonic bladder, but all are unsatisfactory to both patient and physician, result in a lesser quality of life, and may lead to recurrent urinary tract infections and impaired renal function. The intraurethral sphincter prosthesis reported here allows complete drainage of urine with good urinary flow and continence between urinations.

Methods.—The device was designed for women and consists of a valve and pump device operated by an external remote control unit. Produced in a variety of lengths and diameters to allow a close fit to each patient's urethra, the catheter is mounted on an insertion system (pusher and grabber). After the catheter-inserter assembly is inserted into the urethra, it is secured by a fixation method consisting of soft expandable silicone fins at the bladder neck and a flexible flange at the external meatus (Fig 3). A small, hand-held control device is placed on the lower abdomen and the "on" button is pressed. Energy is provided to the pump by a magnetic coupling method. The valve opens when activated, the pump rotates at high speed, and urine is drawn from the bladder. After a series of in vitro studies, the device was tested in 17 patients.

Results.—Women who participated in the trial had a mean age of 56. All had urinary retention caused by atonic bladder. The most common underlying diseases were diabetes mellitus and multiple sclerosis. Insertion of the prosthesis is performed in a simple ambulatory procedure similar to Foley catheterization. The pumping stops and the valve closes when the bladder is completely evacuated. Mastering the insertion procedure took from 1 to 6 days, and no patient reported pain or urethral irritation. Two patients with uninhibited detrusor contractions could not tolerate the device and another discontinued use after 2 weeks because of irritation. The remain-

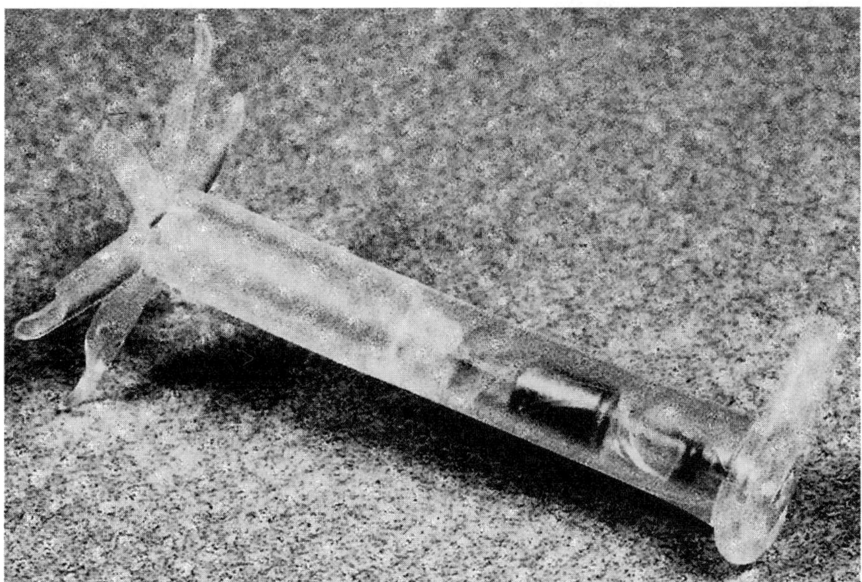

FIGURE 3.—Catheter as configured on insertion, with fins at tip open in a "petal" configuration. (Courtesy of Nativ O, Moskowitz B, Issaq E, et al: A new intraurethral sphincter prosthesis with a self contained urinary pump. *ASAIO J* 43:197–203, 1997. Copyright © ASAIO.)

ing patients used the device for up to 16 months, were dry, and had complete bladder emptying.

Conclusion.—The intraurethral prosthesis tested in these patients is a promising management tool for atonic bladder and may benefit senile and nursing home patients. The implant will have to be replaced after approximately 1 month of use. Its sterile insertion procedure and ability to empty the bladder completely may reduce the rate of urinary tract infections.

▶ This novel device was developed for use in females with atonic bladders. A small pump empties the bladder to completion and the women are continent. Bacteriuria developed in 13 of 15 patients (3 symptomatic). The prosthesis had to be changed every 4–5 weeks because of salt deposits that cause urinary leakage. Follow-up is not long enough to know if the device causes progressive urethral atrophy and intrinsic sphincteric deficiency. The authors state that this device "enhances the quality of life, dignity, and independence of patients," but when intermittent catheterization is technically capable, it would seem to be less cumbersome than this device.

D.E. Coplen, M.D.

11 Urinary Tract Reconstruction and Diversion

Orthotopic Lower Urinary Tract Reconstruction in Women Using the Kock Ileal Neobladder: Updated Experience in 34 Patients
Stein JP, Grossfeld GD, Freeman JA, et al (Univ of Southern California, Los Angeles)
J Urol 158:400–405, 1997   11–1

Introduction.—Orthotopic diversion was originally performed only in males. With increased understanding of the continence mechanism in females, it is now an option for females. The clinical and functional experience with orthotopic reconstruction in 34 females was reported.

Surgical Technique.—The technique of en bloc radical cystectomy with bilateral pelvic iliac lymphadenectomy in females is followed with special attention to certain aspects of the anterior exenteration. It is important to minimize dissection in the region anterior to the urethra to avoid injury to the rhabdosphincter region and corresponding innervation. The pubourethral suspensory ligaments should remain intact because they help maintain an intrapelvic neobladder position, which may contribute to the continence mechanism. The autonomic sympathetic nerves extending from just above the aortic bifurcation, caudally off of the abdominal aorta, common iliacs, and sacral promontory are usually sacrificed. The autonomic neurovascular bundles along the lateral aspect of the uterus and vagina are typically removed down to the level of the bladder neck. This dissection denervates the bladder neck and proximal urethra, making them ineffective parts of the continence mechanism. The rhabdosphincter region and corresponding innervation from branches off of the pudendal nerve produce continence. After vaginal dissection, the vaginal cuff is closed at the apex and suspended to Cooper's ligament to prevent vaginal prolapse or enterocele. An intact anterior vaginal wall can provide additional support to the proximal urethra if invasion does not require its removal. Vaginal reconstruction may be required to preserve sexual function.

Results.—The rates of perioperative deaths, and early and late complications were 0%, 11% (4 patients), and 9% (3 patients), respectively. Three patients died of metastatic bladder cancer and 1 died of unrelated causes. One patient required conversion of the orthotopic reservoir to a cutaneous diversion. All the remaining 29 patients were alive without evidence of disease at final follow-up (median, 30 months). The intraoperative frozen section of the distal surgical margin (proximal urethra) reliably assessed the proximal urethra for tumor in all 29 specimens removed for transitional cell carcinoma. Twenty-nine patients (88%) had complete daytime continence and 27 (82%) had nighttime continence. Twenty-eight patients (85%) were able to void to completion, and 5 (15%) needed some type of intermittent catheterization to empty the neobladder. Patient satisfaction was excellent.

Conclusions.—Careful selection of appropriate female patients for orthotopic diversion is important and should include preoperative evaluation of the bladder neck and intraoperative frozen section analysis of the distal cystectomy margin. Close follow-up is imperative in all women undergoing orthotopic diversion.

▶ This manuscript is important because it further delineates some guidelines for the appropriate selection of female patients for orthotopic lower urinary tract reconstruction. It also describes, in a stepwise manner, the dissection of the vagina and bladder neck that will allow preservation of continence without compromising excision of the cancer.

The authors do not exclude patients with tumor that involves the bladder neck from an orthotopic reconstruction, although tumor at this location is an important risk factor for later urethral tumor involvement. Analysis of historical series disclosed that only about 50% of patients with tumor involving the bladder neck have urethral involvement. In fact, in a contemporary series of patients, only 1 of 6 patients with tumor near the bladder neck had urethral involvement. Based on this rather low urethral involvement rate, the authors routinely perform intraoperative frozen section of the proximal urethra and have found it to be an accurate and reliable method to exclude urethral tumor involvement.

The authors believe that multiple factors contribute to the continence mechanism in women undergoing orthotopic diversion and that these include the musculofascial support system of the urethra as well as its rhabdosphincter. The urethral support mechanism is an elaborate musculofascial complex that includes periurethral and perivaginal connective tissue extending from the anterior vaginal wall that surrounds the proximal and mid-urethra in a slinglike fashion. In addition, the pubourethral ligaments are also believed to be important in maintaining the proximal urethra and the neobladder in an intra-abdominal position. The rhabdosphincter extends from the proximal urethra to the membranous urethra, and receives its innervation from branches of the pudendal nerve. Although other authors have suggested that sympathetic nerve-sparing cystectomy was an important adjunct to the maintenance of continence in women, in the current series the authors make no such effort and, in fact, performed extensive lymph node dissections in the region of the aortic bifurcation. It is their opinion that it is impossible to denervate the urethra completely and that the parasympathetic supply to the rhabdosphincter is the most important component of the rhabdosphincter innervation.

This is a nice article to keep on hand when contemplating neobladder formation in women because it also provides guidelines for effective cancer excision of tumors arising on the posterior bladder wall that may necessitate resection of the anterior vaginal wall.

G.L. Andriole, Jr., M.D.

Double Folded Rectosigmoid Bladder With a New Ureterocolic Antireflux Technique
El-Mekresh MM, Hafez AT, Abol-Enein H, et al (Mansoura Univ, Egypt)
J Urol 157:2085–2089, 1997   11–2

Introduction.—Since the first reports appeared in the early 1950s, ureterosigmoidostomy has undergone a number of revisions. The new method for ureterosigmoidostomy reported here involves 2 technical principles: double folding of the rectosigmoid segment to improve continence, and ureteral reimplantation using the extramural serous lined technique.

Methods.—The operation was performed on 64 patients (32 women, 20 men, and 12 children) between 1992 and 1995. Bladder cancer was the most common indication for diversion. During the procedure, the rectosigmoid is folded into an S-shaped configuration and the 2 adjacent limbs of the bowel on either side are joined to form 2 serous lined troughs (Fig 1). Ureters are then passed through wide buttonholes in the mesocolon and laid down into a corresponding trough. Implanted ureters are covered by an approximation of the mucosal edges of the trough so that each trough is transformed into an extramural serous lined tunnel. The anterior wall of the pouch is closed (Fig 2) and the dome fixed to the posterior parietal peritoneum.

Results.—There was 1 postoperative death, the result of a massive pulmonary embolism, and 6 patients died within 8 months of local recurrence, distant metastasis, or both. During a mean follow-up period of 19 months, all of the remaining 57 patients were continent during the day with a voiding frequency of 2 to 4 times. Four children experienced nocturnal enuresis but have responded to treatment with imipramine hydrochloride. Overall, upper urinary tract function was maintained or improved in 95% of patients. All patients received prophylactic alkalization.

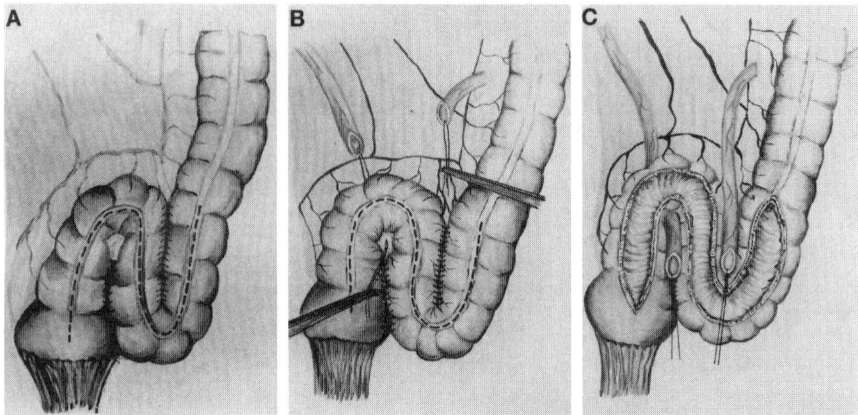

FIGURE 1.—**A,** S-shaped configuration of rectosigmoid. **B,** adjacent limbs of bowel are joined to create 2 serous lined troughs. **C,** ureters are passed through mesocolon and placed into tunnels. (Courtesy of El-Mekresh MM, Hafez AT, Abol-Enein H, et al: Double folded rectosigmoid bladder with a new ureterocolic antireflux technique. *J Urol* 157:2085–2089, 1997.)

Conclusion.—The technique for ureterosigmoidostomy reported here folds the rectosigmoid twice and reimplants the ureters by using the extramural subserous tunnel. This minimizes the chance of obstruction and can be employed in both normal and dilated ureters. The procedure offers an alternative to orthotopic bladder substitution when the urethra cannot be used.

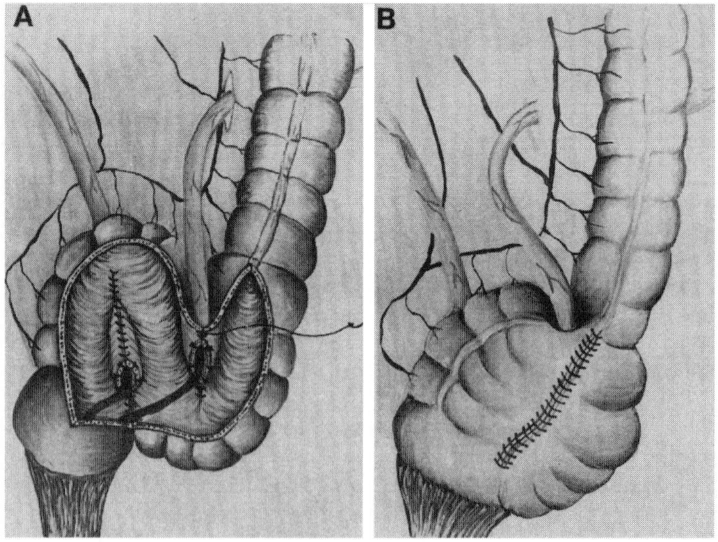

FIGURE 2.—**A,** stented ureterocolic anastomosis and closure of mucosal edges to cover implanted ureters. **B,** anterior wall of pouch is closed. (Courtesy of El-Mekresh MM, Hafez AT, Abol-Enein H, et al: Double folded rectosigmoid bladder with a new ureterocolic antireflux technique. *J Urol* 157:2085–2089, 1997.)

▶ This article describes a surgical technique that should be applicable to women and selected men and children who require radical cystectomy. It employs a double-folded rectosigmoid pouch with the extramural subserous tunnel reimplant that has previously been shown to minimize both obstruction and reflux. This is the type of ureteral reimplant I routinely employ in all of my neobladders and continent urinary diversions, and it is well illustrated in Figures 1 and 2. Additional information is available on this useful form of uretero-intestinal anastomosis.[1, 2]

G.L. Andriole, Jr., M.D.

References

1. Abol-Enein H, Ghoneim MA: A novel uretero-ileal reimplantation technique: The serous lined extramural tunnel: A preliminary report. *J Urol* 151:1193, 1994.
2. Abol-Enein H, Ghoneim MA: Further clinical experience with the ileal W-neobladder and a serous-lined extramural tunnel for orthotopic substitution. *Br J Urol* 76:558, 1995.

The Ileocaeco-Urethrostomy With Multiple Transverse Taeniamyotomies for Bladder Replacement: An Alternative to Detubularized Neobladders. Morphological, Functional and Metabolic Results After 9 Years' Experience
Alcini E, Racioppi M, D'Addessi A, et al (Universita' Cattolica del Sacre Cuoro, Rome)
Br J Urol 79:333–338, 1997   11–3

Background.—In the authors' technique of orthotopic bladder substitution, an ileocecal segment is used without detubularization. Transverse cecal teniamyotomies are used to reduce tension of the intestinal wall and, thus, internal pressure of the bladder substitute (Fig 1). A previous report described good results in the first 4 years' experience with this technique. The long-term follow-up results of ileoceco-urethrostomy with multiple transverse teniamyotomies for bladder replacement were reported.

Methods.—Over an 8-year period, 60 men with infiltrating bladder carcinoma underwent orthotopic bladder substitution by ileoceco-urethrostomy with multiple transverse teniamyotomies. The patients mean age was 63 years. By avoiding detubularization and sectioning of cecal teniae, the procedure sought to achieve a nearly spherical reservoir with good initial capacity that did not overdilate with time. With experience, the mean operative time was about 3.5 hours. The patients were followed for a mean of 34 months; follow-up included physical examinations, laboratory tests, and imaging studies. Fifty-six patients with at least 6 months of follow-up were assessed for continence.

Results.—There were few early complications. Voiding cystography revealed late ureteric reflux in 10% of patients, but this did not cause any clinical or functional problems. Twelve percent of patients had stenosis at the uretero-ileal anastomosis. Diurnal continence, with socially acceptable

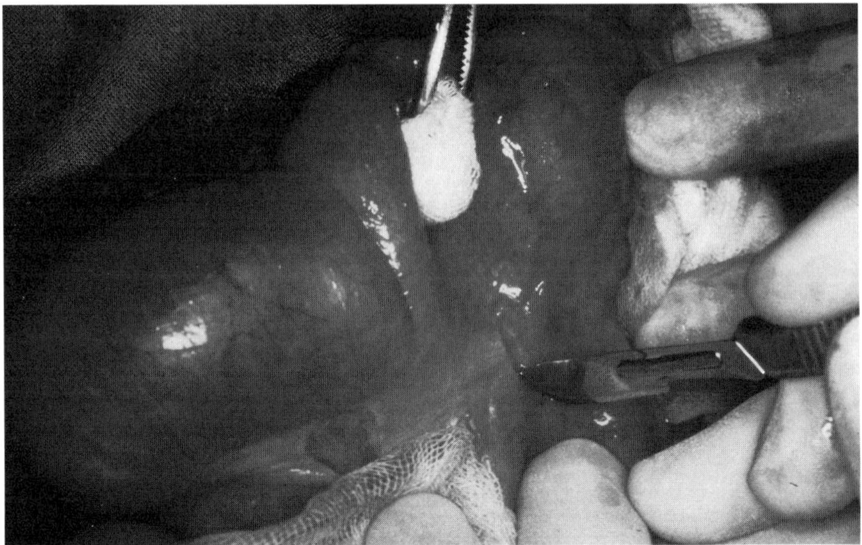

FIGURE 1.—Teniamyotomies are quick, easy to perform, and completely section the longitudinal muscular layer down to the submucosal layer, thus allowing wall tension to be reduced. They are performed with the reservoir filled with about 100 mL of saline to allow good exposure of the submucosal layer. (Courtesy of Alcini E, Racioppi M, D'Addessi A, et al: The ileocaeco-urethrostomy with multiple transverse taeniamyotomies for bladder replacement: An alternative to detubularized neobladders. Morphological, functional and metabolic results after 9 years' experience. *Br J Urol* 79:333–338, 1997.)

intervals between micturitions, was obtained in all patients. The percentage of patients achieving nocturnal continence was 79% for those with a follow-up of less than 3 years and 86% for those followed for longer than 3 years. At 5 years' follow-up, mean reservoir capacity was 469 mL, which is in the physiologic range. The mean maximum internal pressure was 48 cm H_2O and the mean postmicturition residual volume 28 mL. None of the patients required self-catheterization. All metabolic variables remained within the range of normal.

Conclusion.—Many characteristics of the cecum—including receptive relaxation, the presence of teniae, and the ileocecal sphincter—contribute to its value for bladder replacement. Like detubularization, teniamyotomies can reduce wall tension and internal pressure and achieve a near-spherical shape. The difference is that teniamyotomies leave the circular muscle intact. This preserves good basal tone, allowing optimal emptying and avoiding problems related to deterioration of the reservoir.

▶ This manuscript presents an interesting form of orthotopic urinary diversion using a relatively short ileocecal segment that is rendered into a low pressure reservoir by spacing multiple taeniamyotomies. This technique certainly seems to require less operative time than the standard techniques of detubularization. The follow-up of patients is relatively long, and urodynamic studies show relatively low resting pressures and small postvoid residuals without upper tract deterioration. This appears to be an attractive form of orthotopic diversion.

G.L. Andriole, Jr., M.D.

Bladder Autoaugmentation in Adult Patients With Neurologic Voiding Dysfunction

Stöhrer M, Kramer G, Goepel M, et al (Univ Hosp Essen, Germany)
Spinal Cord 35:456–462, 1997
11–4

Background.—Patients with neurogenic voiding dysfunction that does not respond to conservative treatment are candidates for surgery. Although several types of procedures are available, these authors recommend bladder autoaugmentation, which converts part of the bladder into a yielding section that mimics a diverticulum. This report describes the results of bladder autoaugmentation in 50 patients.

Methods.—Since 1992, bladder autoaugmentation was performed in 50 patients as an elective procedure for the treatment of high detrusor pressure, decreased compliance, or both. X-ray videography and clinical findings were used to assess results.

Results.—Among the 50 patients who underwent bladder autoaugmentation procedures, there was 1 bladder rupture and 5 treatment failures.

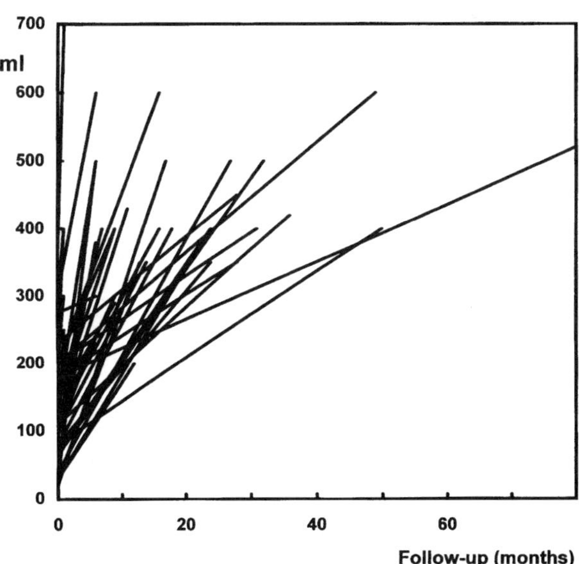

FIGURE 3.—Preoperative data and data at last follow-up on maximal capacity for 37 patients. Follow-up durations between 2 weeks and 80 months. (Courtesy of Stöhrer M, Kramer G, Goepel M, et al: Bladder autoaugmentation in adult patients with neurologic voiding dysfunction *Spinal Cord* 35:456–462, 1997.)

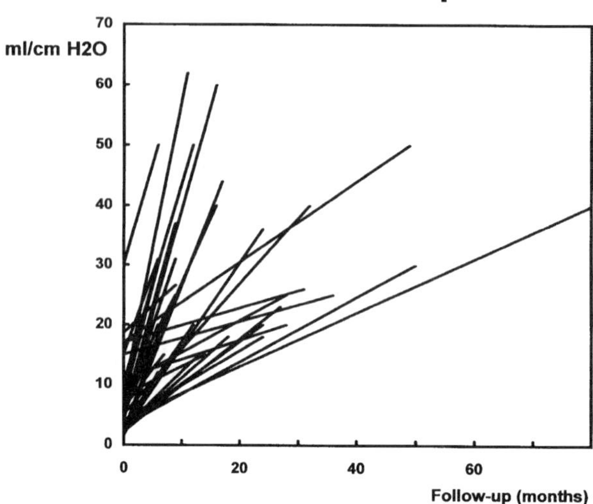

FIGURE 4.—Preoperative data and data at last follow-up on detrusor compliance for 34 patients. Follow-up durations between 3 and 70 months. (Courtesy of Stöhrer M, Kramer G, Goepel M, et al: Bladder autoaugmentation in adult patients with neurologic voiding dysfunction. *Spinal Cord* 35:456–462, 1997.)

For those stable patients with at least 6 months of follow-up, on average, the maximal cystometric capacity increased from 121 mL to 406 mL (Fig 3), detrusor compliance increased from 6.1 mL/cm H_2O to 29.3 mL/cm H_2O (Fig 4), maximal voiding pressure decreased from 86.4 cm H_2O to 50.9 cm H_2O, and residual urine increased from 20 mL to 76 mL. Anticholinergic treatment was sometimes necessary in the early postoperative phase to repress hyperreflexic contractions. About 60% of the patients in this series required intermittent catheterization after the procedure.

Conclusions.—On the basis of their experience, these authors recommend bladder autoaugmentation as the therapy of choice for patients with low-capacity, high-pressure bladders who do not respond to conservative treatment. This procedure does not preclude subsequent enterocystoplasty or deafferentation. This procedure will be most advantageous for those patients who understand that improvement may be delayed and who are willing to perform intermittent catheterization.

▶ Autoaugmentation averts the interposition of intestinal segments in the urinary tract of patients with low-capacity, high-pressure bladders by creating an artificial diverticulum. Long-term improvement has not been seen in most series, presumably because of fibrosis or detrusor smooth muscle regrowth. The authors failure rate was 15% with very short follow-up. An indwelling catheter was left in place for only 48 hours after the procedure, so perhaps the early distention of the bladder prevents contraction of the diverticulum. Detrusor smooth muscle removal is preferential to myotomy. The patients require intermittent catheterization, but this procedure does not preclude subsequent augmentation cystoplasty if it fails to improve bladder dynamics.

D.E. Coplen, M.D.

Long-term Metabolic Advantages of a Gastrointestinal Composite Urinary Reservoir
Austin PF, DeLeary G, Homsy YL, et al (Univ of South Florida, Tampa)
J Urol 158:1704–1708, 1997 11–5

Background.—Using a moderate-sized stomach flap as a composite reservoir with ileum or colon offers the metabolic advantages of the stomach while avoiding the detrimental effects of the hematuria-dysuria syndrome. If the stomach segment used is too large, hematuria-dysuria syndrome may occur; if too small, it cannot counteract the intestinal absorptive properties of chloride that lead to metabolic acidosis. The long-term metabolic effects of a gastrointestinal composite reservoir were investigated.

Methods.—The study included 9 patients undergoing creation of a gastrointestinal composite urinary reservoir for continent urinary diversion: a gastroileal reservoir in 7 cases and a gastrocolonic reservoir in 2. Four patients had a preexisting conduit associated with metabolic acidosis; 5 had preexisting metabolic acidosis or short-bowel syndrome. The reconstructions used a moderate-sized (8 × 4 cm) segment from the greater curvature of the stomach. A tapered and reimplanted segment of ileum was used as the anti-incontinence segment. Serum pH, serum electrolytes, and urinalysis were measured before and after the reconstruction. Postoperative serum gastrin measurements were performed as well. The patients were followed for a mean of 54 months after surgery.

Results.—At follow-up, all patients had serum electrolyte neutrality. The serum pH increased from a mean of 7.36 before reconstruction to 7.40 afterward. Serum bicarbonate increased from 22.3 to 25.14, whereas urine pH was unchanged. Mildly acidic urine with ulcerative skin changes at the stoma site was observed in 1 patient. Short-term measurements showed elevated serum gastrin levels in 3 patients; however, all patients had normal serum gastrin levels at long-term follow-up. Urolithiasis and symptomatic urinary tract infection developed in 1 patient with persistently alkaline urine.

Conclusion.—Patients with a composite urinary reservoir constructed of intestinal segments and a moderate-sized gastric segment have serum electrolyte neutrality on long-term follow-up. The composite gastroileal or gastrocolonic reservoir may offer metabolic advantages over ileal and colonic reservoirs associated with hyperchloremic metabolic acidosis, without the harmful effects of extreme urinary acidity. Composite reservoirs may have important advantages for patients with preexisting metabolic acidosis or short-bowel syndrome.

▶ Gastric segment use in bladder augmentation has been associated with hematuria, dysuria, and in patients with normal sensation, significant discomfort in the native bladder. Intestinal segments are associated with hyperchloremic metabolic acidosis. This long-term metabolic follow-up of patients with combined gastric and intestinal reservoirs indicates a potential metabolic advantage while avoiding potential complications of gastric reservoirs in patients with preexisting metabolic abnormalities.

D.E. Coplen, M.D.

Twenty-Year Experience With Jejunal Conduits

Fontaine E, Barthelemy Y, Houlgatte A, et al (René Descartes Univ–Paris V, Boulogne, France)
Urology 50:207–213, 1997   11–6

Purpose.—In intestinal conduit urinary diversion, use of jejunum and colon may avert some of the morbidity associated with use of ileal conduit. Jejunum can avert the use of irradiated or diseased ileum or colon; however, in as many as two-thirds of patients jejunal conduit syndrome, a distinctive electrolyte imbalance, will develop. The authors have a long experience with the jejunal conduit, having used it for all indications of incontinent urinary diversion since 1985. They report their results with jejunal conduit urinary diversion, focusing on long-term renal function and possible electrolyte imbalance.

Patients.—Jejunal conduits were used for urinary diversion in 50 patients over an 18-year period. In each patient, a 10- to 12-cm jejunal loop was placed transperitoneally. Eighteen patients underwent pelvic irradiation before the urinary diversion procedure. The patients were followed up for a median of 26 months, with 22 patients followed up for >5 years. Creatinine clearance and excretory urography were used to evaluate renal function and the anatomy of the upper urinary tract.

Outcomes.—Revision surgery was required in 16% of patients. There were several different complications related to urinary diversion, including renal calculi in 12% of patients, parastomal hernia in 6%, pyelonephritis in 4%, ureterojejunal obstruction in 4%, and stomal prolapse in 2%. The rate of electrolyte imbalance was only 4%, and the problem was easily managed with 4 gm of sodium bicarbonate. Of the patients followed up for >5 years, none had a significant decline in creatinine clearance. However, 2 of the 22 had >20% reduction in creatinine clearance as a result of ureterojejunal obstruction. Hydronephrosis occurred in 1 of 42 ureterojejunal units and increased in 2. Two units showed new renal scarring, and 2 showed progressive scarring.

Conclusions.—This experience demonstrates good results with jejunal conduits for urinary diversion. The technique of placing a short jejunal conduit transperitoneally gives reliable results with good long-term renal function. Problems with electrolyte imbalance are rare and easily corrected. The ability to use jejunal conduit even after pelvic irradiation is a major advantage.

▶ While the use of jejunum is indicated when other bowel segments have been irradiated, concern with electrolyte abnormalities has limited its use. Electrolytes and water passively diffuse across the jejunal mucosa. The metabolic abnormality associated with jejunal conduits is a hypochloremic, hyperkalemic metabolic acidosis. It is treated with fluid replacement and oral salt (sodium chloride and sodium bicarbonate). In this series, only 2 of 50 patients developed electrolyte abnormalities when a very short (10– to 12-cm [4-inch]) segment was used. The transverse colon is also a viable alternative in irradiated patients.

D.E. Coplen, M.D.

12 Interstitial Cystitis/ Voiding Dysfunction

Improvement in Interstitial Cystitis Symptom Scores During Treatment With Oral L-Arginine

Smith SD, Wheeler MA, Foster HE Jr, et al (Yale Univ, New Haven, Conn)

J Urol 158:703–708, 1997   12–1

Background.—Interstitial cystitis is a chronic, difficult-to-treat disease. It is associated with reduced urinary nitric oxide synthase activity. Nitric oxide may play an important role in the symptoms and immunologic responses of interstitial cystitis. L-Arginine, the substrate for nitric oxide synthase, was tried as a treatment for interstitial cystitis.

Methods.—The study included 10 patients who met the National Institutes of Health diagnostic criteria for interstitial cystitis. Their average age was 56 years, and their average duration of symptoms was 13.5 years. All patients received 6 months of treatment with oral L-arginine, 1.5 gm/day. The patients were followed up closely to assess their symptoms of interstitial cystitis.

TABLE 3.—A Comparison of the Effects of L-Arginine Treatment on Interstitial Cystitis Symptoms, Urinary Nitric Oxide Synthase Activity, and Cyclic Guanosine Monophosphate Levels

	Duration of L-arginine Treatment*	
	1 Mo.	6 Mos.
Voiding pain	Decreased significantly	Decreased significantly
Lower abdominal pain	Decreased significantly	Decreased significantly
Vaginal/urethral pain	Decreased significantly	Decreased significantly
Urinary frequency/day	Not significant	Decreased significantly
Urinary frequency/night	Not significant	Decreased significantly
Urinary nitric oxide synthase activity (pmole./min./mg.)*	Increased significantly	Increased significantly
Urinary cyclic guanosine monophosphate (μmol./mg. creatinine)*	Not significant	Increased significantly

*Nitric oxide synthase activity and cyclic guanosine monophosphate levels were measured in urine from 8 of 10 patients, and in the 6-month column they are averaged for months 2–6.

(Courtesy of Smith SD, Wheeler MA, Foster HE Jr, et al: Improvement in interstitial cystitis symptom scores during treatment with oral L-arginine. *J Urol* 158:703–708, 1997.)

Results.—Treatment produced significant improvement in symptoms. Urinary voiding pain, lower abdominal pain, and vaginal and urethral pain all decreased significantly (Table 3). Mean urinary frequency decreased during the day from 13 to 8 times, and during the night from 5 to 2 times. L-Arginine treatment also decreased pain with walking and sexual activity. There were no side effects of L-arginine. All patients wished to continue taking L-arginine after the end of the study.

Conclusions.—Oral L-arginine appears to be an effective long-term treatment for interstitial cystitis. It achieves significant reductions in symptoms including pain and urinary frequency. The authors are conducting a double-blind trial to confirm the effectiveness of oral L-arginine for interstitial cystitis.

▶ Nitric oxide is a potent smooth muscle relaxant. Studies by these authors show a decrease in nitric oxide synthase activity in patients with interstitial cystitis.[1] In theory, L-arginine increases nitric oxide and cyclic guanosine monophosphate production, rectifying bladder permeability concerns and increasing bladder relaxation. This nonrandomized, unblinded study shows early promise in the treatment of interstitial cystitis.

D.E. Coplen, M.D.

Reference

1. Wheeler MA, Smith SD, Saito N, et al: Effect of long-term oral L-arginine on the nitric oxide synthase pathway in the urine from patients with interstitial cystitis. *J Urol* 158:2045–2050, 1997.

Pseudodyssynergia (Contraction of the External Sphincter During Voiding) Misdiagnosed as Chronic Nonbacterial Prostatitis and the Role of Biofeedback as a Therapeutic Option
Kaplan SA, Santarosa RP, D'Alisera PM, et al (Columbia Univ, New York)
J Urol 157:2234–2237, 1997   12–2

Introduction.—Several causes have been attributed to chronic nonbacterial prostatitis, including bladder outlet obstruction. Many men who are treated for presumed chronic nonbacterial prostatitis have a significant rate of recurrent symptoms, suggesting that multifactorial underlying mechanisms may cause the symptoms. Accurate diagnosis is necessary and sophisticated urodynamic evaluation has been advocated. In men with misdiagnosed chronic prostatitis, contraction of the external urinary sphincter during voiding was analyzed as a cause of voiding dysfunction.

Methods.—Video urodynamic studies of 43 men (23–50 years old) with chronic voiding dysfunction secondary to pseudodyssynergia were analyzed retrospectively. Several criteria were used to diagnose pseudodyssynergia, including brief and intermittent closing of the membranous urethra during voiding detected by electromyography and fluoroscopy, and electrical activity of the external sphincter during voiding in the absence of

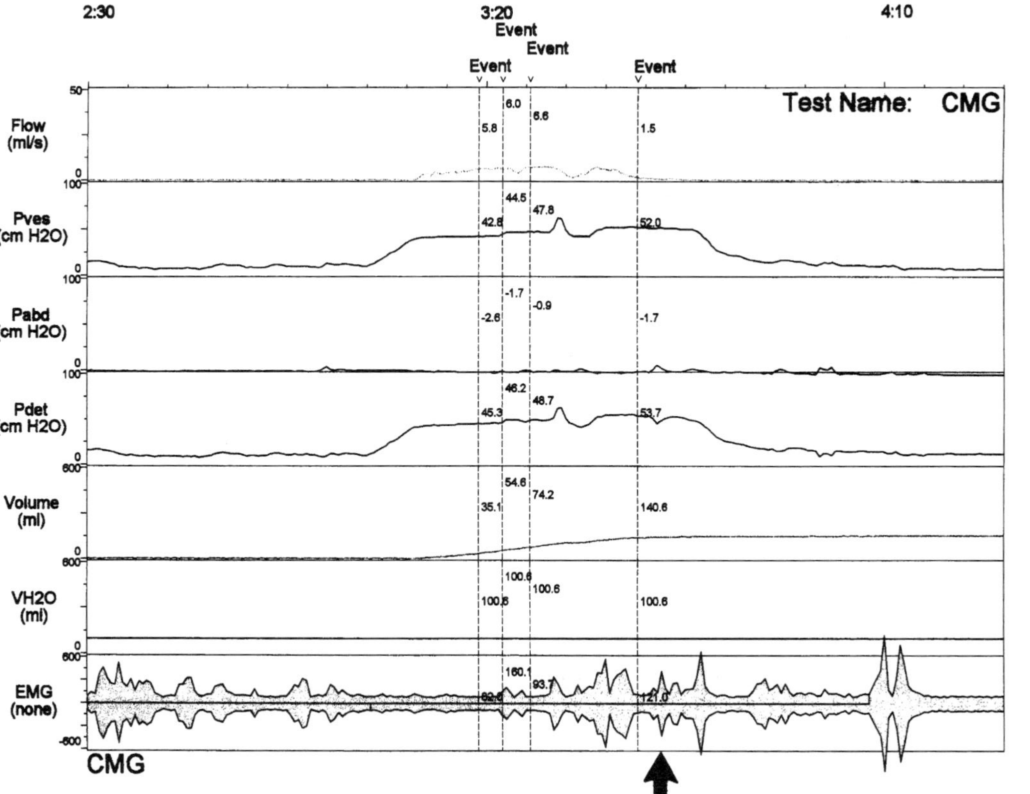

FIGURE 1.—Dyssynergic pattern of voiding. Patient has prolonged detrusor contraction (*Pdet*) with intermittent increases in electromyographic (*EMG*) activity. *ml/s* mL/per second; *Pves*, bladder pressure; *Pabd*, abdominal pressure; *VH20*, volume infused; *CMG*, cystometrogram. (Courtesy of Kaplan SA, Santarosa RP, D'Alisera PM, et al: Pseudodyssynergia (contraction of the external sphincter during voiding) misdiagnosed as chronic nonbacterial prostatitis and the role of biofeedback as a therapeutic option. *J Urol* 157:2234–2237, 1997.)

abdominal straining (Fig 1). Patients with bacterial infection or excessive leukocytes in expressed prostatic secretions were excluded.

Results.—There were 39 men who were firstborn (91%). Symptoms had a duration of 17–146 months (mean, 43.6 months), and the men took antibiotics for 53–186 days (mean, 67.6 days). There was no success with the empirical trials of α-blockers. The mean detrusor contraction duration was 132.8 ± 27.7 seconds; the mean detrusor pressure at maximum flow was 46.3 ± 13.7 cm water; the mean maximum flow rate was 13.3 ± 4.2 mL/second; and the mean American Urological Association symptom score plus or minus standard deviation was 17.5 ± 3.7. In 35 patients (83%), behavior modification and biofeedback were successful in decreasing symptoms at 6 months.

Conclusion.—Functional bladder outlet obstruction is sometimes misdiagnosed as chronic nonbacterial prostatitis. In these cases, urodynamics can help in diagnosing and predicting success with behavior modification and biofeedback.

▶ In many ways, chronic nonbacterial prostatitis is similar to interstitial cystitis, a diagnosis given to a symptom complex that may have many different causes. These authors use video urodynamics to document intermittent closure of the membranous urethra during micturition. Most of the patients had long-standing symptoms that were most likely learned behaviors, perhaps in response to bona fide prostatitis years earlier. No attempt was made to quantify obstructive or irritative symptoms. The American Urological Association symptom score improved in these men after biofeedback. The authors do not give details of the "failed" short trial of α-blockers that was used in all patients. Some of my colleagues have used low doses of imipramine with success in these men.

D.E. Coplen, M.D.

13 Urothelial Cancer

Long-term Follow-up of Cytostatic Intravesical Instillation in Patients With Superficial Bladder Carcinoma: Is Short-term, Intensive Instillation Better Than Maintenance Therapy?
Schwaibold H, Pichlmeir U, Klingenberger H-J, et al (Univ of Hamburg-Eppendorf, Germany)
Eur Urol 31:153–159, 1997   13–1

Background.—Most intravesical trials of mitomycin C and doxorubicin, used in treatment and prevention of superficial bladder tumors, have short follow-ups, making long-term conclusions about efficacy difficult.

Methods.—Two 3-year protocols, a 20-week protocol of mitomycin C instillation, and a 3-year protocol of doxorubicin instillation to retard disease progression and prevent recurrence in patients with superficial bladder tumors removed by transurethral resection were compared with Cox proportional hazards analysis. In a prospective, randomized, parallel-group multicenter trial, 419 patients were studied after a median of 57 months (range of survivors, 6 to 107 months).

Results.—Overall rates were 22.7% for recurrence and 9.8% for progression. Time to recurrence was related to recurrence status before treatment. The intensive, long-term mitomycin arm contained the lowest proportion of progression of recurrent tumors. Crude differences in recurrences and progressions were not statistically significant. Short-term mitomycin (every week for 20 weeks) achieved the same results as long-term (43 instillations in 3 years) mitomycin or doxorubicin.

Conclusions.—Both mitomycin C and doxorubicin are effective in preventing recurrence, even in high-risk patients (those with previous recurrence). Initial intensive mitomycin C instillation, combined with long-term maintenance, delays recurrence significantly among high-risk patients, supporting more intensive (closer to therapeutic than prophylactic) chemotherapeutic instillation, at least in high-risk groups.

▶ This interesting study evaluated 4 intravesical chemotherapeutic regimens and suggests that intensive therapy is more likely to reduce tumor recurrence or the development of invasive disease. To me, this underscores the importance of intensive, regular instillations of intravesical therapy, and patients whose weekly infravesical instillations are interrupted for any reason should probably be restarted so that they may enjoy the full benefit of the treatment.

G.L. Andriole, Jr., M.D.

Long-term Efficacy of Intravesical Bacillus Calmette-Guerin for Carcinoma In Situ: Relationship of Progression to Histological Response and p53 Nuclear Accumulation
Ovesen H, Horn T, Steven K (Univ of Copenhagen)
J Urol 157:1655–1659, 1997   13–2

Background.—Intravesical bacillus Calmette-Guerin (BCG) produces a high initial response rate in patients with carcinoma in situ of the bladder. However, in many of these patients the disease will progress, and most will die of transitional cell carcinoma. Histologic and chromosomal markers are needed to identify patients at high risk for disease progression. Two possible markers were evaluated: the histologic response to intravesical BCG and the prevalence of p53 nuclear accumulation.

Methods.—The study included 60 consecutive patients with carcinoma in situ: 13 with primary and 47 with secondary carcinoma in situ. All patients received 6 weekly treatments with intravesical BCG; those who did not respond received an additional 6 treatments at 2-week intervals. None received maintenance therapy. The patients were followed up for a median of 48 months. The prevalence of p53 nuclear immunoreactivity before and after treatment was assessed by immunohistochemical analysis using antibody PAb 1801. The 2 potential markers were assessed for their influence on clinical outcome.

Results.—Sixty-four percent of patients had a complete histologic response to intravesical BCG; by 4 years, this rate had dropped to 54%. The complete response rate was 85% in patients with primary carcinoma, vs. 57% in those with secondary carcinoma. The disease progression rate was 45% overall: 26% in patients with a complete histologic response to BCG vs. 77% in those with partial response or no response. Primary carcinoma had a progression rate of 8%, compared with 57% for secondary cancer. Progression occurred in 40% of patients who received only 1 course of BCG, 62% of those receiving 2 courses, and 89% of those in whom both courses failed.

Twenty-six patients expressed p53 nuclear immunoreactivity before treatment. In 73% of these patients, p53 immunoreactivity converted from positive to negative after intravesical BCG treatment. The complete response rate in this group was 68%. The disease progression rate was 90% in patients who had p53 nuclear accumulation after treatment, vs. 37% without this finding. Three patients who still had p53 nuclear reactivity after BCG had a complete response to treatment. In all 3, disease progressed, indicating a molecular genetic change occurring before histologic change. The progression rate was lowest (21%) in patients who had a complete response and no p53 nuclear accumulation after intravesical BCG treatment.

Conclusions.—Response to intravesical BCG and presence of p53 nuclear accumulation are both relevant prognostic factors in patients with carcinoma in situ of the bladder. Conservative follow-up, including cystoscopy and cytologic examination, is appropriate for patients with a persistently complete histologic response to BCG and no p53 nuclear reactivity after treatment. All other patients should be considered for cystectomy.

▶ This study provides additional evidence that abnormal p53 protein accumulation is an adverse prognostic marker, even among patients in whom conventional histologic and cytologic responses have been observed. Up to 90% of patients with persistent, abnormal p53 accumulation after BCG therapy experience later recurrence of carcinoma in situ or progressive transitional cell carcinoma. Unfortunately, the number of such patients in this study is small, and a larger series is necessary to confirm this finding.

G.L. Andriole, Jr., M.D.

Oral Bropirimine Immunotherapy of Bladder Carcinoma In Situ After Prior Intravesical Bacille Calmette-Guérin

Sarosdy MF, Manyak MJ, Sagalowsky AI, et al (Univ of Texas, San Antonio; George Washington Univ, Washington, DC; Univ of Texas, Dallas; et al)
Urology 51:226–231, 1998   13–3

Objective.—Intravesical bacille Calmette-Guérin (BCG) is the treatment of choice for carcinoma in situ of the bladder. For those who cannot tolerate the procedure, cystectomy or intravesical therapy with an investigational drug are the only options. Bropirimine, an oral immunomodulator, has shown promise in the treatment of transitional-cell carcinoma in situ (CIS). The efficacy of bropirimine in patients with bladder CIS after prior BCG therapy was investigated in a multicenter phase II trial that included patients who were intolerant of BCG.

Methods.—Bropirimine (3.0 g daily in 3 equal doses) was self-administered by 86 patients with CIS (74 male) who had received at least 12 instillations of BCG (60 patients) or who were intolerant of BCG (26 patients). Patients were followed monthly and toxicity was assessed at each visit. Biopsies and cytologic examinations were performed every 3 months.

Results.—Thirteen resistant and 8 intolerant patients were not evaluable. Fourteen resistant patients (30%) had a complete response and 2 other resistant patients were free of CIS by biopsy. Seven BCG-intolerant patients had a complete response. The overall response rate was 24%. The number of complete responses was not correlated with the number of prior BCG treatments. The duration of complete response ranged from 65 to 810 days, with 12 responders remaining disease-free. Recurrent disease developed in 9 patients after 65 to 486 days. Toxicity was reported in all patients, with the most common adverse reactions being headache, asthenia, and nausea. Thirteen patients discontinued the drug because of adverse reactions. Four nonresponders (6%) progressed to invasive or metastatic disease.

Conclusion.—Bropirimine may serve as an alternative treatment to cystectomy for patients with bladder cancer who have failed or are intolerant to BCG therapy.

▶ In this study, the authors took high-risk patients with bladder cancer with persistent CIS and treated them with bropirimine, an orally administered immunotherapeutic agent. About one third of the patients have experienced a complete response for up to 2½ years. This agent, because it is thought to promote endogenous production of interferon, may be associated with unacceptable side effects, including general feelings of malaise, headache, and flu-like symptoms of nausea and myalgia.

This seems to be a promising therapy for patients who have failed BCG. However, further investigation will be necessary to determine whether it is associated with durable responses and how it would compare with standard therapies for recurrent CIS, such as intravesical mitomycin C or radical cystectomy.

G.L. Andriole, Jr., M.D.

Allium sativum **(Garlic) Treatment for Murine Transitional Cell Carcinoma**
Riggs DR, DeHaven JI, Lamm DL (West Virginia Univ, Morgantown)
Cancer 79:1987–1994, 1997   13–4

Introduction.—Immunotherapy with Bacillus Calmette-Guérin (BCG) is an effective intravesical treatment for superficial bladder carcinoma, but toxicity may limit the widespread use of BCG in patients with transitional cell carcinoma of the bladder. There have been various reports of the benefits of *allium sativum* (AS) (garlic) in the treatment of malignancies. Using the MBT2 murine bladder carcinoma model, investigators examined the therapeutic effect of AS.

Methods.—Female C3H/HeN mice were randomized into 6 groups before the induction of MBT2 bladder tumors. Four groups received subcutaneous immunizations of AS (25 mg, 12.5 mg, 6.3 mg, and 3.1 mg) on days 1, 3, 5, and 7 after tumor transplantation. Negative controls were given saline on the same schedule, and positive controls were treated with BCG 10^7 colony-forming units on days 1 and 7 after tumor transplantation.

Results.—Subcutaneous AS significantly reduced tumor volume compared with saline control in the initial experiment, but the frequency of immunizations was reduced because of treatment-related death. The second experiment yielded similar results, and the cumulative AS dose was reduced for the third experiment. Compared with saline control, mice that received 5 weekly immunizations of AS (5 mg, 5 mg, 1 mg, 1 mg, and 1 mg; cumulative dose of 13 mg) exhibited significant reductions in tumor incidence and tumor growth and increased survival. This treatment schedule did not result in treatment-related deaths. Oral administration of AS was also effective in reducing tumor volume in a dose-dependent manner. Mice treated with 500 mg oral AS had significant reductions in both tumor volume and mortality.

Conclusion.—Subcutaneous AS had a highly significant and reproducible antitumor activity in a murine model of transitional cell carcinoma of the bladder, but repeated injections caused treatment-related death. Oral AS, however, was both safe and effective and may offer a new therapy for this malignancy.

▶ This article will resonate in this era of "natural" medicine. Garlic has been reported to be beneficial in a wide variety of circumstances, including the reduction of serum cholesterol levels, inhibition of platelet aggregation, and as an anti-viral agent. This article explores its potential use to stimulate tumorolytic activity via the immune system. The authors used a poorly differentiated but highly immunogenic strain of murine bladder cancer and showed that subcutaneous and oral therapy was associated with significant reductions in tumor outgrowth. Whether this treatment should be administered orally or topically is not known, and tantalizing evidence also exists that beyond its immunostimulatory capacity, garlic may have direct cytolytic effects on some tumor cells. The exact agents within garlic that account for these stunning results are not yet known.

G.L. Andriole, Jr., M.D.

Gemcitabine: A Promising New Agent in the Treatment of Advanced Urothelial Cancer

Moore MJ, Tannock IF, Ernst DS, et al (Princess Margaret Hosp, Toronto; Tom Baker Cancer Centre, Calgary, Canada; Ottawa Regional Cancer Centre, Canada; et al)
J Clin Oncol 15:3441–3445, 1997   13–5

Objective.—Gemcitabine is a new chemotherapeutic agent for a variety of solid tumors. The response rate to gemcitabine in patients with advanced, previously untreated urothelial cancer was investigated in a phase II study.

Methods.—Gemcitabine (1,200 mg/m^2) was given by IV infusion over 30 minutes on days 1, 8, and 15 of a 28-day cycle to 41 outpatients (median age, 71 years; 10 women) with no previous therapy within 1 year of the present study. Patients received 3 treatment cycles. Toxicity and responses were recorded.

Results.—There were 28 patients with grade 2 and 14 patients with grade 3 toxicity according to World Health Organization criteria. No patient experienced grade 4 toxicity. There were 3 complete responses and 6 partial responses among the 37 evaluable patients. Median survival in these patients was 8 months. Four patients were in remission at 14, 23, 24, and 31 months, and 17% of patients were alive at 24 months. Sixteen patients received other chemotherapeutic regimens in addition to the study drug.

Conclusion.—Gemcitabine is a promising therapeutic agent for treatment of advanced urothelial cancer. Toxicity is acceptable.

▶ Gemcitabine is a cytosine analogue with structural similarities to cytarabine. Gemcitabine is active against a variety of solid tumor lines and requires intracellular activation to its triphosphate derivative which subsequently inhibits DNA synthesis. In this trial, 41 patients with advanced transitional cell carcinoma received gemcitabine. There was an overall response rate of 24.3% with 3 complete responses. This treatment was generally well tolerated, and most patients received the entire dose of therapy without interruption. Because of this promising safety profile and significant efficacy, further studies of gemcitabine in combination with other agents such as cisplatin, are now being designed. This agent may be an alternative to MVAC (methotrexate, vinblastine, doxorubicin, and cisplatin) or CISCA (cisplatin, cyclophosphamide, and doxorubicin).

G.L. Andriole, Jr., M.D.

Bladder Preservation by Combined Modality Therapy for Invasive Bladder Cancer
Kachnic LA, Kaufman DS, Heney NM, et al (Harvard Med School, Boston)
J Clin Oncol 15:1022–1029, 1997   13–6

Objective.—Because radical cystectomy is curative in no more than 50% of patients with muscle-invasive bladder cancer, bladder-conserving methods have been employed to decrease morbidity and associated quality-of-life problems after cystectomy. Using maximal transurethral resection (TURBT), systemic multidrug chemotherapy, and chemoradiation has allowed selected patients to have bladder conservation and the highest likelihood of cure.

Methods.—Between 1986 and 1993, 106 consecutive patients (34 women) aged 38–88 years, with stages T2–T4,Nx,M0 bladder cancer, had TURBT, neoadjuvant chemotherapy with methotrexate, vinblastine, and cisplatin (MCV), followed by 2 additional courses of cisplatin combined with 39.6 Gy pelvic external-beam radiation. Response was defined as T0 if no tumor was visible on cystoscopy, and results of biopsy and urine cytology were negative. Patients were followed up for an average of 4.4 years with cystoscopy, biopsy, manual examination, and urine cytology every 3 months for 2 years and every 6 months thereafter. Abdominal and pelvic CT scans were performed after initial irradiation, at 3 months after final treatment, and every 6–12 months thereafter.

Results.—There were 39 patients who completed the protocol as specified and 46 who completed it with minor deviations. There were 21 patients who were unable to complete the protocol without substantial deviations. There were 76 completers who did not require cystectomy and 70 who had a T0 response. Five-year rate of freedom from recurrence among the 76 completers was 79%; 42 (55%) have been continuously free of bladder tumors, and 21 (28%) had a relapse treated with TURBT and intravesical drug therapy. Fifteen of the latter were tumor-free 13–97 months later, 2 had persistent superficial tumors, and 13 had invasive recurrence. Five-year overall rates of survival and survival with intact bladder are 52% and 43%, respectively. The 5-year overall survival rates for patients with T2 vs. T3 and T4 disease were 63% and 45%, respectively. Rates of freedom from distant metastases were 79% and 57%. For patients with hydronephrosis compared to those without ureteral obstruction, 5-year overall survival rates were 40% and 56% and rates of freedom from distant metastases were 42% and 73%. There were 17 patients with a T0 response who experienced local recurrence and underwent salvage cystectomy.

Conclusion.—Transurethral resection, chemotherapy, and radiation therapy can preserve the bladder in selected patients with muscle-invasive bladder cancer. The overall 5-year survival rate is 52%, and 43% of patients surviving to 5 years have a functioning bladder.

▶ This manuscript presents 5-year actuarial survival data for patients treated with a bladder-sparing protocol for invasive bladder cancer. The 52% overall survival at 5 years approximates what one might expect from a cystectomy series; however, only 43% of patients at 5 years survive with their bladder in place. This bladder preservation protocol differs from others in that patients are sequentially monitored with repeat TURBTs and only patients who are free of disease after 4,000 cGy and 2 cycles of chemotherapy are treated with consolidation radiation therapy and additional chemotherapy.

It must be emphasized that patients entering this protocol were highly selected (recruitment of 106 patients took place over approximately 7 years), and there is considerable systemic toxicity associated with chemotherapy and external beam irradiation. This experience has resulted in the author's statement that "at this time radical cystectomy is the treatment of choice in this country for invasive bladder cancer." The authors are examining lower doses of chemotherapy administered over shorter periods of time, which reduce toxicity and allow outpatient administration of this therapy.

G.L. Andriole, Jr., M.D.

Invasive Bladder Cancer: Treatment Strategies Using Transurethral Surgery, Chemotherapy and Radiation Therapy With Selection for Bladder Conservation
Shipley WU, Zietman AL, Kaufman DS, et al (Harvard Med School, Boston)
Int J Radiat Oncol Biol Phys 39:937–943, 1997   13–7

Background.—In many types of malignancies, combined-modality therapy is used for preservation of the involved organ. In the United States, radical cystectomy is standard treatment for invasive bladder cancer. However, recent reports have shown good results with combined-modality treatment. The results have been especially encouraging in patients with clinical T2 and T3a disease who do not have obstruction of the ureter by the tumor. Recent reports of bladder-conservation therapy for invasive bladder cancer are reviewed.

Combined-modality Treatment for Invasive Bladder Cancer.—Bladder-conservation therapy usually includes transurethral resection of the bladder tumor, followed by chemotherapy and radiation therapy. After induction, chemotherapy, cystoscopy, and rebiopsy are performed to assess the histologic response. A complete response requires that rebiopsy of the tumor site be negative and urine cytologic studies show no tumor cells. If this is the case, a consolidation course of chemotherapy and radiation is given. If induction chemotherapy does not bring a complete response, then immediate cystectomy is performed. On their own, radiation, transurethral resection of the bladder tumor, and multidrug chemotherapy offer primary tumor local control rates of 20% to 40%. In combination, these approaches can yield complete response rates of 65% to 80%. Of the patients with complete responses, 75% to 85% will remain free of recurrent invasive bladder tumors. Overall 5-year survival is about 50%, and 5-year survival with the bladder intact is 40% to 45% (Table 5). The survival results are comparable to those achieved with radial cystectomy for patients of similar age and clinical stage.

Discussion.—Good results have been reported with bladder-conserving therapy for patients with invasive bladder carcinoma. When administered by an experienced, multimodality team of urologists, medical oncologists, and radiation oncologists, this approach offers a real alternative to radical cystectomy. More research is needed to identify those patients who will have local failure after conservative surgery and chemoradiotherapy, and to test promising new chemotherapy agents and adjuvant therapy combinations.

▶ This article summarizes the literature about using bladder-conserving strategies for patients with muscle invasive bladder cancer. It is striking to me that in all series reviewed, only a minority of patients have a 5-year survival with the bladder intact (see Table 5). What we need to know are the characteristics of the patients who do well with these types of approaches, so that these strategies can be selectively offered. Until that is accomplished, however, it is difficult to recommend these approaches with very

TABLE 5.—Recent Results of Various Combined Modality Therapies for Survival and for Survival With Bladder Preserved

Series	Treatment	No. of patients	5-Year survival	5-Year survival with bladder preservation
Dunst (6, 43)	TURBT, concurrent cisplatin and XRT	79	52%	41%
Tester (55, 57)	concurrent cisplatin and XRT	42	52%	42%
Tester (57)	MCV and concurrent cisplatin and XRT	91	62%†	44%†
Kashnic (23)	TURBT, MCV, concurrent cisplatin and XRT	106	52%	43%
Given (12)	TURBT, MCV plus, in 49 patients (53%), concurrent cisplatin and XRT	93	51%	18%
Srougi (52)	M-VAC and partial cystectomy	30	53%	20%
Sternberg (53)	TURBT + M-VAC but without cystectomy in 31 patients	64	—*	33%*
Scher (44) and Schultz (46)	M-VAC and conservative surgery	111	48%	21%

*Median follow-up 30 months at time of report
†Based on 4-year data
Abbreviations: XRT, external beam irradiation; *MCV*, methotrexate, cisplatin, vinblastine; *M-VAC*, methotrexate, vinblastine, adriamycin, cisplatin; *TURBT*, transurethral resection of tumor.
(Courtesy of Shipley WU, Zietman AL, Kaufman DS, et al: Invasive bladder cancer: Treatment strategies using transurethral surgery, chemotherapy and radiation therapy with selection for bladder conservation. *Int J Radiat Oncol Biol Phys* 39:937–943. Copyright 1997, with permission from Elsevier Science.)

much enthusiasm, especially given the excellent functional and disease-control capabilities of radical cystectomy and bladder-substitution surgery.

G.L. Andriole, Jr., M.D.

Radical Cystectomy for Carcinoma of the Bladder: Critical Evaluation of the Results in 1,026 Cases
Ghoneim MA, El-Mekresh MM, El-Baz MA, et al (Cairo Univ, Egypt)
J Urol 158:393–399, 1997   13–8

Introduction.—A series of 1,026 patients who underwent radical cystectomy for bladder malignancy at a Cairo (Egypt) center was analyzed for prognostic factors affecting survival. Median follow-up time was 4 years.

Methods.—From 1969 to 1990, 764 men, average age 47.6 years, and 262 women, average age 43 years, underwent radical cystectomy at the study institution. All had invasive carcinoma of the bladder and underwent urinary diversion. Cystectomy specimens were analyzed for pathological staging of the tumors and histopathological typing and grading. Patients were followed on a regular schedule for evidence of treatment failure.

Results.—Forty patients (4%) died postoperatively in the hospital. Causes of death included hepatorenal failure, septic shock, intestinal obstruction, pulmonary embolism, heart failure, and fecal fistula. Advanced stage disease (greater than P3) was present in 81% of patients at diagnosis. Half of the squamous tumors, which accounted for 59% of cases, were low grade. Other tumor types identified were transitional carcinoma (22.2%) and primary nonurachal adenocarcinoma (11.4%); the remaining 73 cases (7.1%) had pathological features categorized as mixed or unclassified. Regional lymph node involvement was detected in 188 (18.3%) cases. Most excised specimens (85.3%), particularly squamous tumors, showed bilharzial eggs. The overall 5-year disease-free survival rate was 48.1%. Multivariate analysis determined that tumor pathological stage and grade and nodal disease had a statistically significant impact on survival. During follow-up there were 331 cases of treatment failure—198 from local recurrence, 107 from distant metastasis, and 26 from both.

Discussion.—Radical cystectomy can be performed with low morbidity and offers good locoregional control for patients with muscle invasive bladder cancer. Approximately half of cases will achieve an overall 5-year disease-free survival.

▶ This large cystectomy series is notable for the high prevalence of bilharziasis (between 80% and 85% regardless of pathological type) and for the young age of the patients (43 ± 8 years). It is eye-opening that the overall 5-year survival rate among these patients is only 48%. Significant predictors of survival were final pathological stage, grade, and the presence of metastases to the regional lymph nodes. These results must be interpreted with caution, however; first, these patients obviously had very aggressive tumors that may not be directly comparable with those observed in North Americans; second, adjuvant and neoadjuvant therapies were only infrequently administered and could conceivably have improved the survival figures.

G.L. Andriole, Jr., M.D.

Does Prostate Transitional Cell Carcinoma Preclude Orthotopic Bladder Reconstruction After Radical Cystoprostatectomy for Bladder Cancer?
Iselin CE, Robertson CN, Webster GD, et al (Duke Univ, Durham, NC)
J Urol 158:2123–2126, 1997   13–9

Objective.—Prostate transitional cell carcinoma is a risk factor for urethral recurrence after cystoprostatectomy. Whether preservation of the urethra placed these patients at increased risk for recurrence was reviewed in 81 men who underwent cystoprostatectomy and orthotopic bladder replacement with urethral preservation.

Methods.—Between February 1984 and June 1996, 70 of 81 men who underwent cystoprostatectomy and orthotopic bladder replacement were followed for an average of 35 months. Patients received physical examinations, urinary cytology, and imaging studies at 6-month intervals.

Results.—Four patients had adenocarcinoma, 1 had mixed carcinoma, and 65 had transition cell carcinoma. There were 48 patients alive with no evidence of disease and 5 dead without disease at last follow-up. Eight of 53 patients without disease had transitional cell carcinoma of the prostate. Six of 17 patients with recurrence had transitional cell carcinoma of the prostate, and 13 died of their disease. One of these patients with stromal invasive disease had urethral recurrence at 1 month, had distant pelvic recurrence at 3 months, and died at 5 months. Urethral recurrence apparently was not the cause of death in this patient because of the time frame from urethral to pelvic recurrence.

Conclusion.—There was only 1 death in this group in a patient who had urethral recurrence that was not apparently the cause of death. Urethral resection does not appear to increase the risk of urethral recurrence in patients with prostate transitional cell carcinoma and bladder cancer.

▶ There has been a debate concerning urethrectomy for patients undergoing radical cystectomy for transitional cell tumors of the bladder. This issue has become important now that orthotopic bladder substitution is a fairly routine procedure. Historically, urethral recurrence rates for men who had transitional cell carcinoma involving the prostate have ranged between 17% and 39%. In this study, the authors show that urethral recurrence is uncommon—only 7% among men who had transitional cell carcinoma involving the prostate. In the authors' opinion, the presence of transitional cell carcinoma beyond the bladder neck does not require urethrectomy unless the distal prostatic resection margin is positive. This has been my approach to managing such patients. However, I continue to perform careful urethroscopy on all patients with neobladders on a 6- to-12 month basis.

G.L. Andriole, Jr., M.D.

Ureteral Carcinoma In Situ at Radical Cystectomy: Does the Margin Matter?

Silver DA, Stroumbakis N, Russo P, et al (Mem Sloan-Kettering Cancer Ctr, New York)
J Urol 158:768–771, 1997
13–10

Objective.—Intraoperative frozen-section examination of the ureteral margin to ensure complete tumor removal is recommended when malignant change of the ureteral urothelium is found because this malignant change is believed to be an adverse prognostic factor. A series of patients undergoing radical cystectomy was evaluated to determine the clinical significance of concomitant ureteral carcinoma in situ and the usefulness of intraoperative frozen-section examination.

Methods.—A pathologic review of 401 specimens from patients having radical cystectomy from January 1989 through December 1994 found 31 (7.7%) patients (3 women) aged 43–86 years with carcinoma in situ in the distal ureter. Fifteen patients were treated for Calmette-Guerin bacillus. Patients were studied annually for an average of 31.8 months. Positive urinary cytologic findings, recurrence of cancer, and cancer-specific survival were outcomes.

Results.—Positive margins were found in 21 patients. Of the 30 patients on whom frozen sections were prepared, 15 (50%) had positive margins, and 5 (16.5%) had carcinoma in situ undetected initially. Cancer recurred at the ureteroenteric anastomosis in 1 patient and proximal transition cell carcinoma in 2, all of whom had positive urinary cytologic findings. Average intervals to positive cytologic findings and upper tract disease were 38 and 49 months. The incidence of upper tract recurrence among patients with concomitant ureteral carcinoma in situ has been variously reported to range from 8% to 20% (Table 3).

Conclusion.—Upper tract recurrence and positive cytologic results were not related to ureteral margin status. The bladder tumor not the ureteral carcinoma in situ is prognostically significant at radical cystectomy.

TABLE 3.—Concomitant Ureteral Carcinoma in situ and Upper Tract Recurrence

References	No. Cases	% Upper Tract Recurrence	Interval to Recurrence (mos.)	Series Followup (mos.)		
				Mean	Median	Range
Johnson et al	6	16.6	9	31	24	8–66
Batista et al	12	8	53	24.5	—	4–72
Schoenberg et al	5	20	Not specified	—	67	3–148
Present series	31	9.6	49	31.8	22	2–74

(Courtesy of Silver DA, Stroumbakis N, Russo P, et al: Ureteral carcinoma in situ at radical cystectomy: Does the margin matter? *J Urol* 158:768–771, 1997.)

▶ This is another series showing that it is probably not necessary to obtain frozen sections of the ureteral margin during a radical cystectomy. This occurs because the frozen section may be falsely negative (approximately 17% of the time in this series) and follow-up of patients with proved ureteral carcinoma in situ does not disclose a higher rate of upper tract transitional cell carcinoma (see Table 3). On the basis of these data, the authors recommend that frozen sections are unnecessary at the time of surgery and that patients with upper urinary tract carcinoma in situ, irrespective of their margin status, may be monitored expectantly with urinary cytology and upper tract imaging.

G.L. Andriole, Jr., M.D.

The Clinical and Histological Features of Transitional Cell Carcinoma of the Bladder With Microcysts: Analysis of 12 Cases
Paz A, Rath-Wolfson, Lask D, et al (Rabin Med Ctr, Campus Golda, Petah-Tiqva; Tel-Aviv Univ, Israel)
Br J Urol 79:722–725, 1997   13–11

Introduction.—Transitional cell carcinoma (TCC) of the urinary bladder with microcysts may present diagnostic difficulties, for TCC must be differentiated from adenocarcinoma, cystitis glandularis, cystitis cystica, or nephrogenic adenoma. Twelve cases of microcystic TCC of the bladder were reviewed for histological features and clinical course of the disease.

Methods.—The 12 patients represented 1.2% of 940 patients with TCC of the bladder diagnosed at the study institution over a 5-year period. Patients were 8 men and 4 women, mean age 71 years. Tumor specimens were prepared for analysis and the slides reviewed for proportion of microcysts in the TCC. Clinical data were obtained from patient records and follow-up reports.

Results.—Low-grade TCC was present in 1 patient and high-grade TCC in 11; 6 patients had tumor invasion of the lamina propria and 3 had muscle invasion. Tumors were located on the trigone in 7 cases and on the lateral bladder walls in 5. None of the patients had metastatic disease at diagnosis and the 3 patients with stage T2 tumors had no previous bladder tumors. Three patients, 1 with stage Ta and 2 with stage T1 tumors, are alive with recurrences; all recurrent tumors had microcysts. Microcysts ranged from 5 to 40 μm in diameter, and their number showed no correlation with grade or stage of bladder TCC. A pink eosinophilic material in the center of many microcysts (Fig 1) stained positively with both Alcian blue and periodic acid-Schiff. Second primary tumors, including 3 colon carcinomas, were present in 6 patients.

Discussion.—Microcystic TCC was present in about 1% of this series of patients with TCC. The diagnosis of typical TCC was obvious in all 12 cases, but the cases showed a higher percentage of high-grade and high-stage tumors than would be expected. Because 6 of the 12 patients had a

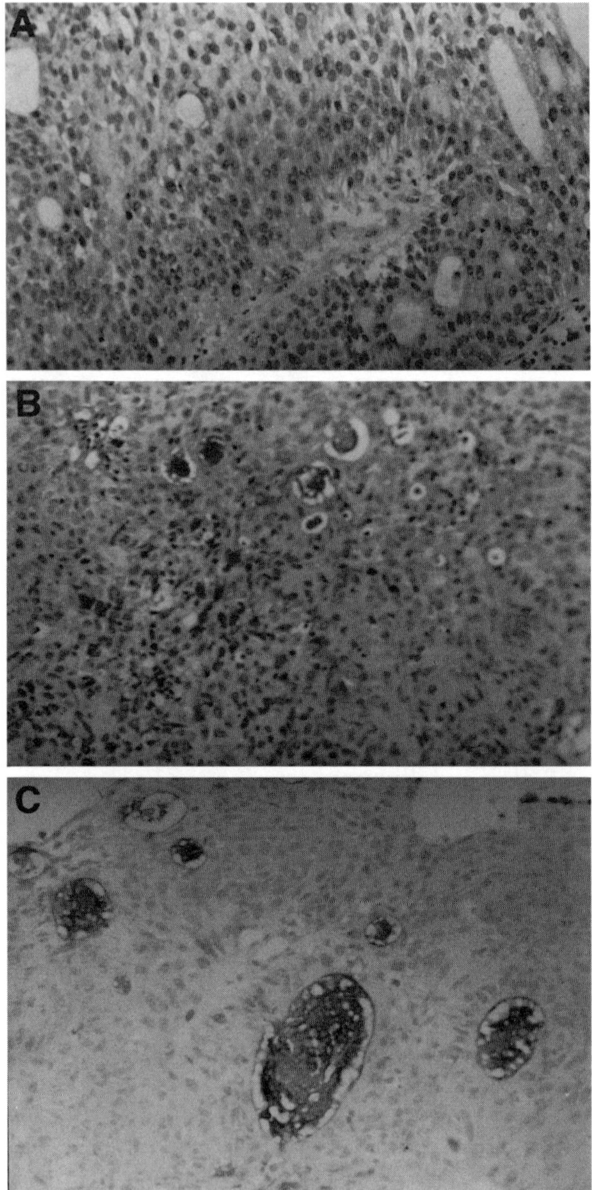

FIGURE 1.—Transitional cell carcinoma with gland-like lumina: **a,** stained with hematoxylin and eosin X 250; **b,** stained with periodic-acid Schiff X 250; **c,** stained with Alcian blue X 250. (Courtesy of Paz A, Rath-Wolfson L, Lask D, et al: The clinical and histological features of transitional cell carcinoma of the bladder with microcysts: Analysis of 12 cases. *Br J Urol* 79:722–725, 1997.)

metachronous tumor, patients with microcystic TCC should be screened for asymptomatic tumors of the colon.

▶ Microcyst formation (or gland-like lumina) may occur in about 1% of patients with transitional cell carcinoma of the bladder. This article reviews 12 cases showing that the majority of the patients had either high-grade or high-stage tumors, and that approximately half of the patients had a coexistent second primary malignancy, most often colonic in origin. This entity should be easily distinguishable on routine staining, and its presence may alert the urologist to look for a second malignant process.

G.L. Andriole, Jr., M.D.

14 Benign Prostatic Diseases

The Effect of Finasteride on the Risk of Acute Urinary Retention and the Need for Surgical Treatment Among Men With Benign Prostatic Hyperplasia
McConnell JD, for the Finasteride Long-term Efficacy and Safety Study Group (Univ of Texas, Dallas; Univ of Wisconsin, Madison; Johns Hopkins Med Institutions, Baltimore, Md; et al)
N Engl J Med 338:557–563, 1998   14–1

Introduction.—Finasteride is reported to improve urinary symptoms in men with benign prostatic hyperplasia (BPH). It is not known to what extent the benefit is sustained or whether finasteride decreases the incidence of related events, particularly the need for surgery and development of acute urinary retention. The long-term effects of finasteride on the symptoms of BPH and the incidence of important outcomes related to taking the drug were assessed in 3,040 men with moderate to severe BPH in a 4-year, double-blind, randomized, placebo-controlled trial.

Methods.—Patients were randomized to receive either finasteride 5 mg daily or placebo for 4 years. Patients were followed-up every 4 months for symptoms scores (scale of 1 to 34), side effects, and measurement of urinary flow rate. Measurement of serum prostate-specific antigen was performed every 4 months for 1 year and every 8 months thereafter. Patients underwent a yearly physical examination and magnetic resonance imaging of the prostate. A subgroup of men underwent measurement of prostate volume.

Results.—Complete data was available for 2,760 men. During the 4-year assessment period, 152 of 1,503 (10%) men in the placebo group and 69 of 1,513 (5%) men in the finasteride group had surgery for BPH. Seven percent of males in the placebo group developed acute urinary retention, compared with 3% in the finasteride group. Mean decreases in symptom scores were significantly greater in the finasteride group than the placebo group (3.3 vs. 1.3). Finasteride significantly improved urinary flow rate and reduced prostate volume.

Conclusion.—Treatment with finasteride for 4 years decreased symptoms and prostate volume, increased urinary flow, and lowered the prob-

"

ability of surgery and acute urinary retention in men with symptoms of urinary obstruction and prostatic enlargement.

▶ This article further refines our understanding of the role of 5-alpha reductase inhibition in the natural history of BPH. These data are very necessary as during the last several years, a variety of studies have been reported that seemingly presented conflicting information regarding the efficacy of finasteride. I think this large and long-term study does allow us to conclude that properly selected patients benefit from finasteride therapy. They experience improvement in their urinary symptoms that is sustained for more than 4 years, and they have significantly reduced rates of elective surgical procedures or of experiencing urinary retention. Moreover, although the data were not presented in this article, it has been reported that use of finasteride preserves the use of serum PSA as a marker for prostate cancer if one doubles the PSA value of a finasteride-treated patient. These findings should be carefully considered by all physicians and patients who are contemplating medical management of BPH.

G.L. Andriole, Jr., M.D.

Prostate Tissue Composition and Response to Finasteride in Men With Symptomatic Benign Prostatic Hyperplasia

Marks LS, Partin AW, Gormley GJ, et al (Univ of California, Los Angeles; Brotman Med Ctr, Culver City, Calif; Johns Hopkins Univ, Baltimore, Md; et al)

J Urol 157:2171–2178, 1997

14–2

Introduction.—Epithelial cells are the locus of the androgen receptor in the prostate. Prostate response to finasteride varies; this may be because prostate tissue composition is not uniform. A man with an epithelial-rich prostate may respond differently to finasteride than a man with an epithelial-poor prostate. A possible relationship between prostate epithelial composition and finasteride responsiveness in men with symptomatic benign prostatic hyperplasia (BPH) was assessed in a randomized, placebo-controlled, double-blind trial.

Methods.—Forty-one men with symptomatic BPH were randomly assigned to 6 months of treatment with either finasteride or placebo (26 and 15 patients, respectively). Patients were followed up using urinary symptom score, flow rate, serum prostate specific antigen levels, dihydrotestosterone levels, transrectal ultrasound, MRI for whole and zonal prostate volumes, and morphometry of prostate sextant biopsies (separated into inner and outer gland segments to measure the percent epithelium, stroma, and glandular lumen).

Results.—Patients in the finasteride group had nonsignificant decreases in symptom scores and increasing flow rates and significant decreases in prostate specific antigen (48%), dihydrotestosterone (74%), and prostate volume (21%). There was a 55% decrease in inner gland epithelium with

TABLE 2.—Prostate Tissue Components Before and After Finasteride (26 Patients) or Placebo (13) Treatment

	Median % Epithelium	Median % Stroma	Median % Lumen	Median Stroma-to-Epithelial Ratio
Overall prostate				
Before:				
Placebo	14.8	59.1	27.4	4.4
Finasteride	12.6	63.2	23.4	4.7
After:				
Placebo	12.8	59.4	26.8	4.2
Finasteride	9.7	59.0	30.5	5.5
Inner gland (mostly transition zone)				
Before:				
Placebo	15.0	51.0	30.0	3.2
Finasteride	13.5	60.5	28.0	4.4
After:				
Placebo	12.0	54.0	30.0	4.8
Finasteride	6.0*	63.4	28.5	10.3*
Outer gland (peripheral zone)				
Before:				
Placebo	25.0	45.0	35.0	2.0
Finasteride	25.5	44.0	32.0	2.6
After:				
Placebo	18.0	44.0	31.0	2.4
Finasteride	19.5	46.0	34.5	3.4

*After finasteride treatment a resulting decrease in epithelial composition and increase of stroma-to-epithelial ratio is statistically significant in the inner gland ($P < 0.01$) but not the outer gland or overall prostate.

(Courtesy of Marks LS, Partin AW, Gormley GJ, et al: Prostate tissue composition and response to finasteride in men with symptomatic benign prostatic hyperplasia. *J Urol* 157:2171–2178, 1997.)

little effect on stroma or lumina in the finasteride group (Table 2). There was a linear correlation between pretreatment inner-gland epithelial content and prostate volume decreases caused by the drug.

Conclusions.—Finasteride caused major suppression of prostate epithelium, which was most pronounced in the inner gland. A finasteride-induced prostate volume reduction was predictable by quantification of epithelial tissues of the inner gland. The inner prostate seems to be anatomically and functionally different from the outer prostate.

▶ This is an interesting study that has demonstrated the differences between the transition zone and peripheral zone of the prostate with regard to baseline stroma-to-epithelial ratios, and also posttreatment changes in this ratio as induced by finasteride. As shown in Table 2, finasteride results in slightly more than a 50% reduction of transition zone epithelium, thereby resulting in more than a doubling of the stroma-to-epithelial ratio (from 4.4 to 10.3). On the other hand, peripheral zone tissue exhibits a more modest 20% reduction in percentage of epithelium, and therefore has a much smaller change in stroma-to-epithelial ratio (from 2.6 to 3.4). It is tantalizing that studies have now demonstrated that type 2, 5α-reductase in the prostate is located mainly in the stroma of the transition zone. One may therefore speculate that inhibition of this activity in the stroma results in a *local* effect on dihydrotestosterone production, with the most profound androgen deprivation occurring in the nearby epithelium. The primacy of the transition zone of the prostate as the location for androgen-stimulated functions such as hypertrophy and prostate specific antigen (PSA) production is also supported by other accumulating studies in the literature showing that serum PSA correlates closely with the calculated volume of the transition zone of the prostate more so than with the estimated volume of the peripheral zone, and that patients who undergo resection of the transition zone during a transurethral resection of the prostate usually have a substantial and significant reduction in their serum PSA. Therefore, there are now several accumulating lines of evidence to suggest that the peripheral and transition zones of the prostate are really quite distinct biologically.

G.L. Andriole, Jr., M.D.

Unique Preclinical Characteristics of GG745, a Potent Dual Inhibitor of 5AR

Bramson HN, Hermann D, Batchelor KW, et al (Glaxo Wellcome Research Inst, Research Triangle Park, NC; Inspire Pharmaceuticals Inc, Durham, NC)
J Pharmacol Exp Ther 282:1496–1502, 1997   14–3

Background.—Selective type 2 5α-reductase inhibition with finasteride is an effective treatment for benign prostatic hyperplasia. Even greater reductions in dihydrotestosterone (DHT) might be achieved using a drug that could inhibit both the type 1 and type 2 enzymes. The authors have identified GG745 as a potent inhibitor of both 5α-reductase isoenzymes. They tested its pharmacokinetic and pharmacodynamic properties in rats, dogs, and humans.

Findings.—The preclinical studies found that in rats GG745 affected DHT-driven prostatic growth in a way similar to finasteride, which is also a dual 5α-reductase inhibitor in this species. However, GG745 appeared to be the more potent of the 2 inhibitors. The terminal half-life of GG745 was much longer than that of finasteride in both rats and dogs. The accumulated data were used to calculate GG745 doses likely to reduce DHT levels in humans. Single-dose studies of GG745 in humans suggested a terminal half-life of approximately 240 hours. A single GG745 dose of greater than 10 mg produced a greater reduction in DHT levels than a single 5 mg dose of finasteride.

Conclusion.—As a dual 5α-reductase inhibitor, GG745 produces lower serum DHT levels than single 5α-reductase isoenzyme inhibitors, such as finasteride. At the maximal doses used in this study, GG745 decreases DHT level by more than 90%. More research will be needed to see whether the greater reduction of serum DHT leads to clinical benefit.

▶ This study provides preclinical data on a dual inhibitor of 5α-reductase that is being actively investigated in men with benign prostatic hyperplasia. This compound is different from finasteride in that it appears to inhibit both type I and type II 5α-reductase; consequently, the level of serum DHT reduction attained by administration of this agent is in excess of 90%, whereas finasteride reduces serum DHT levels by approximately 70%.

Whether the further reduction of serum DHT levels will be translated into greater efficacy in ameliorating the symptoms of benign prostatic hyperplasia is not known, but one may hypothesize that because DHT is the most potent androgen in the prostate, nearly complete abrogation could be associated with more profound prostatic involution. Hopefully, early clinical studies in patients with benign prostatic hyperplasia will be available soon, so the benefit and any potential added morbidity from nearly complete DHT abrogation will be known.

G.L. Andriole, Jr., M.D.

Doxazosin for Benign Prostatic Hyperplasia: Long-term Efficacy and Safety in Hypertensive and Normotensive Patients
Lepor H, Kaplan SA, Klimberg I, et al (New York Univ, Columbia Univ, New York; Pfizer Central Research, NY; et al)
J Urol 157:525–530, 1997   14–4

Objective.—The prevalence of benign prostatic hyperplasia (BPH) increases with age and is almost 50% in men aged 60–80 years. A recent study demonstrated that the antihypertensive drug doxazosin also increased urinary flow in normotensive and hypertensive men. Results of a study of safety and sustained efficacy of doxazosin for long-term treatment of normotensive and hypertensive men with BPH are presented.

Methods.—There were 272 normotensive and 178 mildly to moderately hypertensive men enrolled in a 4-year, open-label, dose titration extension treatment of BPH with 1 mg/d doubling at 2-week intervals to 8 mg/d for normotensive and to as high as 16 mg/d for hypertensive patients, if warranted. Efficacy and safety data were evaluated and compared statistically with baseline values.

Results.—Mean daily doses were 4 mg for normotensive and 6.4 mg for hypertensive patients. Maximum and average urinary flow rates and symptoms improved significantly in the intent-to-treat group. Blood pressure and heart rate decreased significantly in both groups with blood pressure readings decreasing more in the hypertensive group. The incidence of adverse reactions for the long-term study were similar to those for the shorter-term studies and included dizziness, fatigue, hypotension, edema, and dyspnea. Most adverse reactions were mild or moderate, and only 75 patients were withdrawn because of adverse events.

Conclusion.—Doxazosin as treatment for BPH was safe, effective, and well tolerated in normotensive and hypertensive men for up to 48 months. The drug also significantly lowered heart rate and blood pressure in hypertensive patients.

▶ It is hoped that this is the first of many reports we will be seeing soon regarding the medium- and long-term safety and efficacy of medical therapies for BPH. In this study of approximately 450 patients, 131 were followed for more than two years. The data among these patients suggests that the effectiveness of Cardura is maintained; however, there does appear to be a fairly steady number of patients withdrawing from therapy because of either an adverse experience or the perception of lack of efficacy. Obviously this cohort of patients needs to be followed for a longer period of time. Even at that, one must always consider that patients who participate in experimental randomized trials may be especially motivated to continue therapy longer than an ordinary patient would. Therefore, the results of long-term use of medical therapy such as Cardura must always be viewed as a "ceiling" if the data are derived from patients enrolled in an investigational study.

G.L. Andriole, Jr., M.D.

A Multicentric, Placebo-controlled, Double-blind Clinical Trial of β-Sitosterol (Phytosterol) for the Treatment of Benign Prostatic Hyperplasia

Klippel KF, for the German BPH-Phyto Study Group (Dresden Univ, Germany)
Br J Urol 80:427–432, 1997   14–5

Objective.—Treatments for bladder outlet obstruction (BOO) caused by benign prostatic hyperplasia (BPH) should be minimally invasive, economical, low risk, and at least as safe and effective as transurethral resection. Mixtures of plant product constituents, some active and some not, have long been used in European countries to treat BPH, but few have been tested in controlled clinical trials. The results of such a trial of phytosterol, a defined extract of *Pinus, Picea,* or *Hypoxis,* with β-sitosterol as the main constituent, in patients with symptoms of BOO caused by BPH, were assessed.

Methods.—Between October 1993 and September 1994, 177 patients aged 50–80 years, from 13 private urologic centers with BOO caused by BPH were randomly allocated to receive placebo (n = 89) or 130 mg of β-sitosterol (n = 88) daily for 6 months after a 4-week washout period. Symptom score and quality of life were evaluated using the International Prostate Symptom Score (IPSS). To be included, patients had to have an IPSS of 6 or greater and a residual urinary volume of 30–150 mL. The end point was the relative difference in IPSS scores after treatment. Secondary outcomes variables measured included quality-of-life index, postvoid residual urinary volume, and peak urinary flow rate.

Results.—There were 11 withdrawals in each group. The IPSS and secondary variables improved significantly in the sitosterol group, and IPSS improved significantly in the placebo group (Table 3). Improvement was greatest during the first month in both groups, but the advantage with sitosterol increased from 2.6 at 1 month to 4.5 at 3 months and to 5.4 at 6 months.

Conclusion.—Beta-sitosterol is a safe and effective treatment for symptoms of BOO caused by BPH.

TABLE 3.—Primary and Secondary Outcomes After 6 Months of Therapy With β-Sitosterol or Placebo

	Initial	*6 months*	*Difference*
β-sitosterol			
IPSS (points)	16.0 (4.58)	7.8 (4.93)	−8.2 (5.74)
Quality of life			
(points)	3.3 (0.79)	1.4 (0.65)	−1.8 (1.02)
Q_{max} (mL/s)	10.6 (3.33)	19.4 (8.62)	8.9 (8.86)
PVR (mL)	63.4 (29.0)	25.6 (28.8)	−37.5 (37.2)
Placebo			
IPSS (points)	14.9 (5.17)	12.1 (5.56)	−2.8 (4.18)
Quality of life			
(points)	3.1 (0.91)	2.2 (0.98)	−0.9 (0.91)
Q_{max} (mL/s)	11.3 (2.7)	15.7 (6.12)	4.4 (5.87)
PVR (mL)	63.1 (26.36)	59.1 (44.12)	−4.1 (33.57)

Note: Values are mean (SD).

Abbreviations: IPSS, International Prostate Symptom Score; *PVR*, postvoid residual urinary volume; Q_{max}, peak urinary flow rate.

(Courtesy of Klippel KF, for the German BPH-Phyto Study Group: A multicentric, placebo-controlled, double-blind clinical trial of β-sitosterol (phytosterol) for the treatment of benign prostatic hyperplasia. *Br J Urol* 80:427–432, 1997.)

▶ This relatively small, prospective, randomized trial demonstrates superiority of β-sitosterol (a chemically defined extract of phytosterol) over placebo for men with mild to moderate symptoms of BPH. As shown in the accompanying table, the authors observed significant improvements in IPSS, peak urinary flow rates, and postvoid residual urinary volume among the sitosterol recipients in comparison to the placebo recipients. The mechanism of action of this compound is not known, but the authors suggest that its effect on patients with BPH is comparable to that achieved by orthodox medical therapies (5-alpha reductase inhibitors or alpha 1 blockers).

These positive early results are really based upon a rather small subset of patients observed for only 6 months. The true test of an effective therapy for BPH is its ability over the long term to reverse symptoms or eradicate progression of the disease such that specific outcomes (such as surgery or urinary rentention) are averted. Unhappily, there is a dearth of data regarding these solid end points for most medical therapies of BPH, although data from long-term studies suggest that finasteride substantially reduces the probability of surgery or urinary retention if used over a 4-year period of time.[1, 2]

G.L. Andriole, Jr., M.D.

References

1. Andersen JT, Nickel JC, Marshall VR, et al: Finasteride significantly reduces acute urinary retention and need for surgery in patients with symptomatic benign prostatic hyperplasia. *Urology* 49:839–845, 1997.
2. McConnell JD, Bruskewitz R, Walsh PC, et al: The effect of finasteride on the risk of acute urinary retention and the need for surgical treatment among men with benign prostatic hyperplasia. *N Engl J Med* 338:557–563, 1998.

The Safety of Transurethral Prostatectomy: A Cohort Study of Mortality in 9,416 Men

Cattolica EV, Sidney S, Sadler MC (Kaiser Permanente Med Ctr, Oakland, Calif; Kaiser Permanente Med Care Program, Oakland, Calif)
J Urol 158:102–104, 1997   14–6

Purpose.—Transurethral prostatectomy for benign prostatic hypertrophy is a very common surgical procedure. Previous studies have suggested that mortality risk may be higher with transurethral prostate resection vs. open prostatectomy. However, 1 small study found no difference in mortality rate between patients undergoing transurethral prostatectomy and the background population. A larger analysis was performed to compare the mortality rate of transurethral prostate resection with that of the background population.

Methods.—Using HMO data, 2 groups of patients were retrospectively analyzed: 4,708 men undergoing transurethral prostate resection for benign prostatic hypertrophy and a random sample of 4,708 age-matched men undergoing no surgical procedure. Proportional hazards models were used to compare mortality risks for the 2 groups.

Findings.—The mortality risk for patients undergoing surgery vs. no surgery was 0.88, with a 95% confidence interval of 0.82 to 0.95. In each 5-year age group studied—ranging from 55 to over 80 years—the relative risk of mortality ranged from 0.77 to 0.95. Transurethral resection was associated with a slight survival benefit.

Conclusion.—Compared with the background population, men undergoing transurethral prostate resection have no increase in mortality. In fact, this procedure is associated with a slight but significant survival advantage. The data help to establish the safety of transurethral prostate resection and may be taken into account when discussing treatment options with patients.

▶ This study retrospectively compares a cohort of 4,708 men undergoing transurethral resection of the prostate between 1976 and 1984 with an equivalent number of age-matched, randomly selected members of the Kaiser Permanente medical care program who had not undergone surgery for benign prostatic hyperplasia. This large study confirms the fact that transurethral resection does not impart any excess mortality. In fact, men undergoing transurethral resection of the prostate had a relative risk for mortality of only 0.88 compared with men not undergoing this procedure.

This is an important study because the safety of transurethral resection of the prostate has been questioned by earlier investigators who suggested that there was an excess mortality rate for patients undergoing transurethral resection compared with either watchful waiting or open prostatectomy. It is noteworthy that the majority of studies showing an adverse mortality effect in transurethral resection of the prostate were relatively small and more likely to be subject to selection bias than is the present study. This large and well-done study should allay any anxiety that transurethral resection of the prostate is associated with excess mortality.

G.L. Andriole, Jr., M.D.

Does Evaluation With the International Prostate Symptom Score Predict the Outcome of Transurethral Resection of the Prostate?
Hakenberg OW, Pinnock CB, Marshall VR (Repatriation Gen Hosp, Daw Park, Australia)
J Urol 158:94–99, 1997   14–7

Background.—The International Prostate Symptom Score (I-PSS) is commonly used to evaluate the symptoms associated with benign prostatic enlargement. The reliability of the I-PSS in predicting the outcome of transurethral prostectomy was examined.

Methods.—The study group consisted of 105 unselected patients undergoing transurethral prostatectomy who had preoperative I-PSS evaluation. These patients received a follow-up at 3 months with a repeat I-PSS and a flow rate measurement. Pre- and postoperative flow rates were available for 73 and preoperative urinary residual volume was available in 81 of the patients in the study group.

Results.—After surgery, there was significant symptomatic improvement in the group of patients. After 3 months, frequency, urgency, and nocturia had the highest symptom scores. There was a significant correlation between I-PSS and quality of life before and after transurethral prostatectomy. There was a significant correlation between postoperative improvement in flow rate and I-PSS change. Patients with a higher preoperative I-PSS had the most symptomatic benefit from surgery. Among patients with a preoperative I-PSS of more than 17, the positive predictive value of the I-PSS was 87% and the negative predictive value was 71%.

Conclusions.—Preoperative assessment with the I-PSS is valuable in monitoring the symptoms of benign prostatic enlargement. Most patients with a preoperative I-PSS of less than 9 do not benefit from transurethral prostatectomy.

▶ Assessment of quality of life is increasingly important in health care today. Development of standardized tools that allow for evaluation of health status in urology is imperative. The International Prostate Symptom Score is an important effort in this regard. This paper is important because it allows for additional data about the utility of the I-PSS in various clinical settings.

This paper by Hakenberg et al. provides additional information on the validity of the I-PSS, with the results indicating that preoperative I-PSS scores are predictive of postoperative outcomes for men undergoing transurethral resection of the prostate. However, as noted by the authors, the predictive value of the I-PSS is sensitive to the definition of improvement that is used. Additional studies using the I-PSS continue to be reported, with the resultant accumulation of a large data base on I-PSS scores. Similar efforts to evaluate health status and quality of life in other related urologic areas, such as chronic prostatis and prostate cancer, will be extremely important.

C.L. Bennett, M.D., Ph.D.

Adherence to Agency for Health Care Policy and Research Guidelines for Benign Prostatic Hyperplasia
Hood HM, Burgess PA, Holtgrewe HL, et al (Alabama Quality Assurance Found, Birmingham; Health Care Financing Administration, Baltimore, Md; Univ of Kansas Med Ctr, Kansas City)
J Urol 158:1417–1421, 1997
14–8

Introduction.—Transurethral resection of the prostate is a commonly performed surgical procedure. The frequency of transurethral resection of the prostate has declined as an initial method of treating benign prostatic hyperplasia with the use of α-blockers and finasteride. For treatment of symptoms, it has been reported that finasteride is no better than a placebo. There was a 32% drop in frequency of the procedure between 1992 and 1994. To improve case selection, accuracy of diagnosis, and appropriate use of procedure, guideline recommendations from the Agency for Health Care Policy and Research were followed. Adherence to recommendations of the agency were profiled for transurethral resection of the prostate in the treatment of benign prostatic hyperplasia.

Methods.—The American Urological Association and the Health Care Financing Administrations approved measures of care and recommendations developed by Agency for Health Care Policy and Research guidelines. There were 1,828 patients with hyperplasia of the prostate. The reliability and validity were assessed for documentation of indications for a transurethral resection of the prostate, documentation of appropriate preoperative assessment, documentation of indications for an inpatient excretory urogram or sonogram when the procedures were performed, and documentation of surgical time and grams of tissue removed. The results were also determined for these measures of care, and adherence rates were measured as well.

Results.—At least 1 symptom or score, or an anatomical abnormality was documented before surgery in 93% of patients. In 7.5% of patients, an American Urological Association score was documented in the medical record. Urinalysis, a digital rectal exam, and determination of preoperative creatine were the recommendations for preoperative evaluation. In 26% of patients, all of these were documented. In the inpatient setting, 12% had an excretory urogram performed. When sonograms were performed, 36% of indications were documented. When inpatient excretory urograms were performed, 74% had documented indications. In 91% of the prostate patients who had laser transurethral resections of the prostate, surgical time and tissue amounts were documented and recorded.

Conclusion.—In the medical record, there is infrequent documentation of adherence to selected Agency for Health Care Policy and Research guideline recommendations.

▶ Guidelines are being made with increasing frequency by research organizations, specialty societies, and medical providers. The Agency for Health Care Policy and Research (AHCPR) was the original funding source for large-scale guideline projects, but it has since discontinued the effort because of disapproval of some of its guideline efforts by subspecialists. This study by Hood et al. attempts to evaluate adherence rates to 4 quality measures identified in the AHCPR guidelines for benign prostatic hyperplasia evaluation (indications for transurethral prostatectomy, appropriate preoperative assessment, digital rectal examination, and preoperative creatinine). A 4-state sample of inpatient medical records for 1,828 transurethral prostatectomy cases found low rates of documentation for the 4 items, ranging from 7.5% to 26%. However, rather than concluding that urologists do not follow the AHCPR guidelines, one is left questioning the role of reviewing documentation of inpatient medical records for the purpose of the study. It is likely that many of the elements that were evaluated would be preferentially recorded in the outpatient records (such as the type and intensity of symptoms). This study suggests another reason for the unpopularity of the AHCPR national guidelines—the inability to obtain meaningful data for evaluation. However, in prior studies, adherence to guidelines that are passively disseminated has been poor. Successful efforts generally include feedback to individual physicians and other continuous quality-improvement techniques.

C.L. Bennett, M.D., Ph.D.

The Early Postoperative Morbidity of Transurethral Resection of the Prostate and of 4 Minimally Invasive Treatment Alternatives

Schatzl G, Madersbacher S, Lang T, et al (Univ of Vienna)
J Urol 158:105–111, 1997

14–9

Background.—Less invasive alternatives to transurethral resection of the prostate are becoming more popular. This study compared the morbidity of the early postoperative period after transurethral resection of the prostate to the early postoperative period after visual laser ablation, high intensity focused ultrasound, transurethral electrosurgical vaporization, and transurethral needle ablation.

Methods.—Between September 1994 and April 1996, 95 patients with symptomatic benign prostatic hyperplasia participated in this prospective, nonrandomized study. Preoperative evaluation included the International Prostate Symptom Score (I-PSS) quality-of-life question, uroflowmetry, post-void residue, transrectal ultrasonography of the prostate, serum prostate specific antigen level determination, and a multichannel pressure-flow study. On the day of catheter removal, patients were asked to answer 7 questions daily for 6 weeks concerning micturation status. After 6 weeks, patients returned the questionnaire and underwent I-PSS, uroflowmetry, and post-void residue analysis.

Results.—Preoperatively, there was no significant difference in I-PSS, peak flow rate, prostate volume, and bladder obstruction among these 5 groups. After 6 weeks, peak flow rate was most improved in patients who had transurethral electrosurgical vaporization, transurethral resection, and visual laser ablation. I-PSS decreased most after transurethral resection and transurethral electrosurgical vaporization. There was no difference in the rate of adverse events among these 5 groups. The mean duration of catheter drainage was shortest after transurethral needle ablation and longest after visual laser ablation. Daytime frequency, degree of hematuria, and incontinence were similar for all 5 groups. Postoperative dysuria was highest after visual laser ablation and transurethral electrosurgical vaporization. There was no improvement in nocturia after visual laser ablation. The biggest improvement in uroflowmetry occurred after transurethral resection and transurethral electrosurgical vaporization. Patients were more worried after visual laser ablation and transurethral needle ablation.

Conclusions.—This study compared the early morbidity following transurethral prostate resection and transurethral needle ablation, high intensity focused ultrasound, visual laser ablation, and transurethral electrosurgical vaporization. The morbidity of these 5 treatment types was equivalent over the first 6 postoperative weeks. Visual laser ablation appeared to be associated with more morbidity reported by questionnaire than the other 4 procedures.

▶ Assessment of quality of life is increasingly important in health care today. Development of standardized tools that allow for evaluation of health status in urology is imperative. The International Prostate Symptom Score is an important effort in this regard. This paper is important because it allows for additional data about the utility of the I-PSS in various clinical settings.

First, minimally invasive surgery has resulted in dramatic improvements in patient quality of life for persons undergoing cholecystectomy and, more recently, colectomies and other major surgical procedures. Similar advances in the field of minimally invasive surgical procedures in urology have recently begun to be reported. Incorporation of the I-PSS into clinical trials and clinical practice is an efficient and important option, allowing for comparisons with diverse groups of urology patients. The finding by Schatzl et al. that patients who are treated with 4 minimally invasive treatment options have similar overall morbidity as measured by the I-PSS is potentially very important and deserves to be looked at in larger studies and among more practice settings.

C.L. Bennett, M.D., Ph.D.

Transurethral Resection of the Prostate Versus Transurethral Electro-vaporization of the Prostate: A Blinded, Prospective Comparative Study With 1-Year Followup
Kaplan SA, Laor E, Fatal M, et al (Columbia Univ, New York)
J Urol 159:454–458, 1998   14–10

Objective.—For men with symptomatic benign prostatic hyperplasia, transurethral electrovaporization of the prostate may be used as an alternative to prostatectomy. The authors and others have reported good results with this approach, but there have been no long-term studies comparing it with standard transurethral resection. This study prospectively compared transurethral resection of the prostate with electrovaporization.

Methods.—The study included 64 consecutive men with moderate to severe lower urinary tract symptoms. Patients were randomized in equal numbers to undergo transurethral electrovaporization of the prostate or transurethral resection of the prostate. Mean age in these groups was 69 and 73 years, respectively. The 2 groups were compared on a broad range of efficacy, safety, and other variables, including American Urological Association symptom score; peak urinary flow rate; adverse events, including changes in serum hematocrit and sodium; operative time; postoperative catheterization time; hospitalization time; and lost work days. The results were analyzed in blinded fashion.

Results.—One-year follow-up data were available for 61 patients, none of whom required retreatment. Symptom scores decreased by 12.8 points in the electrovaporization group and 12.2 points in the resection group. Peak urinary flow increased by 9.7 and 11.3 mL/sec, respectively. Electrovaporization took a mean of 48 min to perform, compared with 35 min for resection. However, resection was associated with longer catheterization time (67 vs. 13 hr), hospitalization time (3 vs. 1 days), and lost work days (18 vs. 7 days). None of the patients in the electrovaporization group experienced major complications. One patient in the resection group required transfusion, while another had clinical transurethral resection syndrome. Potency was normal in all patients in the resection group and 95% of those in the electrovaporization group. Retrograde ejaculation was normal in 76% and 85%, respectively.

Conclusions.—For men with lower urinary tract symptoms, transurethral resection and transurethral electrovaporization are both efficacious techniques. Both are associated with significant improvements in peak urinary flow, though resection offers greater improvement in this regard. There is no difference in preservation of sexual function. Electrovaporization has a longer operative time, but significantly reduces postoperative morbidity, catheterization time, hospitalization time, and days off work. Longer follow-up is needed to determine the durability of results with electrovaporization.

▶ This article attempts to compare 1-year outcome data on men undergoing either transurethral resection (TURP) or transurethral electrovaporization of the prostate. The men undergoing TURP had more profound improvements in peak urinary flow rate than men who underwent electrovaporization, and surgical time was significantly reduced among those men undergoing TURP. These advantages of TURP were offset by a 1 day longer mean hospital stay for the TURP patients and a slightly longer number of days lost from work. Interestingly, the rates of impotence or retrograde ejaculation were very comparable between both groups, and the overall percentage of men who rated their results as satisfactory or better was 83% and 84%, respectively. I like the way the authors summarized their data, stating that "transurethral electrovaporization is a modification of what is still the best method of treating lower urinary tract symptoms." Moreover, they acknowledge that much longer follow-up from multiple institutions will be necessary.

G.L. Andriole, Jr., M.D.

Transurethral Evaporation of the Prostate for Treatment of Benign Prostatic Hyperplasia: Results in 168 Patients With Up to 12 Months of Followup
Narayan P, Tewari A, Schalow E, et al (Univ of Florida, Gainesville; Dept of Veterans Affairs Med Ctr, Gainesville, Fla; Univ of New Mexico, Albuquerque)
J Urol 157:1309–1312, 1997   14–11

Introduction.—Because of the cost and morbidity associated with transurethral resection of the prostate, treatment of benign prostatic hyperplasia is undergoing intense scrutiny. In more than 2,000 patients with benign prostatic hyperplasia, transurethral laser prostatectomy has been used with good results and an excellent safety profile. Refinement of laser techniques has continued. Simultaneous evaporation and coagulation of the prostate can be achieved with the use of high-power density from a side-firing laser fiber. Results for patients having transurethral evaporation of the prostate were reviewed.

Methods.—Transurethral evaporation of the prostate was performed on 168 patients with symptomatic benign prostatic hyperplasia. A 600 μm internal reflector fiber covered by a quartz glass cap that reflects the Nd:YAG beam at 80 degrees to the fiber axis was used. At the 8, 4, 11 and 1 o'clock positions, the limits of laser ablation at the bladder neck and verumontanum were marked. By lasing at a 45-degree angle to the lobe from the right to the left side and vice versa, the median lobe enlargement was treated. By lasing at the 6 o'clock position deep enough to visualize the bladder neck, ablation was completed. When all median lobe tissue was evaporated, lasing was stopped. Measurements of the peak flow rate, American Urological Association symptom index, and postvoid residual were taken at baseline and at 3-, 6-, and 12-month follow-up.

Results.—There was a statistically significant decrease in mean American Urological Association symptom index at 12 months from 20.6 at baseline to 7.2, representing a 65% reduction. Mean peak flow rate significantly improved from 8.2 cc/sec to 18.2 cc/sec in 12 months. Irritative voiding symptoms were reported in 22.6% of patients; they were cited as the most frequent complication, followed by urinary tract infections, reported by 4.8% of patients. No additional major complications were seen.

Conclusion.—For treatment of benign prostatic hyperplasia, transurethral evaporation of the prostate appears to be safe and effective, according to the 12-month follow-up results.

▶ This manuscript describes a well characterized group of men with benign prostate hyperplasia and/or urinary retention who underwent transurethral evaporation of the prostate using a 600 μm internal reflector fiber and an Nd:YAG laser. The laser energy was transmitted via high-power density with a spot size of 700 μm in a divergence of approximately 15 degrees. This technique of evaporation involves lasing the bladder neck, beginning at the 5 and 7 o'clock positions until the circular fibers of the bladder neck are visible and then continuing to vaporize the middle lobe of the prostate until a flat surface is visualized between the vera montanum and the bladder neck. The lateral lobes were vaporized in the standard manner.

There are a few drawbacks to this technique of transurethral evaporation of the prostate. These include prolonged resection time, especially for larger glands (the authors have estimated it to be 25% to 50% longer than that required for transurethral resection of a comparable-sized prostate). The second consideration is the cost of the procedure because often 2 or, in some cases, 3 fibers are needed for a procedure. Finally, postoperative irritative symptoms occurred in about one quarter of the patients and have been crippling. Until comparative studies regarding this modality and other forms of electrovaporization, including the transurethral needle ablation (TUNA) procedure, are available, it is hard to recommend a specific modality for a given patient with symptomatic benign prostatic hyperplasia.

G.L. Andriole, Jr., M.D.

Transurethral Microwave Thermotherapy for Benign Prostatic Hyperplasia: Clinical Outcome After 4 Years
Hallin A, Berlin T (Huddinge Univ, Sweden)
J Urol 159:459–464, 1998   14–12

Objective.—Transurethral microwave thermotherapy is a new treatment for symptomatic benign prostatic hyperplasia (BPH). Although outcomes have been favorable, the effect of this procedure on prostatic tissue is not fully understood. Pretreatment variables that predict a favorable outcome were discussed.

Methods.—Prostatron and Prostasoft 2.0 software were used in 1992 to administer transurethral microwave thermotherapy to 187 men (average age, 68 years) with BPH. Urodynamic measurements and Madsen score were determined at baseline and annually for 4 years. An actuarial survival plot was constructed. A questionnaire assessing health status and satisfaction with the procedure was mailed to the 98 patients remaining in the study after 2 years. At 4 years, 56 patients remained in the study. Two hours after the procedure, 34% were unable to void and an additional 6% had urinary retention after being released. All were treated with indwelling catheters. The 2 patients who continued to be unable to void underwent transurethral prostatic resection.

Results.—At 1 year, 62% of patients were satisfied, but at 4 years, only 23% were satisfied. Madsen scores increased and urine flow decreased with time. The median time to a supplemental BPH treatment, according to Kaplan-Meier calculations, was 45 months. Preoperative factors predictive of favorable outcome were urine flow greater than 10 mL/sec and an irritative score of less than 5.

Conclusion.—Patients with milder symptoms of BPH are most likely to benefit from transurethral microwave thermotherapy. Satisfaction rates after 4 years were 23%, and two thirds of patients needed supplemental BPH treatment.

▶ This relatively large and long-term study should place in perspective transurethral microwave thermotherapy as performed with the Prostatron and Prostasoft 2.0 equipment. Overall, about two thirds of the patients received additional treatments for BPH, and only 23% of the initial treatment group were satisfied with their voiding pattern 4 years later. Subgroup analysis suggested that the patients most apt to be satisfied with this treatment were those who had relatively higher preoperative urinary flow rates and relatively lower irritative symptoms. Therefore, the men who respond best to this treatment are those who are objectively less in need of treatment at all. It is important to consider that other microwave therapies may be associated with better responses, especially as higher energy sources are applied to the prostate.

G.L. Andriole, Jr., M.D.

Holmium:YAG Laser Resection of the Prostate: Preliminary Experience With the First 400 Cases
Cresswell MD, Cass CB, Fraundorfor MR, et al (Tauranga Hosp, New Zealand)
N Z Med J 110:76–78, 1997   14–13

Background.—Although several minimally invasive techniques for the treatment of benign prostatic hyperplasia have been introduced, none has proven as effective as electrosurgical transurethral resection of the prostate (TURP). Coagulation prostatectomy with the neodymium:YAG laser quickly gained popularity but required the patients to use an indwelling catheter for several weeks and often caused severe irritative symptoms. A new laser technique exploiting the vaporizing and cutting properties of the holmium:YAG (Ho:YAG) laser has been developed. Initial experience with this technique was reported.

Methods.—The study included 411 patients (mean age, 66 years) undergoing laser prostatectomy with the Ho:YAG laser. In the latter part of the experience, an 80-watt Ho:YAG-only laser machine was used. In the surgical technique, an end-firing 550µ fiber was used to excise prostatic tissue by following the prostatic capsule, as in TURP. The resulting pieces of prostate were removed from the bladder at the end of the procedure. The bladder was drained with a 20F catheter, which was removed the next morning. Almost all patients were voiding within a few hours. For this study, the patients' preoperative and postoperative symptom scores and flow rates were evaluated.

Results.—Before laser prostatectomy, the patients had a mean prostate US volume of 56 mL. The procedure took a mean of 44 minutes. The mean American Urological Association symptom score improved significantly, from 24 to 5. At 6 months' follow-up, mean peak urinary flow rate had improved from 8 to 23 mL/sec. Ninety-four percent of patients were discharged the day after surgery. Symptoms of dysuria and urgency, less severe than with Nd:YAG prostatectomy, were present during the first week. Complications were reduced compared with electrosurgical TURP.

Conclusion.—Initial results suggest that Ho:YAG laser prostatectomy is an effective treatment for benign prostatic hyperplasia. Like other laser procedures, it offers low morbidity; like TURP, it provides prompt symptomatic relief. The authors are in the process of performing a prospective, randomized trial of Ho:YAG laser prostatectomy.

▶ This manuscript describes yet another alternative to standard TURP for patients with moderate-to-severe benign prostatic hyperplasia. This technique appears to have several advantages over other TURP alternatives in that it does remove prostatic tissue and patients nearly always leave the hospital within 24 hours and voiding. The authors are to be congratulated for the wisdom of planning a prospective, randomized, urodynamically based trial comparing TURP and Ho:YAG laser resection of the prostate.

G.L. Andriole, Jr., M.D.

15 Tumor Markers

Prospective Longitudinal Evaluation of Men With Initial Prostate Specific Antigen Levels of 4.0 NG./ML. or Less
Harris CH, Dalkin BL, Martin E, et al (Univ of Arizona, Tucson; Tucson Veterans Affairs Med Ctr, Arizona)
J Urol 157:1740–1743, 1997
15–1

Introduction.—There is ongoing controversy over the use of screening programs for early detection of prostate cancer. A single prostate-specific antigen (PSA) measurement is sensitive and specific for the detection of prostate cancer; however, positive and negative predictive values are low. With repeated measurements, it might be possible to identify patients with elevated serum PSA levels who are at greater or lesser risk of cancer. There are few data on how serum PSA levels change over time in men without prostate cancer. This issue was addressed by making repeated serum PSA measurements over time in men with an initial PSA of 4 ng/mL or less and no evidence of prostate cancer.

Methods.—The study included 760 healthy men, aged 50 to 80 years, who were participating in a prostate cancer detection study. All patients had an initial serum PSA value of 4 ng/mL or less with normal or suspicious results on digital rectal examination. All underwent prostate biopsy, with normal results. The men were entered into a prospective, serial PSA monitoring study, with serum PSA measurements made every 4 months for 3 years. For men whose serum PSA values became abnormal (i.e., higher than 4 ng/mL), the data were analyzed to see whether serial monitoring or PSA velocity could identify an at-risk group requiring prostate biopsy.

Findings.—The initial PSA value was 2 ng/mL or less in 559 subjects. Just 3 of these men had a persistently abnormal PSA for the subsequent 3 years, and 1 was found to have prostate cancer. The PSA value increased at a velocity of 0.8 ng/mL/year or greater during the first year in 48 subjects. This rate of increase was sustained for 3 years in only 1 of the subjects. The PSA value was 2.1 to 4.0 ng/mL in 201 subjects. The PSA became abnormal in 85 men in this group, but only 37 met the criteria for biopsy. Twenty-three biopsies were performed; the positive rate was only 35%. In the group of 201 men with higher PSA values, 24 had a PSA velocity of 0.8 ng/mL/year or greater at 1 year. This rate was sustained over 3 years in just 4 of the subjects. These 4 patients all met high-risk PSA criteria, and all proved to have prostate cancer.

Conclusion.—When the serum PSA value is 2 ng/mL or less, there is a low risk that the PSA will become abnormal or that cancer will develop within 3 years. Such patients may not require annual PSA monitoring. For subjects whose PSA is between 2.1 and 4.0 ng/mL, annual PSA monitoring is clinically indicated. For men whose PSA rises above 4 ng/mL, serial monitoring plus interval testing can identify a high-risk subgroup in need of biopsy. For men with initially normal PSA levels, analysis of PSA velocity does not aid in cancer detection.

▶ This study provides some interesting new information regarding the use of PSA tests to screen men for prostate cancer. Men with a PSA of 2 ng/mL or less and a nonspecific digital rectal examination are at low risk for development of an abnormal PSA or cancer (0.5% or less) within the subsequent 3 years of follow-up. Therefore, it seems reasonable to consider that men in this category may be monitored with serum PSA measurements every 2 years rather than annually as may be currently practiced.

In contrast, men with a PSA level between 2.1 and 4.0 ng/mL have an approximate 35% risk of cancer if their PSA rises to more than 4. These patients appear to be best monitored on an annual basis. In this study, for neither group of men (those with an initial PSA of 2 ng/mL or less or those whose PSA was between 2.1 and 4.0 ng/mL) did PSA velocity of more than 0.8 ng/mL/year sustained for more than 1 year add useful information. Consideration of these findings may result in more cost-effective use of total PSA as a screening tool.

G.L. Andriole, Jr., M.D.

Influence of Finasteride on Free and Total Serum Prostate Specific Antigen Levels in Men With Benign Prostatic Hyperplasia

Pannek J, Marks LS, Pearson JD, et al (Johns Hopkins Med Inst, Baltimore, Md; Hybritech Inc, San Diego, Calif; Merck Research Labs, Rahway, NJ; et al)
J Urol 159:449–453, 1998   15–2

Purpose.—Patients with benign prostatic hyperplasia (BPH) taking finasteride show about a 50% reduction in serum prostate-specific antigen (PSA) levels. It has been suggested that the "true" PSA value can be calculated simply by doubling the observed level, thus allowing PSA to be used for prostate cancer screening despite finasteride treatment. However, there are few data on how finasteride affects the molecular forms of PSA, particularly the unbound or free forms. This randomized, placebo-controlled study examined the effects of finasteride on total and free serum PSA levels.

Methods.—The study included 40 men with symptomatic and histologically confirmed BPH. Their mean age was 64.5 years. The patients were randomized to receive 6 months of treatment with finasteride, 5 mg/day, or placebo. The response, in terms of prostate volume, was evaluated by

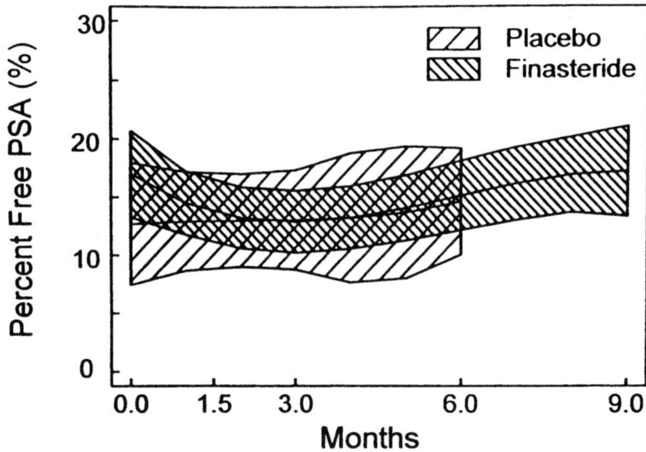

FIGURE 3.—Mixed effects regression plots show estimated mean percent free PSA (solid middle line) and 95% confidence intervals (diagonal hash) for placebo and finasteride treated groups. *Abbreviation: PSA*, prostate-specific antigen. (Courtesy of Pannek J, Marks LS, Pearson JD, et al: Influence of finasteride on free and total serum prostate specific antigen levels in men with benign prostatic hyperplasia. *J Urol* 159:449–453, 1998.)

transrectal ultrasound. The effects of the 2 treatments on serum free and total PSA levels were compared in blinded fashion, using archived serum samples stored at 70°C.

Results.—Mean total PSA level decreased from 3.0 ng/mL to 1.5 ng/mL after 6 months of finasteride treatment. Levels were unchanged in the placebo group. The finasteride group showed a significant reduction in PSA density, but the placebo group did not. Mean percent free PSA was 13%–17% at baseline and was unchanged by either treatment (Fig 3).

Conclusions.—Men taking finasteride for BPH show an average 50% reduction in total PSA serum levels, but no change in percent free PSA. These data may aid in interpreting PSA measurements made for prostate cancer screening in men being treated with finasteride. More information is needed on the use of percent free PSA to detect the development of cancer. Men with BPH show wide variation in PSA levels, and this range may be even greater in men receiving finasteride.

▶ This is 1 of a few articles characterizing the effect of finasteride on free and total serum PSA levels. While it has been well recognized that total serum PSA levels decrease by an average of about 50% during therapy with finasteride, it is a relatively recent observation that the percent of free PSA does not change significantly. Therefore, the same cut-points for percent free PSA that apply to men not receiving finasteride are equally applicable to those who are.

G.L. Andriole, Jr., M.D.

Biologic Variability of Prostate-specific Antigen and Its Usefulness as a Marker for Prostate Cancer: Effects of Finasteride
Oesterling JE, and the Finasteride PSA Study Group (Mayo Clinic, Rochester, Minn; et al)
Urology 50:13–18, 1997   15–3

Purpose.—Treatment with finasteride not only shrinks the prostate gland but also decreases serum prostate-specific antigen (PSA) levels by about half. It is possible for benign prostatic hyperplasia (BPH) and prostate cancer to be present at the same time; thus information on how to read PSA levels in patients treated with finasteride is needed. The effects of finasteride on PSA levels were assessed in men with BPH and men with both BPH and prostate cancer.

Methods.—The study included 149 men participating in a 6-month placebo-controlled trial of finasteride treatment. Seventy-two patients had BPH alone, and 77 had both BPH and prostate cancer. The latter group was studied to assess finasteride's effects on PSA in patients with BPH and latent prostate cancer. In each group, the percent change in PSA values and the number of subjects crossing over from low (1.0 to 3.9 ng/mL) to high (4.0 to 10.0 ng/mL) levels were assessed. For patients receiving finasteride, PSA measurements were doubled for interpretation in keeping with the manufacturer's recommendation.

Results.—For most BPH patients with low baseline PSA levels, PSA remained at less than 4.0 ng/mL, regardless of whether they received placebo or finasteride. Of patients with a high baseline PSA level, 6% of the finasteride group versus 62% of the placebo group crossed into the low range. For most patients with BPH and prostate cancer who received placebo, PSA level stayed in the same range as at baseline. However, nearly one third of finasteride-treated patients who started at low PSA levels crossed into the high range. However, most patients who started at high PSA levels stayed in the high range during finasteride treatment.

Conclusions.—For patients with BPH—with or without coexisting prostate cancer—PSA levels can cross from the low range to the high range with either finasteride or placebo treatment. For patients taking finasteride, the PSA value can be doubled, according to the manufacturer's recommendation. This permits a proper reading of PSA values without masking the presence of prostate cancer. Prospective, long-term studies of this issue are needed.

▶ This nicely done study comparing men with BPH and another group of men with BPH and prostate cancer treated with placebo or finasteride demonstrates that the finasteride decreased PSA levels in both groups by approximately 50%. The PSA levels among finasteride-treated BPH and cancer patients crossed from the low to high PSA ranges appropriately. Therefore, there did not appear to be any significant impact of finasteride in compromising the utility of serum PSA measurements to diagnose or follow prostate cancer. This issue has also been addressed by a much larger study that will soon be reported supporting the conclusion that finasteride does not impair the sensitivity of PSA testing.

G.L. Andriole, Jr., M.D.

Expression of P-Cadherin Identifies Prostate-specific-antigen-negative Cells in Epithelial Tissues of Male Sexual Accessory Organs and in Prostatic Carcinomas: Implications for Prostate Cancer Biology
Soler AP, Harner GD, Knudsen KA, et al (Lankenau Med Research Ctr, Wynnewood, Pa; Bryn Mawr Hosp, Pa)
Am J Pathol 151:471–478, 1997   15–4

Objective.—Cadherins, a family of calcium-dependent cell-cell adhesion glycoproteins, segregate cells to form tissues during embryonic development. P-cadherin is expressed in epithelial tissues in proportion to the proliferative potential of cell populations. E-cadherin expression is reduced in prostatic tumors with tumor progression and correlates with poor prognosis. The expression of E-, N-, and P-cadherin in radical prostatectomy specimens was examined to determine distribution and prognostic significance in prostate cancer.

Methods.—Tissue distribution of cadherins and prostate-specific antigen (PSA) were determined immunohistochemically in radical prostatectomy specimens and in nontumor male accessory organs.

Results.—Epithelia of nontumor prostate glands, ejaculatory ducts, and seminal vesicles expressed E-cadherin predominantly at the plasma membrane. N-cadherin was not detected. P-cadherin expression was selectively found in the epithelial cells of the seminal vesicles and the ejaculatory ducts and distributed throughout the cytoplasm. In prostate tissue, P-cadherin was found only in basal cells of prostatic acini, hyperplastic basal cells, and in luminal secretions of atrophic glands. Prostate-specific antigen was not detected in most of the P-cadherin-positive epithelial tissues. Most tumors expressed E-cadherin, although not uniformly. N- and P-cadherins were not found in the majority of tumors. Tumor cells did not express both P-cadherin and PSA, suggesting that they are involved in different mechanisms of cell regulation. P-cadherin but not E-cadherin or N-cadherin was useful as a marker of prostate cancer. In contrast to normal prostate tissue, malignant tissue lacks basal cells, which apparently have an inhibitory effect on the growth of prostate cancer. Heterogeneous expression of PSA is usually associated with high grade cancers. Prostate-specific antigen level after irradiation yields unreliable results. P-cadherin is possibly expressed only in androgen-insensitive epithelial tissue. E-cadherin levels have been correlated with the presence of various tumors.

Conclusion.—P-cadherin may be a useful marker of prostate cancer progression in patients with low PSA levels.

► This manuscript is representative of the emerging understanding of the cadherins and their role in diagnosing or estimating prognosis of localized prostate cancer. The cadherins are a multigene family of calcium-dependent cell adhesion molecules with several distinctive members that include E-cadherin, N-cadherin, and P-cadherin. E-cadherin is the prime mediator of intercellular adhesion in epithelial cells and earlier clinical studies have generally demonstrated that loss of E-cadherin expression is associated with poor survival and higher Gleason Score.[1-5] These authors look at expression of P-cadherin in epithelial tissues and suggest that its expression identifies cell populations with proliferative potential and its expression decreases as cells differentiate. The majority of studies including this one on the role of cadherins in patients with prostate cancer have been performed on tissue specimens using immunoperoxidase techniques. Whether these molecules are detectable in the serum and whether the biopsy of a given prostate cancer is representative of the entire tumor are yet to be determined. But, for now, it appears that the cadherin molecules are important and may find a role in our armamentarium to diagnose, stage, and estimate the progression of prostate cancer.

G.L. Andriole, Jr., M.D.

References

1. Richmond PJM, Karayiannakis AJ, Nagafuchi A, et al: Aberrant E-cadherin and α-catenin expression in prostate cancer: Correlation with patient survival. *Cancer Res* 57:3189–3193, 1997.
2. Otto T, Rembrink K, Goepel M, et al: E-cadherin: A marker for differentiation and invasiveness in prostatic carcinoma. *Urol Res* 21:359–362, 1993.
3. Umbas R, Schalken JA, Aalders TW, et al: Expression of the cellular adhesion molecule E-cadherin is reduced or absent in high grade prostate cancer. *Cancer Res* 52:5104–5109, 1992.
4. Cheng L, Nagabhushan M, Pretlow TP, et al: Expression of E-cadherin in primary and metastatic prostate cancer. *Am J Pathol* 148:1375–1380, 1996.
5. Umbas R, Isaacs WB, Bringueier PP, et al: Decreased E-cadherin expression is associated with poor prognosis in patients with prostate cancer. *Cancer Res* 54:3929–3933, 1994.

Evaluation of NMP22 in the Detection of Transitional Cell Carcinoma of the Bladder

Stampfer DS, Carpinito GA, Rodriquez-Villanueva J, et al (Boston Univ; Massachusetts Gen Hosp, Boston; MD Anderson Cancer Ctr, Houston)
J Urol 159:394–398, 1998   15–5

Objective.—Nuclear matrix protein (NMP22) is a marker for transitional cell carcinoma. Recently, the NMP22 test kit was approved by the Food and Drug Administration for detection of occult or rapidly recurring disease after resection of bladder cancer. The sensitivity and specificity of the kit as a diagnostic aid was evaluated at 3 investigational sites.

Methods.—Levels of NMP22 in 288 urine samples were compared with cystoscopy and biopsy results in 231 patients (65 women), with an average age of 68 years, with bladder transitional cell carcinoma. Because NMP22 levels are not normally distributed, nonparametric methods were used for statistical analyses.

Results.—Biopsy specimens were positive in 66 and negative in 171 of 288 cystoscopies. Fourteen cases were eliminated because of inconclusive or incomplete data. Median NMP22 values were significantly higher in the positive outcome group (9.8 units/mL) than in the negative outcome group (3.0 units/mL). An NMP22 value greater than 6.4 units/mL was selected as an optimum reference value to separate positive from negative outcomes. Sensitivity and specificity were 68% and 80%, respectively. When combined with cytology, sensitivity increased to 74% for cytology group 1–positive patients (those with malignant cytology results) and 79% for cytology group 2–positive patients (those with suspicious and dysplastic as well as malignant results). The negative predictive value was 91% for those NMP22–negative alone, 92% for those NMP22 and cytology group 1–negative, and 93% for those NMP22 and cytology group 2–negative. These values were not significantly different.

Conclusion.—Values for NMP22, when a reference value of 6.4 units/mL is used, are significantly more sensitive than cytology for detecting transition cell carcinoma of the bladder, and the analysis is less costly.

▶ In this study, the authors have compared the receiver operating characteristic curves of NMP22 and conventional urinary cytology among patients with a history of bladder cancer who are undergoing surveillance. Using an NMP22 cutoff of 6.4 units/mL was associated with a sensitivity of 68% and a specificity of 80%. This compared with a cytology sensitivity of 43% and a specificity of 92%. High risk for progressive disease (those patients with grade III or T1 tumors) was associated with an NMP22 sensitivity of 90%.

This is another in the accumulating experience of using a variety of markers to detect recurrent bladder cancer without cystoscopy or conventional voided urinary cytology. Theoretically, this technique is cheaper than cytology and is more sensitive. How urinary NMP22 testing will compare with "point of care" tests (such as the Bard BTA [bladder tumor antigen] or the AuraTek FDP [fibrin/fibrinogen degradation product]) is yet to be determined. Clearly, however, 1 or more of these tests may emerge as preferable to both conventional cytology and interval cystoscopy.

G.L. Andriole, Jr., M.D.

Rapid Detection of Bladder Cancer: A Comparative Study of Point of Care Tests
Johnston B, Morales A, Emerson L, et al (Queen's Univ, Kingston, Ont, Canada)
J Urol 158:2098–2101, 1997   15–6

Objective.—Two noninvasive diagnostic tests, Bard BTA (bladder tumor antigen) and AuraTek FDP (fibrin/fibrinogen degradation products), for the detection of bladder cancer were compared in a single-center, prospective trial.

Methods.—After a minimum of 4 weeks washout, urine specimens from 60 patients (average age, 71 years; 20 women) with bladder cancer and 70 patients with nonbladder cancer (average age, 62 years; 26 women) were divided into 2 aliquots. One aliquot was tested in the cytopathology laboratory and the other by blinded investigators using the BTA/FDP/hemoglobin dipstick. Test results were assessed by another blinded investigator.

Results.—Sensitivity, specificity, positive predictive value, negative predictive value, and accuracy were, respectively, 81%, 75%, 79%, 78%, and 78% for FDP; 69%, 68%, 70%, 67%, and 67% for the hemoglobin dipstick; 35%, 90%, 80%, 54%, and 60% for cytology; and 28%, 87%, 70%, 52%, and 56% for BTA.

Conclusion.—The FDP test had the highest sensitivity and the best accuracy in detecting bladder cancer and was simple to perform.

▶ This study compares 2 point-of-care tests: the Bard BTA and the AuraTek FDP. The BTA test is an agglutination test that quantitatively detects the presence of basement membrane proteins in the urine. The FDP test is an immunoassay using monoclonal antibodies that measure urinary FDP. Increased FDP levels in the urine are associated with bladder cancer. Patients with a history of bladder cancer were evaluated with both the FDP and BTA tests as well as conventional cytology and with a hemoglobin dipstick. The FDP testing had the highest sensitivity and overall accuracy in comparison with all the other tests. However, FDP testing could be associated with false positive results, particularly if an inflammatory process—such as interstitial cystitis or recent urolithiasis—was present. More studies such as this comparing the emerging diagnostic tests for bladder cancer will be necessary to accurately establish a role for the various new modalities.

G.L. Andriole, Jr., M.D.

The Use of the Bladder-Tumour Associated Analyte Test to Determine the Type of Cystoscopy in the Follow-up of Patients With Bladder Cancer

Hargreave T, and the United Kingdom and Eire Bladder Tumour Antigen Study Group (Western General Hospitals Trust, Edinburgh, Scotland; et al)
Br J Urol 79:362–366, 1997   15–7

Background.—Bladder tumor-associated high-molecular weight complexes in voided urine can be detected by the rapid bladder tumor-associated analyte test (BTA). In some cases, BTA might allow rigid cystoscopy with general anesthesia to be replaced by a more limited procedure with a local anesthetic.

Methods.—In a multicenter, prospective study, 272 patients with previous transitional cell carcinoma of the bladder who were scheduled for rigid cystoscopy with general anesthesia had BTA performed on a freshly voided urine sample. For negative BTA results only, flexible cystoscopy with local anesthesia was substituted.

Results.—Sensitivity of BTA was 58% and specificity was 86%. Urinary infection and other forms of inflammation were more common among the 25 false positive (FP) results than the true negative (TN) results. False negative (FN) results were obtained in 43 cases, 6 of which involved high-grade tumors. The FN results were more common with low-grade than with high-grade tumors ($P < 0.05$). Flexible cystoscopy was performed in 188 patients (145 TN and 43 FN results) and rigid cystoscopy in 126 (59 true positive, 24 FP, and 43 FN), at a total cost of £114,619 (including tests), instead of the 272 general anesthetic procedures originally scheduled at a total cost of £135,184.

Conclusions.—Most FP results were from inflammation. Previous radiotherapy may also yield FP results; this association requires further study. Use of BTA avoided general anesthesia in 145 patients but missed 6 high-grade tumors; in such cases, finding of a tumor by flexible cystoscopy must immediately be followed up by rigid cystoscopy. The test may allow some patients to undergo flexible cystoscopy, avoiding the stresses and costs of more invasive procedures.

▶ This study highlights the limitations of using the BTA test to monitor patients with superficial bladder cancer. This study exhibited a sensitivity of 58% and a specificity of 86%, which is in the range of other reports using this test. What this particular series highlights, however, are the adverse effects bladder inflammation, urinary tract infection, and a history of radiation therapy have on the BTA test results. Each of these entities may cause false positive BTA results.

G.L. Andriole, Jr., M.D.

16 Prostate Cancer Screening

Early Detection of Prostate Cancer: Serendipity Strikes Again
Collins MM, Ransohoff DF, Barry MJ (Massachusetts Gen Hosp, Boston;
Univ of North Carolina, Chapel Hill)
JAMA 278:1516–1519, 1997   16–1

Objective.—Prostate cancers may be detected by accident. Whether serendipity plays a role in cancer screening was examined by reviewing prostate cancer screening articles for serendipitous results.

Definition of Detection by Serendipity.—Serendipitous discovery of prostate cancer during digital rectal examinations (DREs) would occur if a random biopsy in an area other than the suspicious one revealed prostate cancer. Serendipitous discovery of prostate cancer in prostate-specific antigen (PSA) screening would occur if a random biopsy of a nonpalpable tumor too small to cause elevated PSA levels revealed prostate cancer.

Magnitude of Prostate Cancer Detection by Serendipity.—Serendipity accounted for approximately 25% of prostate cancers detected during DREs and for approximately 25% of prostate cancers detected during PSA screening. Serendipity may be responsible for the detection of prostate cancer in 30%–100% of tumors less than 1.0 cm^3.

Conclusion.—Prostate cancers detected by serendipity may contribute to overestimating the value of DRE and PSA screening. Whether serendipitous detection of smaller prostate cancers makes a significant difference in outcome depends on their importance. If they are indolent, they may encourage overly aggressive treatment. If they are fast-growing, not enough are being found.

▶ This highly publicized article, presents very misleading information, I believe. On the basis of a single autopsy study,[1] the authors have predicted that if the prostate gland is smaller than 80 g and a prostate cancer is smaller than 1 cc, the patient will infrequently have elevated serum PSA levels. In the autopsy study, only 7.7% of cancers smaller than 1 cc were associated with elevated PSA levels. By using this figure and the frequency with which men with suspicious DREs are found to have cancer on biopsy only on the contralateral side, the authors estimate that about one half of the cancers discovered by standard PSA and DRE screening are serendipitous.

The main flaw in this article is that the autopsy study correlating tumor size with serum PSA elevation used serum PSA levels obtained from men in the immediate premortem period. It is well known that hospitalized men have lower PSA values than ambulatory men, and often nutritional issues, sepsis, and other chronic medical conditions may result in functional hypogonadism that may in turn cause spuriously low premortem PSA values. It is unfortunate that this issue has been raised in such a public manner on the basis of a misleading analysis.

G.L. Andriole, Jr., M.D.

Reference

1. Brawn PN, Speights VO, Kuhl D, et al: Prostate-specific antigen levels from completely sectioned, clinically benign, whole prostates. *Cancer* 68:1592–1599, 1991.

American Cancer Society Guidelines for the Early Detection of Prostate Cancer
von Eschenbach A, Ho R, Murphy GP; et al (American Cancer Society Prostate Task Force; Univ of Hawaii, Honolulu; Pacific Northwest Cancer Found, Seattle; et al)
Cancer 80:1805–1807, 1997   16–2

Introduction.—There was a dramatic increase in the incidence of prostate cancer between 1988 and 1992, largely because of the introduction and application of the prostate-specific antigen (PSA) screening. While 5-year prostate cancer survival rates have increased, there is no direct evidence that this screening test has decreased prostate cancer mortality rates. But there is indirect evidence that this screening method accounts for diagnoses of earlier-stage disease.

Guideline Review.—In 1992, the American Cancer Society recommended that a digital rectal exam and prostate screening antigen be performed on men 50 and older. This guideline was reviewed in 1997. At that time, the recommendation was made that both the digital rectal exam and prostate screening antigen be performed annually on men 50 and older, men who have at least a 10-year life expectancy, and younger men who are at high risk.

Research Issues.—Questions that remain to be addressed include the influence of known prostate cancer risk factor on the age at which screening should be initiated; the influence of patient characteristics, prior test outcomes on the optimal screening factor, and risk factors; the psychosocial impact of screening; enhancements to this screening method; new tests which may compliment or serve as alternatives to prostate screening antigen; imaging techniques; biopsy technique; follow-up of negative biopsy; need for more trials; impact for early detection; and the definition of high risk groups.

Conclusion.—When new knowledge becomes available, other revisions will be considered. Health professionals seeking to provide optimal care to asymptomatic men at risk for prostate cancer can use this guideline.

▶ Given the controversy over the costs and benefits of screening, early detection, and treatment of early-stage prostate cancer, developing guidelines for early prostate cancer detection is a formidable task. In 1992, the ACS guidelines for prostate cancer strongly urged annual performance of PSA and digital rectal examination for men 50 years of age and older. Subsequently, many articles were written questioning the utility of this approach. Other studies reported the marked increase in early-stage disease, and suggested that the potential existed for an increased number of cured cases. In 1997, the revised guidelines were less emphatic and recommended offering the PSA and digital rectal examination annually, beginning at age 50, to men who have at least a 10-year life expectancy, and to younger men who are at high risk. The offer should include provision of information about the potential risks and benefits of screening. This revision is important, because it suggests that there is some upper age limit where PSA and digital rectal examination should not be performed. In addition, the Public Health Service guidelines are even less supportive, resulting in continued confusion among primary care practitioners about the preferred approach to prostate cancer screening. The randomized screening trials may be the only way to resolve this uncertainty.

C.L. Bennett, M.D., Ph.D.

The Results of Prostate Carcinoma Screening in the U.S. as Reflected in the Surveillance, Epidemiology, and End Results Program
Smart CR (Natl Cancer Inst, Bethesda, Md)
Cancer 80:1835–1844, 1997   16–3

Introduction.—The introduction of prostate-specific antigen resulted in an increase in the detection of prostate cancer from 106% incidence in 1988 to 189.4% in 1994. Previous studies have suggested that detection of advanced disease in prostate carcinoma is decreased with serial screening. The Surveillance, Epidemiology, and End Results program, which monitors cancer incidence, stage of disease at diagnosis, treatment, and end results, is the basis of most national trends for cancer. Results from this data were analyzed regarding prostate carcinoma to determine the effectiveness of screening.

Methods.—There were 208,234 prostate carcinoma patients diagnosed between 1973 and 1993. To permit observation of long-term trends, the general staging system was used. To indicate the significance of the prostate carcinoma, Grade-incorporating Gleason scores were used. To separate prostate carcinoma deaths from those resulting from other causes, age-adjusted survival rates were used.

Results.—No other malignancy has had as great an increase in incidence as has prostate carcinoma, largely in Grade 2 significant tumors. The detection of advanced disease has decreased. A progressive decrease to near baseline levels occurred after the peak incidence in 1992. Prostate carcinoma accounted for about 38% of all deaths. Deaths from other causes increased with age. Results showed that men older than 69 had a greater rate of death from prostate carcinoma than did men ages 50 to 69 when the results were corrected for death from other causes. Within 5 years of diagnosis, about 61% of deaths from prostate carcinoma occurred. Within 10 years of diagnosis, about 88% of deaths occurred There was a 100% 10-year survival rate for patients treated by radical prostatectomy. For patients treated by radiation, the 10-year survival rate was 78%, and for those treated with other modalities, there was a 33% 10-year survival rate.

Conclusion.—The incidence of distant disease, which influences the mortality rate, was decreased with prostate carcinoma screening of men older than 50, according to the indirect evidence.

▶ While most studies attribute the rise in the annual number of prostate cancer cases to widespread use of prostate-specific antigen testing, the Surveillance, Epidemiology, and End Results database provides empirical data of an increase in cases steadily from 1973 to 1992. The initial increase is undoubtedly related to increased use of transurethral resection of the prostate, while more recent changes are the result of prostate-specific antigen screening. The conclusion of this paper is that annual prostate cancer screening is recommended for men over 50 who have at least a 10-year life expectancy. This recommendation from the Chief of the Early Detection Branch of the National Cancer Institute is even stronger than that of the American Cancer Society or the Public Health Service. The prostate cancer screening controversy continues.

C.L. Bennett, M.D., Ph.D.

Prostate Carcinoma Incidence and Patient Mortality: The Effects of Screening and Early Detection
Brawley OW (Natl Cancer Inst, Bethesda, Md)
Cancer 80:1857–1863, 1997   16–4

Introduction.—New screening and diagnostic technologies have led to a dramatic increase in the rate of diagnosis of prostate carcinoma in the United States. There is concern that a significant number of men will be treated unnecessarily and experience morbidity and complications. Data collected from the Surveillance, Epidemiology, and End Results (SEER) Program of the National Cancer Institute were used to describe national and regional trends in prostate carcinoma incidence and the impact that screening has had in the United States.

Methods.—The SEER Program is a population-based cancer database containing information on all cancers diagnosed among nearly all residents of 9 defined areas in the United States. Data from SEER and demographic data of the U.S. Census are used to make projections of cancer incidence and mortality.

Results.—During the period 1973 to 1994, incidence rates of prostate carcinoma increased for both black and white men, and the increase in mortality rates was slower in both races. Both incidence and mortality rates, however, were significantly higher among blacks. There was a decline in distant disease at diagnosis and an increase in local and regional disease. All of these changes are attributed to increased numbers of men undergoing screening and early detection but are also consistent with lead-time bias, length bias, and a decline in mortality. Incidence rates of prostate carcinoma varied considerably among the 9 SEER regions. Mortality rates have declined in recent years, but the decline has been small compared with the rise in incidence rates. In Connecticut, for example, a state with less screening than the other areas, mortality declined from 25.3 to 23 per 100,000 white men.

Discussion.—Although prostate carcinoma can be diagnosed, it is difficult to distinguish those who need treatment from those who do not need treatment. It is estimated that one third of men who are diagnosed fall into the category of those for whom cure is necessary but not possible. Although the benefits of screening and early detection are theoretically possible, treatment prompted by screening results has clearly caused harm.

▶ While all studies agree that screening can diagnose early stage prostate cancers, overall benefits will occur only if this detection does not represent lead time and length time bias, as described in this article by Dr. Brawley. The paper makes a strong argument that the current evidence of a downward trend in prostate cancer mortality and a large increase in incidence rates during the period 1973–1994 does not allow one to differentiate between bias and true benefits of screening. However, the regional variations in the SEER database show little evidence of differences in prostate cancer mortality, accompanied by large differences in screening and treatment practices. The logical conclusion from these observations is that prostate cancer screening might be expected to cost a lot and increase the detection rate of localized cancers yet not lead to any improvements in overall mortality. The conclusion of the paper, that the benefits of screening and early detection are theoretical but not well supported in the SEER registries whereas the costs and risk are known, is important. This study provides insight that the large scale screening studies will not conclude that screening is effective, nor is it likely to be cost-effective.

C.L. Bennett, M.D., Ph.D.

Future Benefits and Cost-Effectiveness of Prostate Carcinoma Screening
Littrup PJ (Wayne State Univ, Detroit)
Cancer 80:1864–1870, 1997   16–5

Introduction.—Since prostate-specific antigen (PSA) developed widespread recognition and use after 1989, a new era of early detection of prostate cancer has begun. Concerns about the effectiveness of disease-specific mortality reduction and the test performance of PSA have led to concerns of cost effectiveness. A bridge must be made between PSA's diagnostic ability and population-based mortality reduction. A review of current data, modeling efforts, and perspectives on societal impact and costs are necessary to determine estimates of cost-effectiveness for prostate carcinoma screening.

Methods.—Incidence trends in prostate carcinoma in relation to age groups and racial differences were examined in 60,289 men diagnosed with prostate carcinoma. A clinical biopsy series of 2,000 men with more than 900 carcinoma patients was used to assess differences in tumor biology between African-American men and white men. Estimates of treatment, screening efficacy, and costs were evaluated with a review of the literature addressing Markoff modeling.

Results.—Men older than age 70 have seen a decline in the incidence of prostate carcinoma since 1992; however, there was a maintenance of 100% greater incidence of localized disease than in 1989 when PSA screening became more common among men aged 45 to 70. For both groups, the rate of distance disease has decreased by 60%. More cores involved with carcinoma and more carcinoma cores involved with a Gleason score of at least 7 in men age 70 or less with a prostate specific antigen level of 10 ng/mL or less is seen in African-American men. Men choosing radical prostatectomy over watchful waiting if younger than 70 years and with no severe comorbidities showed significant increases in quality-adjusted life expectancy. Similar results of cost per carcinoma and costs per quality-adjusted life-year extension were seen in original cost estimates from benefit-cost analysis and later cost-effectiveness models.

Conclusion.—Significant potential mortality reductions are suggested by current diagnostic trends toward the persistent increased detection of localized prostate carcinoma in younger men, combined with a marked reduction in distant stage disease. There may be greater implications for African-American men, but models of mortality reduction need to be based on further research.

▶ The major debates over prostate cancer screening center around 3 questions: (1) is it effective, (2) is it costly, and (3) is it cost-effective? This discussion summarizes nicely the multiple models of effectiveness of early treatment over watchful waiting for localized prostate cancer, ranging from a loss of 0.3 quality-adjusted life years to a gain of 0.9 quality-adjusted life years for men with well-differentiated cancers who are less than 70 years to a gain of

1.0 to 2.4 quality-adjusted life years for men with poorly differentiated tumors in the same age group. These models provide additional insight into the difficulties of accrual to the national Prostate Intervention versus Observation Trial (PIVOT). For those urologists who feel that the 4 Markoff model-derived estimates described in the paper represent what would be realized in practice, accrual to the PIVOT trial would be difficult. Potential improvements in PIVOT accrual might result if additional support is published for estimates that are more equivocal between watchful waiting and early surgical treatments.

C.L. Bennett, M.D., Ph.D.

The European Randomized Study of Screening for Prostate Cancer: An Update
Standaert B, Denis L (Oncology Centre Antwerp, Belgium)
Cancer 80:1830–1834, 1997

16–6

Introduction.—A huge healthcare problem in the United States is prostate cancer among aging men. It is the second most common malignancy after lung carcinoma among European men. Three tests are used mainly to detect early prostate cancer, but it is not known which should be performed first. The collaborative formation of a multinational randomized screening trial is being pursued by European cancer prevention centers. The name of this trial is the European Randomized Study of Screening for Prostate Cancer and began in 1992. An update of the research study was presented.

Methods.—The trial pooled analyses of ongoing and planned screening programs. The objectives were to demonstrate whether the effect of screening causes specific mortality reduction of at least 20%. The trial attempted to identify the best screening method by selecting the most appropriate combination of available screening tests. The purpose was to identify risk groups who will benefit most from the screening process and to evaluate the quality of life of the participants and the cost-effectiveness of the screening of death. The collaborating centers are in Belgium, Finland, Italy, The Netherlands, and Sweden.

Results.—The types of screening methods used are prostate-specific antigen, digital rectal examination, and transrectal ultrasound. The false-positive rate of transrectal ultrasound as a primary test has been found to be too high to be included in routine screening, and an agreement to eliminate this test as a primary test will go into effect in the near future. Two centers suggest a prostate-specific antigen threshold of 3 ng/mL rather than 4 ng/mL. In the patients whose prostate specific antigen ranges between 4 and 9.9 ng/mL, it is still unknown whether adjustment to prostate volume or age should be made to decrease the number of biopsies taken per carcinoma detected.

Conclusion.—Among the data collected in each center, there are some discrepancies which are related to the key variables selected by each center that cause differences in carcinoma detection rates. Variables include screening tests used, age groups selected, and screening criteria selected per test. The first results of the trial are expected to be reported by the year 2007.

▶ The debate over screening for prostate cancer is one that is carried out internationally. In the United States, answers are expected in 15–20 years, when the National Cancer Institute–sponsored PLCO trial will be completed. In Europe, the European Randomized Study of Screening for Prostate Cancer (ERSPC) is addressing the same question. The first study results of this trial are expected in the year 2007, with collaborations from 5 European countries and including results from 180,000 men over a 10-year screening period, with a goal of reducing prostate cancer–specific mortality by 20% or more. In contrast to the U.S. effort, the European studies represent a collaboration of efforts from Belgium, Finland, Italy, The Netherlands, and Sweden, with each country having different eligibility criteria and indications for biopsy. However, the collaboration has resulted in uniform definitions for end points, trial types, recruitment, and methods for assessing mortality. Four of the 5 studies involved randomization after consent was signed, with Sweden opting for a randomization before consent. By 2007, initial results from Europe are expected.

C.L. Bennett, M.D., Ph.D.

Observations on the Early Detection of Prostate Cancer From the American Cancer Society National Prostate Cancer Detection Project
Mettlin CJ, for the Investigators of the American Cancer Society National Prostate Cancer Detection Project (Roswell Park Cancer Inst, Buffalo, NY; Northwest Hosp, Seattle; MD Anderson Cancer Ctr, Houston; et al)
Cancer 80:1814–1817, 1997   16–7

Introduction.—To evaluate the yield of a combined modality intervention applied to well men for the purpose of early detection of prostate cancer, the American Cancer Society National Prostate Cancer Detection Project was begun in 1987 as a multidisciplinary project. During 10 years of this project's intervention and follow-up, findings concerning the efficacy of early detection as a prostate cancer control strategy have been reported.

Methods.—Prostate-specific antigen, transrectal ultrasound, and digital rectal examination were used to test 2,999 well men ages 55–70 annually. On men with suspicious findings, biopsies were performed and a review of pathologic findings was conducted. The detection yield of multimodality testing and the comparative sensitivity and specificity of the different tests were the initial study outcomes. Patient quality of life and survival were the longer term outcomes.

Results.—Across the years of intervention, the cancer detection rate declined significantly. A lower sensitivity was found for digital rectal examination than for transrectal ultrasound or prostate-specific antigen. There was a lower specificity of transrectal ultrasound than for digital rectal examination. At the time of diagnosis, fewer than 9% of the cancers detected were clinically advanced. After an average follow-up of 54 months, 94% of patients who had cancer detected were alive. After surgery, death occurred in 1 patient. Prostate cancer was the cause of 2 deaths, and 11 deaths were not related to prostate cancer or its treatment.

Conclusion.—High levels of early detection with infrequent adverse outcomes are yielded by a combined modality approach to prostate cancer detection. To evaluate long-term morbidity and mortality, continued follow-up is necessary. Although prostate cancer mortality rates in the United States have declined 6.3%, it is still not known whether the increased use of early detection interventions are involved in this trend.

▶ In addition to large-scale randomized trials evaluating the potential benefits of early screening for prostate cancer (such as the United States' PLCO study or the European Randomized Studies for Screening for Prostate Cancer), there is the ACS-NPCDP effort. This study, while not randomized, is an attempt to evaluate the yield and impact of periodic examinations for early detection of prostate cancer. The project was begun in 1987, before widespread use of the PSA test. As with many of the ongoing U.S. efforts, the majority of participants were white (88%). Detection rates using transrectal ultrasound (for years 1–6), digital rectal examination (for years 1–8), and PSA (for years 1–8), decreased steadily over time, from 2.8% in year 1 to 0.6% in year 8 for the men who participated in 5 consecutive years of screening. Of interest is that the screening effort identified a preponderance of localized cancer, and 90% of the tumors had a Gleason score of 7 or less. This study suggests that aggressive and annual screening programs will identify cancer that is primarily localized, but it raises the question again of the benefits of screening. How would these patients with excellent histologies fare under expectant management strategies (of whom only 12% opted for this approach)? The authors raise the question of whether the current downward trend in prostate cancer deaths is indeed because of the increased use of early screening.

C.L. Bennett, M.D., Ph.D.

Prostate Carcinoma Screening in the County of Tyrol, Austria: Experience and Results

Reissigl A, Horninger W, Fink K, et al (Univ of Innsbruck, Austria)
Cancer 80:1818–1829, 1997   16–8

Introduction.—Prostate-specific antigen-based screening is considered to be the most effective screening method for men referred to urologic care settings because of signs and symptoms of the diseases. However, it is not known how useful this test is on asymptomatic men. A mass screening project was performed in Tyrol, Austria. The experience and results of different prostate carcinoma screening projects using total prostate-specific antigen (PSA) as the initial test was summarized as well as different diagnostic tests to improve specificity.

Methods.—Seven projects were studied: results of mass screening with PSA as the initial test, comparison of different PSA cutpoints, PSA study in blood donors, incidence and significance of transitional zone carcinoma, determination of the ratio of free and total PSA in volunteers to define the optimal range of total prostate specific antigen and to determine the appropriate cutpoints for percent free prostate specific antigen within this range, evaluation of the diagnostic benefit of prostate specific antigen transitional zone density, and prostate specific antigen screening and percent of incidental prostate carcinoma.

Results.—Of the 21,078 volunteers, 8% had elevated PSA levels and 48% had biopsies. Of these biopsies, 25% were positive, and 135 men had radical prostatectomy. Of the 135 pathologically staged lesions, 95 (70%) were organ-confined. An 8% increase in the number of biopsies and the detection rate of organ-confined disease resulted with a PSA cutoff of 2.5 ng/mL in men age 45–49 and 3.5 ng/mL in men age 50–59. Twelve percent of men who were asymptomatic blood donors had elevated PSA levels, and of these, 22% had prostate carcinoma detected and radical prostatectomy. In men with negative rectal examination findings and visible prostate zones on 3-dimensional transrectal ultrasound, 28.8% had biopsies positive for carcinoma and 28.5% had carcinoma that originated in the transitional zone only. About 37% of negative biopsies could be eliminated by using a percent free PSA of 18% as a biopsy criterion in men with an elevated PSA serum level. There were 24.4% of negative biopsies that could be avoided without missing the detection of a single carcinoma by using a PSA transitional zone density of more than 0.22 ng/mL/cc as a biopsy criterion. The years after PSA-based screening were established, the incidence of T1a Grade 1 and 2 carcinomas rose from 3.1% to 4.6%, and for T1a Grade 3 and T1b carcinoma, the incidence declined from 2.3% to 1.03%.

Conclusion.—The detection rate of clinically significant and organ-confined tumors is increased with PSA screening. An additional diagnostic benefit is provided with percent free PSA and PSA transitional zone density over total PSA.

▶ Prostate-specific antigen testing in the United States has resulted in a dramatic shift in the distribution of stage at diagnosis for prostate cancer, with less than 20% of patients having metastatic disease at diagnosis. This study illustrates similar results from Tyrol, Austria. The PSA-based screening in Tyrol increased the detection rate of clinically significant and organ-confined tumors with additional benefits from transitional zone density and percent free PSA. However, left unanswered is the major question—does the change in distribution of the stage at diagnosis for prostate cancer translate into better overall survival for prostate cancer patients? This dilemma continues in Europe as well as in the United States.

C.L. Bennett, M.D., Ph.D.

The Early Detection of Prostate Carcinoma With Prostate Specific Antigen: The Washington University Experience
Smith DS, Humphrey PA, Catalona WJ (Washington Univ, St Louis)
Cancer 80:1852–1856, 1997
16–9

Introduction.—The only feasible option for reducing prostate carcinoma morbidity and mortality is earlier screening. The prostate-specific antigen (PSA) and digital rectal examination are the 2 most widely used screening tests. In terms of reduction of prostate carcinoma mortality, the impact of PSA is still unknown, although it is known that the screening method has contributed to an increase in prostate carcinoma incidence rates and a favorable shift in disease stage at the time of diagnosis. A longitudinal screening protocol has been conducted since 1989, and the intermediate results are evaluated.

Methods.—There were 30,000 men older than age 60 who were screened with PSA or PSA in combination with digital rectal examination at 6-month intervals. Those with results suspicious for cancer were recommended to have a biopsy. Screening test results, proportion of men recommended to have biopsy, those who had a biopsy, and carcinoma detection rates were reported. For a subset of men who had radical prostatectomy and for whom complete embedding and microscopic examination of the surgical specimen was performed, the pathologic features of screen-detected carcinoma were reported.

Results.—Prostate specific antigen levels greater than 4.0 ng/mL were seen in about 10% of the volunteers, and digital rectal examination results that were suspicious for cancer were seen in 3% to 10% of volunteers. Biopsy was recommended for 9% to 20% of volunteers, and the procedure was actually given to 8% to 13% of the volunteers. For carcinoma detection, the positive predictive value ranged from 25% to 33% across studies. Clinicopathologic features of significant carcinoma were seen in the majority of the subset of men for whom surgical specimens were completely embedded.

Conclusion.—Screening with PSA, PSA in combination with digital rectal examination, or both has resulted in encouraging intermediate outcomes. Reasonable positive predictive values were demonstrated and carcinomas were detected at an earlier age with these screening tests. The pathologic characteristics of medically significant carcinoma are seen on the majority of screen-detected tumors.

▶ In one of the largest screening programs in the country, the Washington University investigators provide conclusive evidence that a broad-based early detection program with PSA testing with or without digital rectal examination will detect clinically significant but localized prostate cancers. Almost three fourths of patients with detected cases of cancer opted to undergo a radical prostatectomy. As with many studies, this large scale effort is limited by including only those individuals who chose to participate.

Also, almost 90% were white, leaving unanswered the question about the generalizability to the black population.

C.L. Bennett, M.D., Ph.D.

Determinants of Prostate-Specific Antigen Test Use in Prostate Cancer Screening by Primary Care Physicians
Austin OJ, Valente S, Hasse LA, et al (Univ of Cincinnati, Ohio)
Arch Fam Med 6:453–458, 1997   16–10

Introduction.—Prostate cancer is the second leading cause of cancer death in American men. An intervention in prostate cancer screening that has unproved efficacy and that may even be harmful to patients is the prostate-specific antigen (PSA) test, yet many primary care physicians use this test as a screening tool for prostate cancer. By analyzing primary care physician's self-reported reasons for performing this screening test, a better understanding of the rationale for this trend was obtained.

Methods.—There were 408 primary care physicians who responded to a survey that included questions on beliefs, attitudes, knowledge, and reasons for PSA prostate cancer screening. The following questions were included: Are you currently using PSA as a screening test for prostate cancer? Which of the following best describes your feeling about the PSA test in prostate cancer screening? (Responses ranged from a very poor screening test to a very good screening test.) Do you feel age should be an important factor in considering PSA screening?

Results.—The PSA test for screening was used often or always by 55% of the respondents. The strongest direct predictor of use was physicians' reported belief that PSA screening is the standard of care in one's community, according to multiple regression analysis. Physicians' feelings about the test, patient requests for the test, age of the patient, and recommendation of specialty or other organizations were the other direct predictors of PSA test use.

Conclusion.—More than half of primary care physicians surveyed reported regular screening, although PSA prostate cancer screening has yet to be proved definitely effective in decreasing mortality or morbidity from the disease. Changes in physician behavior probably will be difficult to achieve because the rationale for such screening seems to be multifaceted.

▶ Prostate cancer screening is among the most controversial cancer screening tests today. Screening guidelines exist from both the American Cancer Society and the United States Public Health Service; however, those from the United States Public Health Service are not nearly as supportive. This study, which represents survey responses from a random sample of physicians (family practice and internal medicine) from Ohio, illustrates the disagreement over PSA testing. The study had an excellent response rate (60%), with a 51% rate of usable surveys. Of note, while 43% of the physicians knew that the American Cancer Society recommended screening, only 20% knew that the United States Public Health Service did not. Just over half were frequent users of the PSA test, one quarter sometimes used the test, and only one sixth rarely or never used the test. Also, of note, physicians who knew about the opposing recommendations were less supportive of the test. However, the strongest predictor of use is the physician belief that the standard of care includes a PSA. This raises some concern about PSA use in the near future. President Clinton is proposing legislation that is supporting reimbursement for prostate cancer screening tests. If enacted, it is likely to lead to widespread acceptance that the PSA test is the standard of practice and result in significant increase in tests and prostate cancer diagnoses as a result.

C.L. Bennett, M.D., Ph.D.

Sons of Men With Prostate Cancer: Their Attitudes Regarding Possible Inheritance of Prostate Cancer, Screening, and Genetic Testing
Bratt O, Kristoffersson U, Lundgren R, et al (Lund Univ, Sweden; Helsingborg County Hosp, Sweden)
Urology 50:360–365, 1997

16–11

Introduction.—In recent years, the concept of hereditary predisposition for prostate cancer has emerged. There is an intensive search being conducted for genes associated with hereditary prostate cancer. Although no genes have yet been identified, a linkage to the long arm of chromosome 1 was recently discovered. No study concerning the related psychological aspects or attitudes regarding cancer risk notification has been published, despite the current attention paid to familial prostate cancer. Attitudes toward genetic information and screening of men whose fathers have prostate cancer were investigated.

Methods.—There were 65 men with prostate cancer and their 100 unaffected sons who responded to a mailed questionnaire and were interviewed by telephone. Data about the fathers' disease were collected, as well as sociodemographic data.

Results.—Worries about having an increased risk of prostate cancer resulting from possible inheritance was expressed by 60 of the sons. Wanting to know whether prostate cancer was inherited was expressed by 90% of the sons, who also were positively inclined to have screening and genetic testing, particularly if there were multiple instances of prostate cancer in the family. Sons with less than 12 years of education, with worries about inheritance, with younger age, with a father treated with curative intent, and with children of their own, especially if sons, had a greater frequency in wanting to know whether prostate cancer could be inherited. Less than 12 years of education and worries about inheritance were associated with an interest in genetic testing.

Conclusion.—An interest in knowing whether the disease could be inherited was expressed by a large majority of healthy men with a family history of prostate cancer, and they were positively included to have screening and genetic testing. In families with multiple patients of prostate cancer, genetic counseling and a screening program could have beneficial psychological effects.

▶ With the recent recognition of families with high rates of prostate cancer comes additional concerns over patient attitudes toward cancer, screening, and testing. These issues have been evaluated extensively for individuals who are at risk for Huntington's chorea, breast cancer, and colon cancer. Not everyone endorses getting the genetic information and dealing with the consequences, and many prefer not to know. In this study from Sweden, these issues are evaluated with respect to prostate cancer. Of interest, this study is from a country that has not actively promoted prostate cancer screening or treatment. It found a general level of support for screening sons of affected men. However, 25% of the sons who had 12 years or more of education were more likely to consider screening visits negatively.

C.L. Bennett, M.D., Ph.D.

17 Prostate Cancer

Fifteen-Year Survival in Prostate Cancer: A Prospective, Population-based Study in Sweden
Johansson J-E, Holmberg L, Johansson S, et al (Örebro Med Centre, Sweden; Uppsala Univ, Sweden; Harvard Univ, Boston)
JAMA 277:467–471, 1997   17–1

Objective.—The course of prostate cancer is highly variable, and the prognosis of an individual patient is impossible to predict. With the rise of screening and aggressive treatment of early disease, the risk of overdiagnosis and overtreatment is expected to increase. The natural history of initially untreated early-stage prostate cancer was studied, including an analysis of long-term survival by stage, grade, and patient age.

Methods.—The prospective cohort study included 642 consecutive patients in whom prostate cancer was diagnosed between 1977 and 1984. All cases were diagnosed at 1 Swedish hospital with a strictly defined catchment area. The patients' mean age was 72 years, and all were followed up until 1994. Three hundred patients had localized disease, T0 to T2. One hundred eighty-three had locally advanced prostate cancer, T3 to T4, and 159 had distant metastases at diagnosis. The proportion of patients who died of prostate cancer was calculated, with the 15-year survival rate corrected for other causes of death.

Results.—Prostate cancer accounted for 201 of 541 deaths. Eleven percent of patients with localized disease died of prostate cancer. The corrected 15-year survival rate in this group was 81%, whether treatment was deferred (deferred in 223 of 300 patients). The corrected 15-year survival rate was 57% for patients with locally advanced disease and 6% for those with distant metastases.

Conclusions.—"Watchful waiting" is associated with good long-term survival for patients with localized prostate cancer. In this group, initial radical treatment appears to prevent few deaths. Taking such an aggressive approach to all patients would lead to considerable overtreatment of early stage prostate cancer. The situation is different for patients with locally advanced or metastatic disease, who need aggressive therapy in an attempt to improve their prognosis.

▶ The natural history of prostate cancer is a matter of worldwide debate. While many have quoted the Swedish experience of excellent long-term survival rates of untreated early-stage patients with prostate cancer, long-term follow-up has not been published. In this study, with a 15-year follow-up of 642 patients with prostate cancer seen in Sweden, long-term survival was the same for those who had early-stage disease and delayed treatment vs. those with initial therapy. These data are in contrast to the data reported from Britain in the recent Medical Research Council trial (better survival with early treatment) but support the theory behind the ongoing Prostate Cancer Intervention Versus Observation Trial (PIVOT) trial. Additional support for the PIVOT trial is needed in the United States. If not, one of the most important study questions in the United States may never be answered. (The Europeans are also conducting a similar trial and might answer the question for us.)

C.L. Bennett, M.D., Ph.D.

The Natural History of Prostate Carcinoma Based on a Danish Population Treated With No Intent to Cure

Borre M, Nerstrøm B, Overgaard J (Aarhus Univ, Denmark)
Cancer 80:917–928, 1997   17–2

Objective.—Although prostate cancer is the second most common cancer in Western males, its etiology is still largely unknown. In Denmark, the traditional approach to treatment has been conservative. This approach coupled with an extensive personal and cancer registry makes possible a detailed study of the natural course of the disease.

Methods.—Between January 1, 1979, and December 31, 1983, 719 patients aged 49–96 years, in Aarhus County received a diagnosis of prostate cancer, which was classified retrospectively according to the International Union Against Cancer (UICC) 1992 system. Patients were retrospectively studied from diagnosis to death, a median of 15 years.

Results.—Age was significantly related to overall death but not to disease-specific death. There were 265 (37%) patients whose cancer was diagnosed incidentally and 58 (8%) in which it was diagnosed at autopsy. Median duration of symptoms until diagnosis was 1.7 years. The most common symptom at presentation was prostatism. Of the 224 (31%) patients with organ-confined disease (T1a-T2, Nx, MO*), cancer was diagnosed at autopsy in 16. Overall and disease-specific survival rates at 10 years for this group were significantly higher than for patients with non–organ-confined disease (Fig 3). Overall and disease-specific survival rates at 10 years were significantly higher for patients with G1 (well differentiated) tumors than for those with moderately (G2) or poorly (G3) differentiated tumors. Metastatic potential was dependent on tumor size and differentiation. Erythrocyte sedimentation rate was an independent predictor of overall and disease-specific survival. Only 17 (2%) of the patients were alive at last follow-up, and 62% had died of their disease. Disease-specific survival rates were 80% at 1 year, 38% at 5 years, and 17% at 10 years. T classification, degree of differentiation, and erythrocyte

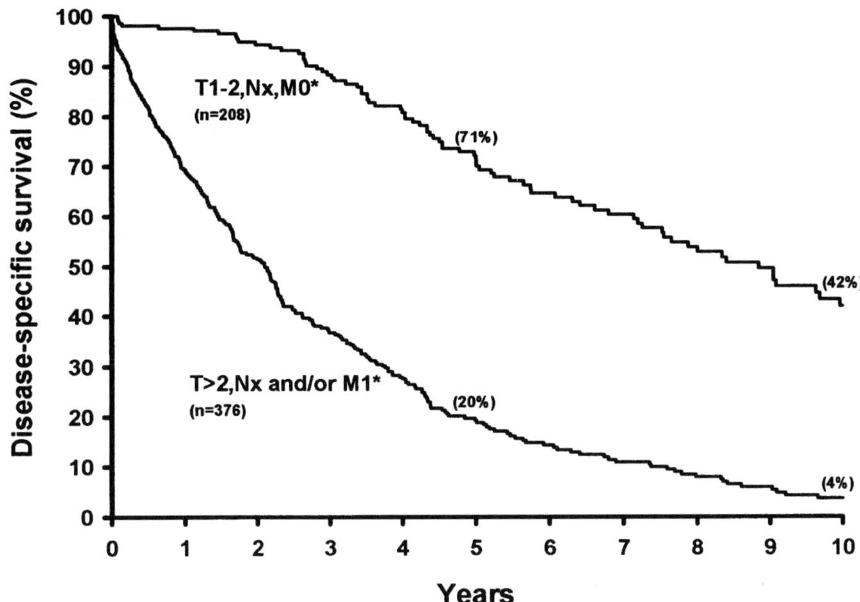

FIGURE 3.—Disease specific survival in 584 patients with known TM* classification at diagnosis: clinically organ-confined disease (208 T1–2, Nx, MO* classified patients) and non–organ-confined disease (376 T greater than 2, Nx, and/or M1 classified patients). (Courtesy of Borre M, Nerstrøm B, Overgaard J: The natural history of prostate carcinoma based on a Danish population treated with no intent to cure. *Cancer* 80:917–928, copyright 1997. American Cancer Society. Reprinted by permission of Wiley-Liss, Inc., a subsidiary of John Wiley & Sons, Inc.)

sedimentation rate at diagnosis were significant predictors of disease-specific death.

Conclusion.—Whereas 62% of patients with prostate cancer suffer and die of their disease, 31% do not. It is important to use prognostic indicators to identify patients who will benefit from early aggressive intervention.

▶ This is another study from Scandinavia following up a cohort of men discovered to have prostate cancer between the years 1979 and 1983. Examination of 200 patients with clinically organ-confined prostate cancer (stage T1 or T2, Nx, M0) showed that 41% died of prostate cancer, resulting in a 10-year disease-specific survival of only 42% (see Fig 3). This is yet another study demonstrating that early-stage prostate cancer is not a "toothless lion," especially if discovered among men who have an expected survival exceeding 10 years.

G.L. Andriole, Jr., M.D.

Prospective Evaluation of Men With Stage T1c Adenocarcinoma of the Prostate

Carter HB, Sauvageot J, Walsh PC, et al (Johns Hopkins Univ, Baltimore, Md; James Buchanan Brady Urological Inst, Baltimore, Md; Johns Hopkins Hosp, Baltimore, Md)

J Urol 157:2206–2209, 1997   17–3

Introduction.—Some prostate cancers detected by prostate specific antigen (PSA) testing are quite small and organ confined. Previously reported criteria used to identify men with the smallest tumors were prospectively applied to help patients with stage T1c prostate cancer in choosing treatment options. The study also evaluated the ability of pretreatment parameters to predict tumor significance in stage T1c disease.

Methods.—The study group included 336 men with stage T1c prostate cancer who were seen between October 1994 and April 1996. Radical prostatectomy was performed in 240 patients, 20 had radiation therapy, and 76 were treated expectantly. Criteria predictive of a significant stage T1c cancer ($\geq$0.2 cm^3) requiring therapy were: PSA density $\geq$0.15 ng/mL/gm, Gleason score $\geq$7, 3 or more cores involved with cancer, or $\geq$50% involvement of any core with cancer. Expectant treatment was recommended only if none of these conditions were present. Specimens were classified on the basis of size, Gleason score, and capsular penetration as insignificant, minimal, moderate, or advanced. The pathological characteristics of tumors in these cases were compared to those of a previous series of T1c cancers treated by radical prostatectomy between 1988 and 1992.

Results.—Tumors of the 240 men who underwent radical prostatectomy were classified as insignificant in 17%, minimal in 12%, moderate in 52%, and advanced in 19%. When these patients were compared with those treated between 1988 and 1992, the 1994 to 1996 series had more organ confined cancer (72% vs. 51%) and fewer cases with positive margins (8% vs. 17%), but a stable proportion of insignificant tumors (17% vs. 16%). Although a lesion on transrectal US and $\geq$3 mm of cancer (or Gleason pattern of 4 or 5) within any biopsy core had high positive predictive values (83% and 87%, respectively), the absence of these criteria was not predictive of an insignificant tumor (negative predictive value 22% and 28%, respectively). The highest pretreatment positive and negative predictive values (84% and 63%) were obtained with pretreatment criteria based on a combination of PSA density, Gleason score, number of involved cores, and percentage of cancer within the core. Neither total length of cancer within the biopsy or absence of a lesion on US was predictive of an insignificant tumor.

Conclusion.—The increased use of PSA testing could be expected to lead to the identification of more small tumors. Although these cancers are being identified earlier, the incidence of insignificant tumors does not appear to have increased.

▶ This article reviews a contemporary series of patients with clinical Stage T1c prostate cancer who were counseled to undergo treatment if they had a PSA density of 0.15 ng/mL/g or more, Gleason Score 7 disease or higher, 3 or more cores involved with cancer, or 50% or greater involvement of any single core that showed prostate cancer. Using these criteria, among the men who chose to undergo radical prostatectomy, 16% were discovered on final pathology to have "insignificant" tumors. On the other hand, 3 men who were predicted by these same criteria to harbor insignificant prostate cancer chose to undergo a radical prostatectomy and were discovered to have "significant" tumors on final pathology. This article underscores that despite careful consideration of all clinical variables, it is not possible to define precisely an individual prostate cancer. We must await development of more elaborate molecular markers or of more sophisticated analysis (i.e., neural network) to improve our ability to predict the significance of an individual prostate cancer.

G.L. Andriole, Jr., M.D.

Incidence and Clinical Significance of High-grade Prostatic Intraepithelial Neoplasia in TURP Specimens
Gaudin PB, Sesterhenn IA, Wojno KJ, et al (Johns Hopkins Med Insts, Baltimore, Md; Armed Forces Inst of Pathology, Washington, DC; Univ of Michigan, Ann Arbor)
Urology 49:558–563, 1997   17–4

Introduction.—There is considerable evidence for a relationship between high-grade prostatic intraepithelial neoplasia (PIN) and prostatic adenocarcinoma, particularly when PIN is present in needle biopsy specimens. The significance of high-grade PIN in specimens obtained from transurethral resection of the prostate (TURP) has received less attention.

Methods.—A review of TURP specimens was conducted to determine the frequency with which high-grade PIN is found in specimens without adenocarcinoma of the prostate. Eighty-five cases of PIN 2 and PIN 3 were identified; slides stained with hematoxylin-eosin were reviewed in 82 cases. At low magnification, high-grade PIN consists of prostatic ducts or acini with a micropapillary, papillary, cribriform, or flat architecture. Secretory cells show hyperchromasia, nuclear enlargement, and prominent nucleoli at high magnification.

Results.—Patients had a mean age of 70 at the time of TURP; 74% were 65 or older. Follow-up clinical information was available in 48% of cases. The median post-TURP follow-up time was 52 months. Four patients had died of unrelated diseases and with no evidence of prostate cancer. Repeat TURP or follow-up needle biopsy was performed in 14 (34%) patients, and adenocarcinoma of the prostate was discovered in 8 patients. An additional case was diagnosed at the time of surgery for transitional cell carcinoma of the urinary bladder. The mean time between TURP and diagnosis of adenocarcinoma was 44 months. Patients with focal+ or diffuse high-grade PIN at TURP were more frequently found to have adenocarcinoma that those with focal high-grade PIN, but the difference was not statistically significant. The estimated incidence of high-grade PIN was 2.3% in all TURP specimens and 3.2% in those without invasive carcinoma.

Conclusion.—The finding of high-grade PIN in specimens obtained by means of TURP is relatively uncommon and occurs primarily in men 70 or older. In approximately one fifth of the patients in this series for whom follow-up information was available, adenocarcinoma of the prostate was subsequently diagnosed. The risk of prostatic cancer is less than that associated with high-grade PIN in needle biopsy specimens.

▶ This study reviewed 85 cases of high-grade PIN without co-existent prostate cancer, discovered on transurethral resection of the prostate. Because this was an older series (patients accumulated between 1984 and 1987), preoperative PSA levels were not routinely available and the patients were relatively old (median age of 71 years). Twenty-two percent of the patients were subsequently discovered to have invasive prostate cancer, at a median follow-up of 52 months. The mean time from the discovery of high-grade PIN to the diagnosis of adenocarcinoma was 44 months, with a range of 2 to 180 months. In the aggregate, these results indicate that high-grade PIN is an uncommon occurrence as an isolated finding during transurethral resection of the prostate (2.3% in this series). Moreover, although TURP-detected high-grade PIN does imply an increased risk of developing prostatic carcinoma, high-grade PIN discovered on needle biopsy of the peripheral zone of the prostate is associated with higher rates of later prostate cancer development. This latter statement, however, must be viewed as tentative, since there was no uniform follow-up of the patients in this TURP series and it is conceivable that transurethral resection of the prostate may lead to the discovery of relatively minute amounts of high-grade PIN, while a significant volume of high-grade PIN may need to be present to be detectable with conventional sextant biopsy techniques.

G.L. Andriole, Jr., M.D.

Clinical Significance of High-grade Prostatic Intraepithelial Neoplasia in Transurethral Resection Specimens
Pacelli A, Bostwick DG (Mayo Clinic, Rochester, Minn)
Urology 50:355–359, 1997   17–5

Objective.—Prostatic intraepithelial neoplasia (PIN) is strongly associated with, and is a probable precursor lesion of, prostatic adenocarcinoma. When PIN is found in a prostate biopsy specimen, further examination for invasive cancer is indicated. There are few data on the incidence and clinical relevance of PIN in specimens from transurethral resection of the prostate (TURP), however. To address this question, including correlation with prostate-specific antigen (PSA) concentration and other clinicopathologic factors, a large series of TURP specimens were reviewed.

Methods.—The retrospective study included 698 TURP specimens obtained over a 1-year period. The investigators reviewed a mean of 6 slides per case, noting the presence, extent, and architectural pattern of PIN. In addition to serum PSA concentration, the findings were correlated with patient age, Gleason score, disease stage, and follow-up data. To evaluate outcome, 16 patients with PIN alone were matched by age and serum PSA level with 2 patients with benign prostatic hyperplasia (BPH) alone.

Results.—Benign prostatic hyperplasia was found in 82% of specimens, and adenocarcinoma plus BPH in 18%. The incidence of high-grade PIN was about 4%—nearly 3% among patients with BPH and 10% among those with carcinoma plus BPH. At 3 to 7 years' follow-up, adenocarcinoma developed in 3 of 14 BPH-only patients with PIN. None of this group died of prostate cancer. None of the matched controls without PIN went on to have cancer on follow-up.

Conclusion.—Review of TURP specimens finds a 4% incidence of PIN overall, a 3% incidence in specimens without cancer, and a 10% incidence in those with cancer. About 20% of patients whose TURP specimens show PIN will have adenocarcinoma on long-term follow-up, compared with none of a group of similar patients without PIN. High-grade PIN is an infrequent finding in TURP specimens, and, when found, indicates a significant cancer risk. This finding should be included in the pathology report and should prompt histologic examination of the entire TURP specimen to exclude carcinoma.

▶ This manuscript describes the histologic findings in 698 TURP specimens of which 16 (2.8%) showed BPH and high-grade PIN and 13 (10.2%) disclosed high-grade PIN in association with prostate cancer and BPH. Follow-up of the men with only high-grade PIN disclosed adenocarcinoma in 3 patients (21%) within 7 years. These data confirm that PIN arising in the transitional zone mandates further follow-up in a manner comparable with what would generally be recommended for patients whose high-grade PIN was discovered on needle biopsy of the peripheral zone. Such patients should be remonitored intensively at 3- to 6-month intervals for the first 2 years and annually for life.

G.L. Andriole, Jr., M.D.

The Impact of Systematic Prostate Biopsy on Prostate Cancer Incidence in Men With Symptomatic Benign Prostatic Hyperplasia Undergoing Transurethral Resection of the Prostate
Ornstein DK, Rao GS, Smith DS, et al (Washington Univ, St Louis)
J Urol 157:880–884, 1997   17–6

Introduction.—Up to 20% of men with symptomatic benign prostatic hyperplasia (BPH) undergoing transurethral resection of the prostate will be found to have prostate cancer. Ninety-five percent of cancers detected in this way arise from the transition zone, previous reports suggest. More and more patients with BPH are being treated without surgery, making it important to determine whether transition zone cancers are adequately detected by current biopsy approaches. This study analyzed cancer incidence in transurethral resection specimens among men with BPH, including the impact of preoperative serum prostate-specific antigen (PSA) levels, digital rectal examinations, and systematic needle biopsies.

Methods.—The retrospective study included 85 consecutive men with symptomatic BPH undergoing transurethral resection of the prostate. All patients had elevated serum PSA levels, suspicious results on digital rectal examination, or both. Before prostate resection was performed, 56 of the men had at least 1 set of benign systematic prostatic needle biopsy specimens, i.e., 4 to 6 cores. The incidence of cancer in the resection specimen and the impact of other variables was assessed.

Results.—The incidence of cancer in the transurethral resection specimens was 17% for men without previous biopsy and 16% for those with at least 1 previous benign biopsy. For the men with previous biopsies, the chances of finding cancer in the resection specimen were unaffected by the number of previous biopsies, the PSA concentration, or the PSA density. Eighty-nine percent of cancers detected in this group were stage T1b or greater.

Conclusion.—The incidence of clinically significant prostate cancer among men with symptomatic BPH undergoing transurethral resection of the prostate is at least 15%. This is so even with previous serum PSA screening, digital rectal examination, or previous needle biopsies of the prostate. The findings suggest that, for early diagnosis of prostate cancer in men with BPH, standard transurethral resection is preferred over laser surgery or other ablative procedures.

▶ This article suggests that clinically relevant prostate cancers may be present in the transition zone of the prostate and be detectable only by transurethral resection of the prostate. Fifteen percent of men with symptomatic BPH who have undergone prior evaluation with serum PSA, digital rectal examination, and 1 or more systematic US-guided biopsies have prostate cancer detected by transurethral resection of the prostate. This finding has implications for the use of medical therapy and for invasive therapies that do not resect or histologically examine transition zone tissue, especially among younger men. Whether transition zone–directed transrectal US-guided biopsies would have detected these cancers is not known and is the subject of an ongoing investigation.

G.L. Andriole, Jr., M.D.

Use of Repeat Sextant and Transition Zone Biopsies for Assessing Extent of Prostate Cancer

Epstein JI, Walsh PC, Sauvageot J, et al (Johns Hopkins Univ, Baltimore, Md)
J Urol 158:1886–1890, 1997   17–7

Background.—The combination of needle biopsy and serum prostate specific antigen (PSA) density levels may identify some men with insignificant prostate cancer. In some cases, serial PSA measurements and repeat needle biopsies could be used for follow-up. The repeat needle biopsies might identify larger tumors that were under sampled at first. The information provided by such repeat needle biopsies was analyzed, along with the reasons that some prostate cancers are missed by needle biopsy.

Methods.—The laboratory study used 193 radical prostatectomy specimens from men with nonpalpable prostate cancer. All were stage T1c tumors detected by needle biopsy with an 18-gauge biopsy gun. Sextant and transition zone needle biopsies were performed on each specimen. After serial sectioning, the specimens were totally embedded, mapped, and staged.

Results.—The biopsy positivity rate in the transition zone was just 2%. Repeat sextant transition zone biopsy found no cancer in nearly one third of specimens even though all were positive on preoperative needle biopsy. Factors independently associated with negative repeat biopsy on multivariate analysis were decreased tumor volume, increased gland size, and decreased radical prostatectomy grade. The frequency of organ-confined tumor was 90% for cases showing no cancer on repeat biopsy, 66% for those showing a single cancer focus measuring less than 3 mm, and 58% for those showing larger areas of cancer. Thirty-eight patients had characteristics likely to prompt repeat biopsy, that is, preoperative needle biopsy showing less than 3 mm of non–high-grade cancer on a single core and a PSA level of 10 or less. For this group, the finding of cancer on repeat biopsy was significantly related to extent of disease in the radical prostatectomy specimen. However, of 16 such patients with no cancer on repeat biopsy, 6 had moderate disease on radical prostatectomy.

Conclusions.—Certain extent-of-disease factors are related to the absence of cancer on repeat prostate biopsy. However, these values show considerable overlap among patients. Sextant needle biopsy is of limited value for the evaluation of tumor status in patients opting for watchful waiting or less invasive forms of therapy.

▶ Repeat biopsies of the prostate are often necessary in patients who have a negative initial set of biopsies, in those considering or undergoing watchful waiting, and in those with prostate cancer who have undergone therapy that leaves the prostate in situ. In this study, the authors performed sextant needle biopsies on 193 radical prostatectomy specimens from men with PSA-detected prostate cancer. Twenty-two percent of tumors were located within the transition zone and only 10% of these were discovered on transition–zone-directed biopsies. Overall, 31% of the repeat biopsies showed no cancer. This included 6 patients with histologically significant tumor in the radical prostatectomy specimen.

These findings have significance not just for patients with established prostate cancer who may be considering watchful waiting but also for patients who have received therapy for prostate cancer such as cryoablation or interstitial seed implantation that leave the prostate in situ and in which negative biopsies are used as an outcome parameter. Additionally, this study illustrates that men with BPH, despite negative biopsies of the peripheral zone, have a 10% to 15% chance of significant transition-zone cancer that is also unlikely to be detected by needle biopsy. This may have implications for patients electing medical therapy for BPH or ablative treatments that attempt to destroy the transition zone rather than remove it for histological interpretation.

G.L. Andriole, Jr., M.D.

Characterisitics of Prostate Cancer in Families Potentially Linked to the Hereditary Prostate Cancer 1 (HPC1) Locus

Grönberg H, Isaacs SD, Smith JR, et al (James Buchanan Brady Urological Inst, Marsburg; Johns Hopkins Univ, Baltimore, Md; NIH, Bethesda, Md)
JAMA 278:1251–1255, 1997   17–8

Introduction.—Mutations of prostate cancer susceptibility genes are thought to account for approximately 9% of cases of prostate cancer. Studies of various racial and ethnic groups have suggested that prostate cancer risk may be related to changes in the *HPC1* locus on chromosome 1q24-25. However, it is unknown whether such inherited prostate cancers are clinically different from those occurring in the general population. The prostate cancer phenotypes of patients with hereditary prostate cancer were assessed.

Methods.—Seventy-four North American families with hereditary prostate cancer were identified. Haplotype analysis in the *HPC1* region identified 133 cases of prostate cancer in 33 families as potentially linked, i.e., carrying an altered *HPC1* gene; and 172 cases in 41 families as potentially unlinked. The clinical characteristics of the 2 groups of prostate cancers were compared, including age at diagnosis, tumor stage and grade, primary treatment received, and presence of other cancers. The findings were compared with those of a reference population of prostate cancer patients from the National Cancer Data Base.

Results.—The mean age at diagnosis was 64 years for men in potentially linked families vs. 66 years for those in potentially unlinked families, compared with 72 years in the reference population. Patients from potentially linked families were more likely to have grade 3 cancers. Forty-one percent of these patients had advanced-stage disease, compared with 31% of patients from potentially unlinked families and from the reference population. None of the other clinical variables examined was significantly different between groups. Compared with potentially unlinked families, the potentially linked families had more than the expected number of cases of breast and colon cancer, but not significantly so.

Conclusion.—For the most part, cases of familial prostate cancer potentially linked to the *HPC1* gene are clinically similar to nonfamilial cases. However, the familial cases may be characterized by younger age at diagnosis, higher-grade tumors, and more advanced disease. Many cases of hereditary prostate cancer are not recognized until they are at an advanced stage, underscoring the need for early detection in potential carriers of prostate cancer susceptibility genes. In keeping with current recommendations, men with a family history of prostate cancer should be screened, starting at age 40 years.

▶ There is increasing recognition that approximately 10% of all patients with prostate cancer and as many as half of patients in whom the diagnosis is made at an early age have an inheritable form of the disease. A recent linkage study demonstrated evidence of a major prostate cancer susceptibility locus on chromosome 1.

In this study, 74 North American families with hereditary prostate cancer (defined as 3 or more first degree relatives or 2 or more with diagnosis at age less than 55 years or families with at least 3 successive generations of prostate cancer) demonstrated a few distinguishing characteristics of hereditary prostate cancer. First, approximately 41% presented with advanced disease, which is approximately 10% higher than anticipated. Secondly, these patients tended to be at a younger age at diagnosis; and, thirdly, they had an overall higher tumor grade. Results such as these provide a further rationale for beginning screening of men with a strong family history of prostate cancer, starting before the age of 50 years.

G.L. Andriole, Jr., M.D.

Body Size and Prostate Cancer: A 20-Year Follow-up Study Among 135 006 Swedish Construction Workers
Andersson S-O, Wolk A, Bergström R, et al (Örebro Med Ctr, Sweden; Univ Hosp, Uppsala, Sweden; Univ Hosp; et al)
J Natl Cancer Inst 89:385–389, 1997   17–9

Introduction.—Because hormonal factors have been implicated in the development of prostate cancer, an association between body weight and the risk of prostate cancer might be expected. A retrospective cohort study examined possible associations of adult weight, height, body mass index (BMI), and lean body mass (LBM) with the incidence and mortality rate of prostate cancer.

Methods.—The study cohort consisted of 135,006 Swedish construction workers. Data from their regular health checkups were compiled in a computerized central register beginning with visits in 1971. Information obtained at the index visit during 1971 through 1975 was analyzed. The workers completed a detailed questionnaire before each visit and had their height and weight recorded. Follow-up for the development of prostate cancer continued through 1991.

Results.—Because the risk of prostate cancer is strongly age dependent, the workers were categorized according to age at entry (under 30 years, 30–39, 40–49, 50–59, and 60 and older). Prostate cancer was diagnosed in 2,368 men during follow-up; 708 died of the disease. Overall, each of 4 measurements exhibited a positive association with a risk of prostate cancer. The trend was statistically significant for weight, height, and LBM, but not for BMI. All individual measurements were consistently more strongly related to death from prostate cancer than to the incidence of prostate cancer. The excess risk of death from prostate cancer was statistically significant in all BMI categories above the reference category.

Discussion.—Weight, height, BMI, and LBM were all positively associated with the risk of prostate cancer, and all measurements were more strongly associated with death from prostate cancer. The effects of each anthropometric variable were difficult to determine because the variables were highly inter-related. In addition, the measurements reflect a variety of potentially relevant nutritional, hormonal, and neuroendocrine factors.

▶ The authors used anthropometric measurements derived over a 4-year interval between 1971 and 1975 and correlated them with the incidence of prostate cancer by linkage to the 1991 Swedish National Cancer Register, the Death Register, and the Migration Register. All measures, weight, height, lean body mass, and body mass index were positively associated with the risk of prostate cancer but very strongly related to mortality from the disease. These data suggest that these anthropometric measurements may play a role in the growth of prostate cancer from its earliest latent stages to its more clinically apparent and death-inducing stages. It is conceivable that one day these anthropometric measurements will be included in sophisticated neural network analysis programs that will predict the presence of prostate cancer and its probability of causing mortality.

G.L. Andriole, Jr., M.D.

Prostate Cancer in Nigerians: Facts and Nonfacts
Osegbe DN (College of Medicine, Lagos, Nigeria; Lagos Univ Teaching School, Nigeria)
J Urol 157:1340–1343, 1997   17–10

Background.—Black men in Africa are reported to have a lower incidence of prostate cancer than black men in the United States, and Nigeria is rated globally as a low risk zone for the tumor. Although some studies state that low androgen levels may protect Nigerians from cancer of the prostate, others indicate no difference in androgen levels between Nigerians and other men throughout the world. A prospective study sought to establish the actual incidence of prostate cancer in Nigeria.

Methods.—The study population included men aged 45 or older who were seen for obstructive or irritative urinary symptoms. All underwent a detailed history and physical examination with digital rectal examination. A general blood profile and chemistry studies were also performed. Further tests were ordered in suspicious cases, but prostate-specific antigen tests were not available. Patients with histologically positive prostate cancer and at least 1 year of follow-up were analyzed for clinical features, tumor characteristics, and survival.

Results.—During the study period, 125 patients with a mean age of 68 years had prostate cancer. Based on hospital admissions data and national population statistics, the hospital incidence was 127 per 100,000 cases and the national prostate cancer risk was 2%. Duration of symptoms varied widely, but symptoms lasted for more than 16 months on average. No specific occupation was associated with prostate cancer. Common clinical features were prostatism (93.6%), low back pain (17.6%), and hematuria (16%). Most (86%) patients had advanced stages C and D disease and more than one third of tumors were poorly differentiated or entirely anaplastic. Twenty-eight patients had paraplegia. There were 25 deaths during the initial hospitalization or within 1 year of diagnosis, and approximately 64% of patients died within 2 years.

Discussion.—The incidence of prostate cancer is greatest in black men in the United States, suggesting a genetic predisposition. African black men, however, were reported to have a low incidence of the tumor. This study indicates that the prostate cancer incidence rate in Nigerians may be approximately 13 times greater than previously reported, a finding that supports a common genetic predisposition among black men in both countries.

▶ Environment vs. genetics: the high incidence of prostate cancer among African Americans has often been attributed to a combination of genetics and diet, with the general belief that diet and other environmental issues may be the overriding factors, especially if one considers earlier reports that indigenous black men in Africa experience relatively low rates of prostate cancer. In this prospective study, Nigerian men on an age-adjusted basis have a comparable prostate cancer incidence and stage at the time of discovery as African American men. This suggests that genetics may be a more important factor than environment and diet.

G.L. Andriole, Jr., M.D.

Has There Been a Recent Shift in the Pathological Features and Prognosis of Patients Treated With Radical Prostatectomy?

Soh S, Kattan MW, Berkman S, et al (Matsunaga-Conte Prostate Cancer Research Ctr, Houston; Baylor College of Medicine; Houston; The Methodist Hosp, Houston)
J Urol 157:2212–2218, 1997

17–11

Introduction.—Now that more clinical stage T1c prostate tumors are being detected by means of prostate specific antigen (PSA) testing, there is concern that radical surgery will be performed for cancers of low biologic potential. A series of patients with clinical stages T1 to 3NXM0 prostate cancer treated with radical prostatectomy during a 13-year period was

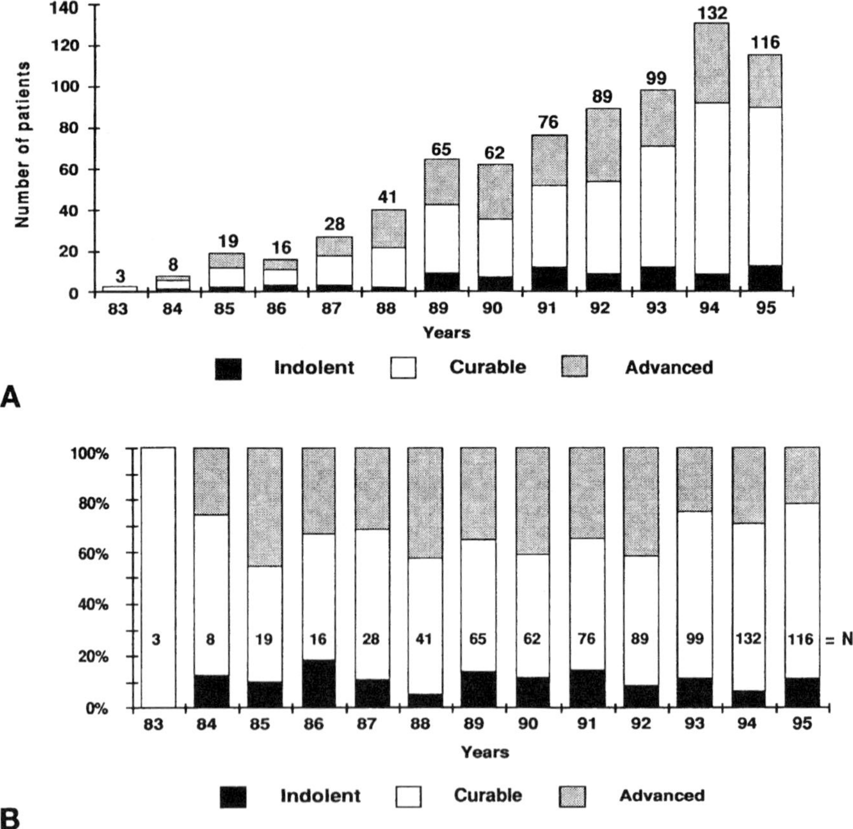

FIGURE 3.—Change in prognostic category with time, defined by pathological features (volume, grade and extent) of cancer in radical prostatectomy specimens. While total number of patients increased, there was no significant change in the proportion of patients with indolent cancer with time. *A,* number of patients each year. *B,* percent of patients. (Courtesy of Soh S, Kattan MW, Berkman S, et al: Has there been a recent shift in the pathological features and prognosis of patients treated with radical prostatectomy? *J Urol* 157:2212–2218, 1997.)

reviewed to determine whether there was a significant change in pathologic features or prognosis over time.

Methods.—Two groups of patients were analyzed. The first included 2,326 patients who underwent staging pelvic lymphadenectomy for clinically localized prostate cancer at a teaching hospital between 1984 and 1995. The 759 consecutive patients in the second group were treated with radical retropubic prostatectomy by a single surgeon between 1983 and 1995; morphometric analysis was possible in 754 cases. Methods of diagnosis, pathologic features, and prognosis of these 754 patients were analyzed by year of diagnosis.

Results.—Analysis of the first patient group indicated a decrease in the proportion with lymph node metastases and an overall shift away from regional stage disease at diagnosis. There was a marked decrease in the proportion of cancers initially detected by means of transurethral detection after 1989, and an increase in nonpalpable cancers detected by means of PSA after 1990. Although there was a marked increase in the annual number of radical prostatectomies over time, preoperative serum PSA, tumor volume, and pathologic stage did not change significantly during the study period. The proportion of patients with Gleason sum 7 cancer increased significantly after 1991. Fewer patients had an advanced cancer at diagnosis during recent years, but there was no increase in the proportion of patients with indolent or clinically unimportant cancers (Fig 3). When the study years were grouped into 3 periods (1983 to 1987, 1988 to 1991, and 1992 to 1995), the actuarial probability of progression after surgery showed no change.

Conclusion.—There were considerable changes in method of detection and number of patients treated each year for prostate cancer, but no changes in pathologic stage or rate of progression were observed in patients treated between 1983 and 1995. These findings suggest that few radical procedures are being performed for small, indolent cancers.

▶ This interesting paper documents the experience of a single surgeon over a 12-year period. The study shows that despite aggressive screening with digital rectal exam, serum PSA testing, and ultrasound-guided biopsies of the prostate, the proportion of cancers discovered that are potentially indolent has not changed. This underscores the fact that current sextant biopsy techniques are generally not capable of finding many small-volume, well-differentiated tumors.

G.L. Andriole, Jr., M.D.

Adjuvant and Salvage Irradiation Following Radical Prostatectomy for Prostate Cancer

Morris MM, Dallow KC, Zietman AL, et al (Harvard Med School, Boston)
Int J Radiat Oncol Biol Phys 38:731–736, 1997   17–12

Objective.—Many patients will have elevated prostate-specific antigen (PSA) levels after radical prostatectomy, as many as half of postoperative patients thought to have organ-confined disease will have more extensive disease, and as many as half of these will have a relapse. Because radiation can be useful in patients who will have relapse, it is important to identify the subgroup of patients who can benefit from this treatment. The durability of benefit derived from salvage irradiation after prostatectomy for pT3NO disease and the possibility of cure were retrospectively assessed.

Methods.—Between 1987 and 1994, 88 patients aged 47–80 years, were treated with adjuvant or salvage irradiation to the tumor bed (total dose of 60–64 Gy) after radical prostatectomy because of high risk of local failure (adjuvant therapy, n = 40) or elevated PSA levels and/or a palpable locally recurrent tumor (salvage therapy, n = 48). Patients were studied for an average of 31 months after irradiation and 44 months after surgery. Complications were recorded. Kaplan-Meier life-table survival analysis was determined. Outcome was biochemical disease-free status (bNED). Biochemical failure was defined as a rise in PSA greater than 10% or detection of a PSA level that was previously undetectable.

Results.—At 3 years after surgery, 88% of adjuvant patients and 68% of salvage patients were bNED. After irradiation, 21 (70%) of 30 patients with persistent PSA elevation and 12 (67%) of 18 patients with later rise of PSA had undetectable PSA levels. After irradiation, 12 of 13 patients with low PSA levels before irradiation had undetectable PSA levels, and 8 were bNED at last follow-up. Patients with higher PSA levels were less likely to achieve undetectable levels after irradiation. Preoperative PSA levels, seminal vesicle status, and preirradiation PSA levels greater than 1.6 were significant predictors of outcome according to univariate analysis. Salvage patients with persistently elevated PSA and those with late rising PSA had a similar outcome at 3 years. On multivariate analysis, only treatment group was an independent and significant predictor of outcome. At 3 years, 77% of adjuvant patients and 60.3% of salvage patients were biochemically disease-free.

Conclusion.—Adjuvant irradiation was more successful than salvage irradiation after radical prostatectomy.

▶ This retrospective analysis addresses a contentious issue, i.e., the management of patients with adverse pathologic findings at radical prostatectomy. In general, the controversy arises because patients with histologic findings suggestive of a higher risk of local failure (extracapsular extension or margin-positive disease) may not ever fail biochemically or clinically. Many such patients will continue to have an undetectable PSA for many years after surgery in the absence of any specific therapy. On the other hand, such patients who are destined to fail are more apt to be salvaged if treated early when a smaller tumor volume is present. Therefore, waiting for such patients to manifest a detectable PSA may result in missing the window of cure.

The results from this study show a benefit to adjuvant radiation therapy over salvage therapy. However, the benefit to adjuvant therapy disappears if patients are treated very promptly after the PSA becomes detectable (i.e., if the PSA is 1.7 or less). It is only among patients whose postradical prostatectomy serum PSA rises above 1.7 that a rather unsatisfactory 3-year biochemical disease-free status of 30% is observed.

In my own practice, I tend to consider the age of the patient, the focality of the adverse histologic finding, and the grade of the tumor to recommend further therapy. I generally monitor focally positive margins or capsular penetration if the Gleason Score is 6 or less and recommend adjuvant radiation therapy for all others.

G.L. Andriole, Jr., M.D.

Radioimmunoscintigraphy With In-111-Labeled Capromab Pendetide Predicts Prostate Cancer Response to Salvage Radiotherapy After Failed Radical Prostatectomy
Kahn D, Williams RD, Haseman MK, et al (Univ of Iowa, Iowa City; Sutter Gen Hosp, Sacramento, Calif)
J Clin Oncol 16:284–289, 1998   17–13

Introduction.—Salvage radiotherapy may be performed to eliminate tumor in the pelvis and prostatic fossa for men with failed radical prostatectomy. For this approach to be successful, the cancer must be confined to the radiation field; however, there is no way to accurately identify those patients whose cancer is still confined to the prostatic fossa. Indium-111-labeled capromab pendetide scanning was studied for its ability to identify patients who would or would not respond to salvage radiotherapy.

Methods.—The study included 32 men with prostate cancer in whom radical prostatectomy had failed. All underwent whole-body scanning with Indium-111-labeled capromab pendetide to assess activity inside and outside the prostatic fossa. Patients then underwent salvage radiotherapy, consisting of at least 60 Gy of radiation administered to the prostatic fossa and immediately adjacent pelvic tissue. The patients were followed for a median of 13 months, with regular measurement of prostate-specific antigen levels. Indium-111-labeled capromab pendetide scan findings and other variables were evaluated for association with durable complete response (DCR), nondurable response, or no response by logistic regression modeling.

Results.—Twenty-three of the 32 patients had normal scan results outside the prostatic fossa. Salvage radiotherapy produced a DCR in 70% of this group, compared with 22% of those who had positive scan results outside the prostatic fossa and pelvis. The study model predicted that 88%

of patients with a normal scan would have a DCR (95% confidence interval, 55%–98%). This probability fell to 62% for men with a positive scan limited to the prostatic fossa (42%–79%) and 27% for men with a positive scan outside the pelvis. None of the other preradiotherapy variables analyzed was significantly associated with the likelihood of DCR.

Conclusions.—For men in whom radical prostatectomy has failed, the results of Indium-111-labeled capromab pendetide scanning can predict the likelihood of DCR to salvage radiotherapy. Durable response is more likely for men who have normal scan results or a scan that is positive outside the prostatic fossa. Patients with a positive scan outside the prostatic fossa may have an initial decline in prostate-specific antigen levels, but this is only temporary.

▶ In my medical community, the ProstaScint Study has not yet found its hour, owing in part to the technique's expense and also to its limited ability to guide effective therapy. In this study, the authors investigated the ability of this imaging modality to identify which men with detectable post-radical prostatectomy prostate-specific antigen would benefit from salvage radiation therapy. An interesting group of patients were the 18 men who had positive scans only in the pelvis. With follow-up ranging between 8 and 31 months, 6 (33%) patients have already failed. This demonstrates that even over a relatively short time, the finding of a negative ProstaScint scan outside the pelvis is not total reassurance that only local disease is present. Moreover, the proportion of those patients with a persistently undetectable prostate-specific antigen will only diminish with longer follow-up. For these reasons, I suspect this scanning will continue to be used very selectively among such patients.

G.L. Andriole, Jr., M.D.

Preservation of the Anterior Urethral Ligamentous Attachments in Maintaining Post-Prostatectomy Urinary Continence: A Comparative Study

Lowe BA (Oregon Health Sciences Univ, Portland)
J Urol 158:2137–2141, 1997   17–14

Objective.—Urinary incontinence is a common treatment-related side effect after total prostatectomy that can significantly affect quality of life. Although many surgeons preserve the anterior urethral ligamentous attachments, there is little evidence to suggest that this results in improved urinary continence. The technique of preserving these structures was described (Fig 1), and urinary continence results in patients with and without preservation of these attachments were prospectively compared.

Methods.—Rate of total continence, time to return of continence, incidence of extra organ disease, and operative blood loss were compared at 1 year in prostatectomy patients undergoing preservation of the anterior urethral attachments (51 patients), resection of the bladder neck (70

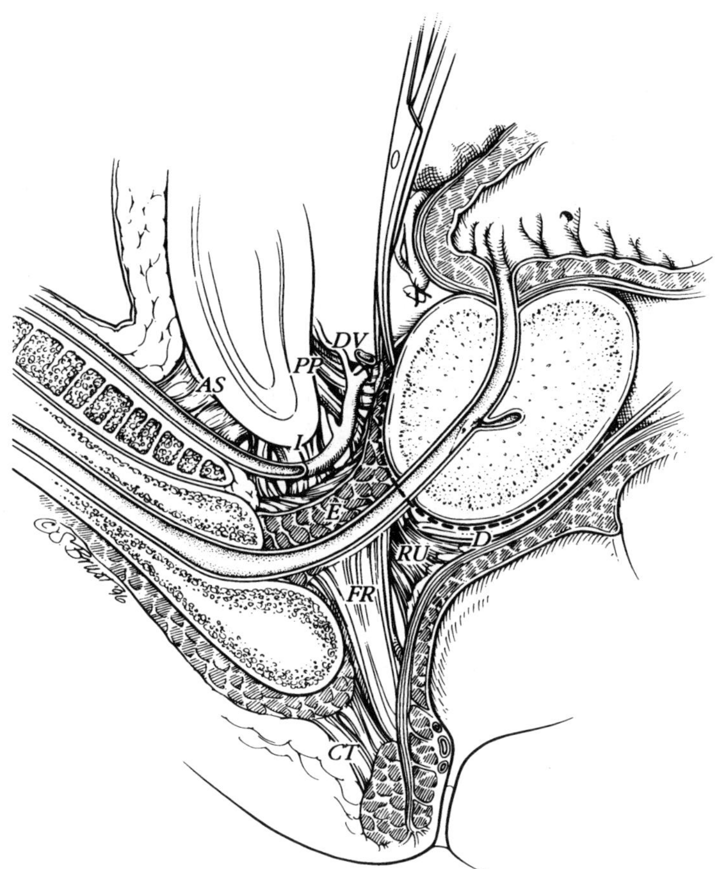

FIGURE 1.—Diagrammatic view of surgical approach to preserve anterior urethral attachments. *Dotted line* indicates plan of surgical dissection. *Abbreviations: AS*, anterior suspensory ligament of penis; *CT*, central tendon; *D*, Denonvillier's fascia; *DV*, dorsal vein of penis; *E*, external urethral sphincter; *FR*, fibrous raphe; *I*, intermediate anterior urethral ligament; *PP*, puboprostate ligament; *RU*, rectourethralis. (Courtesy of Lowe BA: Preservation of the anterior urethral ligamentous attachments in maintaining post-prostatectomy urinary continence: A comparative study. *J Urol* 158:2137–2141, 1997.)

patients), preservation of the bladder neck (55 patients), and dorsal vein gathering (14 patients).

Results.—Total continence was 84.3% at 1 year in the bladder neck resection group, 89.1% in the bladder neck preservation group, 85.7% in the dorsal vein–gathering group, and 100% in the attachments preservation group. In the attachments preservation group, 25.5% of patients had total continence after catheter removal. Total continence at 3 months was 41.4% in the bladder neck resection group, 50.9% in the bladder neck preservation group, and 50% in the dorsal vein–gathering group. Mean quality-of-life scores on a 0 to 100 scale were 82 for the bladder neck resection group, 87 for the bladder neck preservation group, 89 for the dorsal vein–gathering group, and 94 for the attachments preservation group. Clinical staging was similar for all groups. The attachments preservation group had significantly less operative blood loss.

Conclusion.—Preservation of the anterior urethral ligamentous attachments improved speed of attainment of continence, quality of life, and decreased operative blood loss.

▶ This is my current approach to radical prostatectomy and my experience generally is consistent with this report. However, there are some pitfalls with this technique: Specifically, some patients may have a narrow pelvis and relatively proximal insertion of the puboprostatic ligaments on the prostate. This may make hemostasis and complete extirpation of both the anterior and posterior aspects of the apex of the prostate quite difficult. Nonetheless, the early return of urinary continence is more than adequate payback for this potential intraoperative difficulty.

G.L. Andriole, Jr., M.D.

Rectus Fascial Sling Suspension of the Vesicourethral Anastomosis After Radical Prostatectomy

Jorion JL (Clinique St Pierre, Louvain-La-Leuve, Belgium)
J Urol 157:926–928, 1997

17–15

Background.—Urinary incontinence is a side effect of radical retropubic prostatectomy for prostate adenocarcinoma. Fascial sling suspension of the vesicourethral anastomosis could reestablish continence earlier and more reliably.

Methods.—Radical retropubic prostatectomy with a rectus fascial sling suspension was performed in 30 patients (group 2), whose postoperative continence patterns were compared with those of 30 previous patients (group 1).

Results.—At 1 month, 60% in group 2 had complete continence, vs. 33% in group 1 ($P < 0.069$). At 3 months, 93% in group 2 had complete continence, vs. 70% in group 1 ($P < 0.042$). At 6 months, rates were 100% in group 2 and 90% in group 1 ($P < 0.237$). At 9 and 12 months, 93% of group 1 had recovered fully, with no patients in either group totally incontinent. There were 3 related complications in group 2, 2 cases of urinary retention (cleared without treatment) and 1 of evisceration (treated surgically with success).

Conclusions.—Fascial sling suspension after radical retropubic prostatectomy, a simple procedure that adds little operative time, increases early continence. To avoid urinary retention, the sling must be placed to suspend without tension. Because most patients eventually regain acceptable continence regardless of technique, this modification's chief benefit lies in earlier recovery of continence.

▶ This small series describes 30 men who underwent creation of a rectus fascial sling during a radical prostatectomy and compares them to men undergoing radical prostatectomy without a sling. A more rapid return of urinary continence but also higher rates of urinary retention and, in 1 patient, evisceration of the retropubic wound were observed among men undergoing the sling procedure.

Currently, use of techniques that minimize disruption of the periurethral tissues (e.g., preservation of the puboprostatic ligament) will allow some patients to experience immediate return of urinary control. For selected patients in whom the dissection is difficult, it may be reasonable to employ a fascial sling.

G.L. Andriole, Jr., M.D.

Late GI and GU Complications in the Treatment of Prostate Cancer
Schultheiss TE, Lee WR, Hunt MA, et al (Fox Chase Cancer Ctr, Philadelphia)
Int J Radiat Oncol Biol Phys 37:3–11, 1997   17–16

Background.—Radiation therapy for cancer of the prostate is often associated with gastrointestinal (GI) and genitourinary (GU) side effects. This study evaluated the acute and late GI and GU side effects in such patients, and whether early effects can predict late effects.

Methods.—In a 9-year period, 712 patients received radiation therapy for cancer of the prostate at a dose of 65 Gy or more. Acute and late GU and acute GI side effects were graded according to RTOG criteria. Late GI side effects were categorized as grade 2 if they involved moderate diarrhea and colic, 5 or more bowel movements/day, excessive rectal mucus, rectal bleeding requiring 2 or fewer coagulation procedures, and pain requiring nonnarcotic drugs. Grade 3 late GI effects included dysfunction requiring hospitalization (without surgery), rectal bleeding associated with transfusion or more than 3 coagulation procedures, and pain requiring narcotics. Grade 4 late GI effects included surgical intervention, necrosis, perforation, fistula, or life-threatening bleeding.

Findings.—As for acute complications, 246 patients had Grade 2 or higher GI complications, 201 patients had Grade 2 or higher GU complications, and 67 patients had both. Prior treatment of pelvic nodes, use of conformal fields, and diabetes resulted in significantly more acute GI and GU side effects; transurethral prostatectomy (TURP) was associated with fewer acute side effects.

GI effects: For Grade 2 acute complications, diabetes, pelvic nodes, and age under 60 years had significant effects. For Grade 2 late complications ($n = 115$), central axis dose, use of increased rectal shielding, and androgen deprivation before radiotherapy had significant effects. Acute GI complications were predictive of late GI complications. For Grade 3 or higher late complications ($n = 15$), the only significant factor was dose.

GU effects: For Grade 2 acute complications, diabetes, use of conformal fields, TURP, and urinary obstructive symptoms at presentation had significant effects on morbidity. For Grade 2 late complications ($n = 43$), central axis dose, androgen deprivation, and obstructive symptoms at presentation had significant effects. Acute GU complications were predictive of late GU complications. Increasing dose was associated with more late GU complications.

Conclusions.—Acute GI and GU Grade 2 complications are predictive of late complications. Androgen deprivation therapy before radiotherapy and a history of diabetes increased late GI and GU morbidity, and a dose-dependence was observed for both complications. For late Grade 2 or higher GI complications, additional rectal shielding in the lateral fields for the last 10 Gy of treatment was associated with reduced morbidity.

▶ While current assessments of quality of life include formal evaluations with patient self-administered instruments such as the Functional Assessment of Cancer Therapy (FACT) or the European Organization for Research and Treatment of Cancer (EORTC) instrument, earlier studies focused on physician reports of treatment-related toxicities. In one of the largest studies to date, Hanks et al. report on gastrointestinal and genitourinary complications of radiation therapy for prostate cancer. In a study of 712 consecutive patients seen at the Fox Chase Cancer Center, over half of the patients had acute (up to 3 months after completion of treatment) GI or GU complications, characterized by frequency of urination at greater than 1 hour intervals or diarrhea requiring pharmacologic intervention. Almost 15% had late GI or GU complications of Grade 2 or greater. Of interest, the factors associated with late toxicity included central axis radiation dose (both GI and GU), androgen deprivation therapy prior to radiation therapy (GU only), history of obstructive symptoms (GU only), and acute GU side effects (GU only). The study indicates that late GI and late GU toxicities demonstrate a dose response dependence as well as increased frequency with hormonal therapy prior to radiation therapy. As clinicians adopt neoadjuvant hormonal treatment for men who will receive radiation therapy, concern exists about the potential for adverse effects on quality of life. In addition, this study highlights the need to incorporate formal quality-of-life assessments for prostate cancer patients.

C.L. Bennett, M.D., Ph.D

Interstitial Iodine-125 Radiation Without Adjuvant Therapy in the Treatment of Clinically Localized Prostate Carcinoma
Ragde H, Blasko JC, Grimm PD, et al (Pacific Northwest Cancer Found, Seattle; Univ of Washington, Seattle; Northwest Tumor Inst, Seattle; et al)
Cancer 80:442–453, 1997   17–17

Background.—Prostate brachytherapy for prostate carcinoma was popular for a short period in the 1970s after Whitmore et al. introduced a method of retropubic implantation of iodine-125 radionuclides. Follow-up showed that the implant had a high rate of local failure, which was attributed to several causes. In the 1980s, various technological advances helped to correct the original problems of the open-implantation tech-

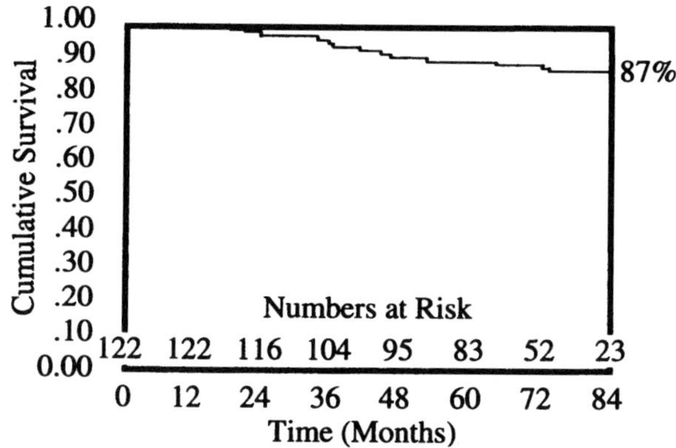

FIGURE 2.—Plot of Kaplan-Meier data to 7 years demonstrates 87% freedom from prostate specific antigen greater than 1.0 ng/mL failure. (Courtesy of Ragde H, Blasko JC, Grimm PD, et al: Interstitial iodine-125 radiation without adjuvant therapy in the treatment of clinically localized prostate carcinoma. *Cancer* 80:442–453, 1997. Copyright © 1997, American Cancer Society. Reprinted by permission of Wiley-Liss, Inc., a subsidiary of John Wiley & Sons, Inc.)

nique. These advances include transrectal ultrasound planimetry for accurate prostate volume determination, transrectal ultrasound and template guidance to help implant the prostate transperineally, radiation treatment planning computers, and the availability of palladium-103 for needle insertion.

Methods.—Iodine-125 radionuclides were implanted in 126 consecutive patients with T1 and T2 prostate adenocarcinoma. The minimum radiation dose was 160 gray. Prebiopsy prostate specific antigen (PSA) values were obtained for all patients. Clinical biochemical and pathologic studies were performed after implantation. Surgical staging was not performed, and androgen deprivation treatment was not used. Morbidity was graded using the Radiation Therapy Oncology Group grading scale. PSA failure was defined as (1) PSA progession of 2 consecutive increases from a nadir value and (2) failure to attain a serum PSA value of 1.0 ng/mL or 0.5 ng/mL. Follow-up was 69.3 months.

Results.—Evaluations were completed in 122 of 126 patients; 4 men died less than 1 year after implantation. At 7 years, overall survival was 77%. No patient died from prostate carcinoma. At 7 years, PSA progression-free survival was 89%. The outcome for PSA less than or equal to 1.0 ng/mL was 87% (Fig 2). When PSA less than or equal to 5 ng/mL was the outcome measure and the PSA values of these patients were compared to the values proposed for disease-free survival after radical prostatectomy, the 7-year disease-free survival was 79%. There were few complications. Post-treatment incontinence occurred only in patients who had undergone transurethral prostate resection.

Discussion.—Patients with T1 or T2 prostate carcinoma treated with iodine-125 prostate brachytherapy had biochemical outcomes similar to outcomes expected from radical prostatectomy and external beam radiation. This single-session outpatient procedure causes minimal morbidity and has high patient acceptance. Although the long, natural history of prostate carcinoma has required 10 to 15 years to assess treatment results, sequential evaluation of serum PSA and biopsy may allow treatment results to be assessed sooner than was thought possible.

▶ This study represents further follow-up of the single institution series of interstitial iodine-125 implants performed between January 1988 and December 1990. This report continues to show outstanding clinical and PSA control rates as exhibited in Figure 2. This report also describes a 5% positive biopsy rate and a 13% indeterminate biopsy rate among the 77 patients who underwent post-treatment biopsy. As shown in Table 8 of the original article, this procedure was associated with very acceptable late complications, especially urinary incontinence, in 5% of patients, but the rate was 12% among men who had undergone a prior transurethral resection of the prostate. Vesicourethral and bulbous urethral strictures occurred in an additional 15% of patients.

Collectively, these results continue to suggest that interstitial therapy appears to be a promising treatment for selected patients with early stage disease. Whether this experience can be replicated at other centers remains to be seen. It is also of concern that only about 10% of the patients have been followed for more than 6 years.

G.L. Andriole, Jr., M.D.

Improved Survival in Patients With Locally Advanced Prostate Cancer Treated With Radiotherapy and Goserelin

Bolla M, Gonzalez D, Warde P, et al (Univ Hosp, Grenoble, France; Akademisch Medisch Centrum, Amsterdam; Princess Margaret Hosp, Toronto; et al)

N Engl J Med 337:295–300, 1997   17–18

Introduction.—The role of external irradiation in patients with locally advanced prostate cancer is uncertain. External irradiation was compared with external irradiation plus goserelin in a prospective, randomized trial of 415 patients with locally advanced prostate cancer.

Methods.—Patients were randomized to receive either radiation alone or radiotherapy plus goserelin (3.6 mg subcutaneously every 4 weeks for 3 years, starting on the first day of irradiation). Patients receiving goserelin also received cyproterone acetate, 150 mg by mouth daily, to inhibit the transient increase in testosterone subsequent to goserelin administration. Both groups of patients received 50 Gy of radiation to the pelvis for 5 weeks and an additional 20 Gy over an additional 2 weeks as a prostatic boost.

Results.—The median patient age was 71 years and the median follow-up was 45 months. Data were available for 401 of 415 patients. There were 198 patients in the radiotherapy group and 203 in the combined-treatment group. Estimates of 5-year survival were 79% and 62% for the combined-treatment and radiotherapy groups, respectively (a significant difference). Freedom from disease at 5 years was significantly higher for the combined-treatment group, compared with the radiotherapy group (85% vs. 48%).

Conclusion.—Five-year overall survival can be significantly improved in patients with locally advanced prostate cancer who receive an analogue of gonadotropin-releasing hormone (goserelin) initiated at the start of external irradiation treatment and continuing for 3 years.

▶ This well-done, relatively large, long-term study further supports preliminary data showing that the combination of radiation therapy and androgen deprivation therapy results in improved local control. Moreover, this combination therapy improved overall survival for patients with locally advanced disease. It is important to note that in this study, androgen ablation therapy was administered for at least 3 years, with some patients continuing on therapy beyond that time. Thus, an important question raised by the study is whether radiation therapy added any benefit to androgen deprivation therapy.

This is an important issue because it is known that even relatively short-term luteinizing hormone-releasing hormone analogue analog therapy may suppress testosterone for a very long time (possibly permanently), especially in men who have experienced radiation injury to their testes during therapy for prostate cancer. Happily, this issue is being evaluated in a randomized study in Canada. Until the results of the study are available, it does appear that combinations of androgen deprivation therapy and radiation therapy should be recommended for patients with locally advanced disease. However, the exact duration of the androgen ablation therapy is not yet established.

G.L. Andriole, Jr., M.D.

Bladder Carcinoma and Other Second Malignancies After Radiotherapy for Prostate Carcinoma

Neugut AI, Ahsan H, Robinson E, et al (Columbia Univ, New York; Northern Israel Oncology Ctr, Haifa)
Cancer 79:1600–1604, 1997   17–19

Background.—Studies have shown that radiation therapy (RT) to the pelvis is associated with an increased risk of bladder cancer and other malignancies. To date, there have been no controlled studies of the risk of second malignancies after RT for prostate carcinoma.

Methods and Findings.—Data on a cohort of patients with prostate carcinoma were analyzed retrospectively. Radiation therapy had been performed in 34,889 and no RT had been performed in 106,872. The RT group had a relative risk of 1.5 for bladder carcinoma after 8 years. The risk in the no-RT group was 1.0. In addition, the RT group had a relative risk of 1.3 for bladder carcinoma. Neither group had an increased risk for rectal carcinoma, acute nonlymphocytic leukemia, or chronic lymphocytic leukemia.

Conclusions.—Patients undergoing RT for prostate carcinoma had an increased risk of bladder carcinoma several years later, but the increase was not dramatic. These patients had no increased risk of rectal carcinoma or leukemia.

▶ This large study used the Surveillance, Epidemiology, and End Results Program database to determine whether radiation therapy for prostate cancer increased the risk for the development of bladder cancer, rectal cancer, or leukemia. In this study, the incidence of bladder cancer among men with prostate cancer who received irradiation therapy was statistically increased after 5 years and rose for patients monitored more than 8 years to a relative risk of 1.5. Previous studies have demonstrated an elevated risk of bladder cancer for other forms of radiation therapy that encompass the bladder, and these included women who received pelvic irradiation for both ovarian and cervical cancer. On the statistical basis, the relative risk for bladder cancer is dramatically increased, but the overall increased risk to an individual patient is rather small. It amounts to a 0.26% per person-year among patients with prostate cancer treated with radiation therapy.

Whether current forms of irradiation therapy (that are delivered more specifically to the prostate and infrequently encompass the bladder and the pelvic lymph nodes) will be associated with similar increased risks for bladder cancer are not known. Urologists should use this information to remind them to diligently evaluate men with radiation-therapy treated prostate cancer who develop hematuria and should not ascribe that hematuria to some benign cause, such as radiation induced cystitis, without fully evaluating the patient.

G.L. Andriole, Jr., M.D.

Treatment Considerations for Persons With Metastatic Prostate Cancer: Survival Versus Out-of-Pocket Costs
Matchar DB, McCrory DC, Bennett CL (Duke Univ, Durham, NC; Univ Med School, Chicago)
Urology 49:218–224, 1997   17–20

Background.—Treatment of metastatic prostate cancer must consider not only the method's effectiveness on patient survival but also the patient's quality of life after treatment. For drug treatments not covered by medical insurance or Medicare, the patient's out-of-pocket expenses can have a significant impact on his quality of life. This study evaluated physicians' perceptions on the use of flutamide (cost: $200–$300/month, which Medicare does not cover) as adjunctive therapy to orchiectomy or medical castration in treating metastatic prostate cancer.

Methods.—Forty-three oncologists and urologists who saw 5 or more patients with prostate cancer each week were convened into 4 focus groups to discuss common problems associated with the disease. Physicians were asked to estimate how much a patient would be willing to sacrifice from survival in order to avoid 5 specific health states associated with the disease (the time tradeoff technique). Physicians also completed a questionnaire addressing how important factors would be in prescribing flutamide: expected improvement in disease-free survival, gastrointestinal side effects, and cost of drug therapy.

Findings.—Every focus group reported that pain and weight loss/anorexia were the strongest influences on quality of life. Depression and urinary obstruction were also reported by more than half the groups. Physicians consistently rated worse health states with lower utility scores. The time tradeoff assessments revealed that physicians with older patients associated each of the 5 health states with better quality of life than did the physicians with younger patients. The out-of-pocket cost of flutamide was the biggest influence on whether it would be prescribed, and this concern was balanced with the drug's ability to extend survival. All physicians showed a similar response, but physicians at HMOs were more sensitive to these factors than those in private or academic practices.

Conclusions.—Physicians were consistent in their assessments of quality of life for patients with metastatic prostate cancer. Physicians treating older patients typically felt that their patients had a better quality of life than physicians treating younger patients. Flutamide's cost is a significant factor in the decision to initiate therapy for all physicians, especially those in an HMO.

▶ Many of the treatments that cancer patients receive are associated with out-of-pocket costs. Especially important in this area are oral pharmaceuticals such as flutamide, bicalutamide, and nilutamide—oral anti-androgens that are not reimbursed by Medicare. In this study, physicians were asked to consider important tradeoffs of treatment benefit vs. out-of-pocket concerns. Of interest, physicians' concerns over out-of-pocket costs were the most important determinant of whether oral anti-androgen therapy would be prescribed. Also, physicians who worked in managed care settings (where out-of-pocket cost concerns for pharmaceuticals are less than in the fee-for-service setting) were more likely to prescribe oral anti-androgens, but they were the most sensitive to out-of-pocket cost considerations. This study is an example of health services research efforts providing good insight into patient care. It also illustrates an example of how variations in patterns of prostate cancer care are likely to be shaped by financial, rather than medical, considerations.

C.L. Bennett, M.D., Ph.D.

Bicalutamide for Advanced Prostate Cancer: The Natural Versus Treated History of Disease
Scher HI, Liebertz C, Kelly WK, et al (Mem Sloan-Kettering Cancer Ctr, NY; Cornell Univ, New York; Zeneca Pharmaceuticals, Wilmington, Del)
J Clin Oncol 15:2928–2938, 1997   17–21

Background.—Hormones play variable roles in different stages of prostate cancer. The optimal time to initiate antiandrogen therapy with bicalutamide, a pure antiandrogen, was determined in patients with various stages of prostate cancer and after various treatments.

Methods.—Bicalutamide, 200 mg/day, was administered to 104 patients with progressive prostate cancer. Tumors were classified as androgen-dependent (androgen-independent). Patients in the androgen-dependent group included 37 who had not received prior hormones and 16 who were either being treated with an intermittent approach or who had been treated with neoadjuvant therapy prior to surgical or radiation treatment. The androgen-independent group was subdivided into 4 groups: those who had a relapse after orchiectomy or gonadotropin-releasing hormone [GnRH] analogue monotherapy (first group, n = 13); those whose disease progressed despite androgen blockade with a GnRH analogue and flutamide, and who either responded (second group, n = 14) or did not respond (third group, n = 12) to flutamide withdrawal; and those whose disease progressed despite 2 hormone treatments exclusive of antiandrogen withdrawal (fourth group, n = 12).

Findings.—Bicalutamide had a much better effect on androgen-dependent tumors as measured by decreases in prostate-specific antigen (PSA) levels (88% vs. 10%, androgen-dependent vs. androgen-independent), an improvement in bone scan (48% vs. 12%, respectively), and regression of soft-tissue disease (37% vs. 0%, respectively). Response to bicalutamide did not differ significantly in the 2 subgroups of androgen-dependent tumors. In the androgen-dependent group as a whole, 5 of 15 patients with rising PSA after a GnRH analogue had a greater than 80% decrease in PSA levels. Of those who did not respond to bicalutamide plus GnRH analogue, bicalutamide withdrawal caused a greater than 80% decrease in PSA levels in 3 patients.

In the patients with androgen-independent tumors, those in the first group (relapse) experienced only a modest benefit from bicalutamide, and those in the fourth group (2 previous hormones) showed no response at all. However, both groups 2 and 3 (previous exposure to flutamide) received benefit, as 38% experienced a greater than 50% decrease in PSA level (no significant difference between groups 2 and 3). Adverse effects in all patients included decreases in libido, difficulty in erections, hot flashes, and breast swelling or tenderness or both.

Conclusions.—Prior hormone exposure had a significant effect on the response to the antiandrogen, bicalutamide. The drug had more effect on androgen-dependent tumors and in those androgen-independent tumors that had been exposed to flutamide. Thus, a patient's prior treatment history had a significant influence on response to therapy, and should be considered in individualizing patient management.

▶ This is an interesting article because it examines several permutations of androgen deprivation therapy for patients with advanced prostate cancer. These issues are becoming increasingly important as novel forms of hormone therapy using 5-alpha reductase inhibitors, and various androgen receptor blockers either alone or in combination are often being used as the initial form of androgen deprivation therapy instead of conventional approaches such as castration and continuous or intermittent luteinizing hormone-releasing hormone analogue administration. This article emphasizes 2 things: patients may respond to a second antiandrogen if they have previously had relapse during therapy with an antiandrogen, even if they have enjoyed a withdrawal response to eliminating the initial antiandrogen. Second, patients who are initially treated with androgen receptor blockers (and in other studies 5-alpha reductase inhibitors alone or in combination with androgen receptor blockers) respond to conventional forms of androgen deprivation subsequently. Although these authors looked mostly at PSA response rather than survival, more studies are necessary to confirm the survival advantages of these approaches of androgen deprivation therapy.

G.L. Andriole, Jr., M.D.

Clinical Benefits of Bicalutamide Compared With Flutamide in Combined Androgen Blockade for Patients With Advanced Prostatic Carcinoma: Final Report of a Double-blind, Randomized, Multicenter Trial
Schellhammer PF, for the Casodex Combination Study Group (Eastern Virginia Med School, Norfolk)
Urology 50:330–336, 1997   17–22

Introduction.—For the treatment of prostate cancer, studies have been conducted comparing combined androgen blockade and the pairing of antiandrogen therapy with medical or surgical castration. Those studies combining an antiandrogen with a luteinizing hormone–releasing hormone analogue have demonstrated a significant benefit for survival. Severe symptoms of gastrointestinal toxicity have been seen with flutamide therapy, the availability of an antiandrogen with equal efficacy but a better profile for gastrointestinal toxicity and a greater convenience than the 3-times-daily dosage schedule would be more advantageous for the patients. An orally active nonsteroidal antiandrogen, bicalutamide, with negligible gastrointestinal intolerance can be taken only once a day. Previous reports have published the results at a median follow-up of 49 weeks and a median follow-up of 95 weeks. This report gave the results after a median follow-up of 160 weeks.

Methods.—There were 813 patients with metastatic prostate cancer randomized in a double-blind fashion 1-to-1 to bicalutamide (50 mg once daily) or flutamide (250 mg 3 times daily), and 2-to-1 to goserelin acetate (3.6 mg every 29 days) or leuprolide acetate (7.5 mg every 28 days).

Results.—For the bicalutamide plus luteinizing hormone–releasing hormone analogue group, the median time to progression and death was 97 weeks; for the flutamide plus luteinizing hormone–releasing hormone analogue group, the median time to progression and death was 180 weeks. The hazard ratio for time to progression for bicalutamide plus luteinizing hormone–releasing hormone analogue to flutamide plus luteinizing hormone–releasing hormone analogue was 0.93; for survival time, the ratio was 0.87. There was generally good tolerance to the therapies. Hot flashes were the most common adverse event in the 2 groups. The bicalutamide plus luteinizing hormone–releasing hormone analogue group had a higher incidence of hematuria than the flutamide plus luteinizing hormone–releasing hormone analogue group (12% vs. 6%). Hematuria did not cause any patients to withdraw from therapy. The flutamide plus luteinizing hormone–releasing hormone analogue group had a significantly higher incidence of diarrhea (26% vs. 12%) and more withdrawals for diarrhea (25 patients vs. 2 patients) than the bicalutamide plus luteinizing hormone–releasing hormone analogue group.

Conclusion.—Compared with flutamide plus luteinizing hormone–releasing hormone analogue, the combination of bicalutamide plus luteinizing hormone–releasing hormone analogue was well tolerated and had equivalent time to progression and survival after a median follow-up time of 160 weeks. Longer median survival was seen in treatment with bicalutamide plus luteinizing hormone–releasing hormone analogue than in treatment with flutamide plus luteinizing hormone–releasing hormone analogue.

▶ Results of this study were reported when 55% of the patients enrolled in the study had died (53% in the bicalutamide plus luteinizing hormone–releasing hormone analogue arm and 57% in the flutamide plus luteinizing hormone–releasing hormone analogue arm). The hazard ratio for death after bicalutamide was 0.87 with 95% confidence intervals ranging from 0.72 to 1.05. The patients receiving bicalutamide appear to have experienced fewer adverse events leading to withdrawal; this was most notable with respect to gastrointestinal function, including higher rates of diarrhea, liver function abnormalities, and nausea and/or vomiting among flutamide-treated patients.

This large study comparing 4 different forms of total androgen blockade must now be evaluated in light of recent reports that there may not be much benefit to adding antiandrogen therapy if orchiectomy is the form of testicular androgen ablation.[1] Why patients in earlier studies who had undergone luteinizing hormone–releasing hormone analogue therapy alone or orchiectomy alone seemed to fare worse than those who underwent similar procedures but who also took an antiandrogen remains enigmatic. For now, however, the weight of emerging evidence seems to suggest that a minority of patients benefit significantly from the addition of an antiandrogen. Moreover, it is not clear whether earlier data suggesting that patients with minimal metastatic disease benefit the most are actually true.

G.L. Andriole, Jr., M.D.

Reference

1. Crawford ED, Eisenberger MA, McLeod DG, et al: Comparison of bilateral orchiectomy with or without flutamide for the treatment of patients with stage D2 adenocarcinoma of the prostate: Results of NCI Intergroup Study 0105 (SWOG and ECOG) *J Urol* 157 (suppl):336, 1997.

Combined Finasteride and Flutamide Therapy in Men With Advanced Prostate Cancer

Ornstein DK, Rao GS, Johnson B, et al (Washington Univ, St Louis)
Urology 48:901–905, 1996   17–23

Background.—Conventional hormone therapy has a high response rate in men with advanced prostate cancer. However, it also has some undesirable side effects—such as decreased libido and impotence, hot flashes, lethargy, and muscle weakness—that are often treatment limiting. Flutamide and other nonsteroidal antiandrogenic agents may be used to limit the side effects of conventional hormone therapy, but they are not as effective on their own. A combination of finasteride and flutamide was tested in men with advanced prostate cancer.

Methods.—The study included 13 men with advanced prostate cancer who had not previously received hormone therapy. Four had stage D2 disease, 1 each had stage D1 and D0 disease, and 7 had rising prostate-specific antigen (PSA) levels after radical prostatectomy or definitive radiation therapy. All patients received finasteride, 5 mg/day. When their serum PSA levels stabilized, flutamide, 250 mg 3 times daily, was added. The tolerability effects of finasteride alone on serum PSA and hormone levels were assessed. Then the effects of adding flutamide were evaluated.

Results.—Finasteride monotherapy lasted for a median of 5 weeks. Serum PSA levels were unchanged with finasteride but decreased by 91% in response to finasteride plus flutamide. With combination therapy, the serum PSA level fell below 4 ng/mL in 85% of patients and became undetectable in 46%. The serum testosterone level was unaffected by finasteride alone, but serum dihydrotestosterone fell by 74%. With the addition of flutamide, serum testosterone decreased by 56%, with no further change in serum dihydrotestosterone. Eighty-five percent of subjects had side effects while receiving combination therapy, including gynecomastia or breast tenderness in 62% and diarrhea in 23%. Impotence was avoided in two thirds of patients. In 5 patients, combination therapy was halted because of flutamide-induced diarrhea or disease progression. This left 8 patients, all with serum PSA levels of less than 4 ng/mL and 4 with undetectable levels. The median duration of combination therapy in this group was 11 months.

Conclusion.—For most men with advanced prostate cancer, the combination of finasteride and flutamide significantly reduces serum PSA levels, often to undetectable levels. This combination therapy preserves potency and is well tolerated, although gynecomastia and diarrhea may occur. Finasteride plus flutamide may be a useful treatment option for patients with advanced prostate cancer who refuse conventional hormone therapy. More study—including longer follow-up and cost-benefit analysis—is needed.

▶ Conventional hormone therapy for advanced prostate cancer is associated with unacceptable side effects especially for men who have asymptomatic manifestations of advanced prostate cancer (for example, biochemical failure after local therapy or minimal stage D disease). Because of this, there has been great interest in developing novel forms of hormone therapy that are oral, easily reversible, and not associated with the typical side effects.

One such approach is to treat men with finasteride and flutamide (or another androgen-receptor blocker). In this small series of patients, men with biochemical failure achieved approximately 97% reduction in their serum PSA levels and 57% achieved an undetectable level. By comparison, men with stage D disease had a mean 81% PSA reduction, and only 33% achieved an undetectable level.

The duration of response to this form of androgen manipulation and the probability of a secondary response to more conventional approaches (such as administration of a luteinizing hormone–releasing hormone analogue) are not presently known, but preliminary evidence suggests that PSA response to this modality will exceed 1 year for most patients, and nearly all will later respond to conventional approaches. If cost and side effects are acceptable, such therapies may be offered more commonly to men with biochemical failure after radical prostatectomy or radiation therapy.

G.L. Andriole, Jr., M.D.

Bone Fractures Associated With Luteinizing Hormone–Releasing Hormone Agonists Used in the Treatment of Prostate Carcinoma
Townsend MF, Sanders WH, Northway RO, et al (Emory Univ, Atlanta, Ga)
Cancer 79:545–550, 1997   17–24

Objective.—Treatment of prostate cancer with luteinizing hormone-releasing hormone agonists (LHRH-a) decreases bone density in men and increases their risk of fractures. The incidence of bone fractures in patients with prostate cancer receiving LHRH-a was established.

Methods.—Medical records were reviewed and telephone interviews were conducted with 224 of 302 patients aged 45–96 years with prostate cancer treated with LHRH-a between 1988 and 1995. Date of first LHRH-a injection, number of monthly injections, age, clinical stage of disease, sites of metastases, and history of bone fracture were determined.

Results.—Since their first injection, 20 (9%) patients had a bone fracture, 19 within 1 month of injection. Nine patients were censored based on fractures occurring within 12 months of starting injections, those resulting from trauma or motor vehicle accidents, or those considered to be pathologic. The remaining 11 (5%) patients had an average treatment time to fracture of 19.6 months, whereas the average for all patients was 22.2 (1–96 months) and for nonfracture patients was 20.8. Ten fractures were treated at hospitals other than the hospitals where LHRH-a was administered, and no fracture information was recorded on the urology clinic chart.

Conclusion.—The incidence of fracture in a cohort of patients with prostate cancer receiving LHRH-a was 9%. The incidence of osteoporotic fractures was 5%.

▶ This is one of a few manuscripts pointing out that patients who receive long-term androgen deprivation experience relatively high rates of fractures (9% of men followed up for a mean of 20.8 months [range, 1 to 96]). This manuscript provides a cautionary tale for use of androgen deprivation among patients with biochemical relapse after failed therapy for early-stage disease. Such patients would be anticipated to receive androgen deprivation for many years. The finding of osteoporotic fractures and other reports describing anemia and overall reduced quality of life from lassitude and weakness suggests that in the future continuous testicular androgen deprivation will probably be avoided. Whether we will use intermittent androgen deprivation or alternative oral forms of androgen deprivation (such as androgen receptor blockers in conjunction with 5-α reductase inhibitors) remains to be seen.

G.L. Andriole, Jr., M.D.

Phase II Trial of Suramin, Leuprolide, and Flutamide in Previously Untreated Metastatic Prostate Cancer
Dawson NA, Figg WD, Cooper MR, et al (Natl Cancer Inst, Bethesda, Md)
J Clin Oncol 15:1470–1477, 1997   17–25

Introduction.—The death rate for cancer of the prostate continues to rise, even though metastatic disease is present in a significantly lower percentage of patients at diagnosis. Current therapy for metastatic prostate cancer results in disease regression in most patients, but responses are not durable. A pilot trial evaluated the efficacy and toxicity of the 3-drug combination of leuprolide, flutamide, and suramin in patients with poorly differentiated stage D1 or any stage D2 prostate cancer.

Methods.—Fifty patients were enrolled in the trial, 48 with stage D2 and 2 with stage D1 disease. None had been treated with prior hormonal therapy or chemotherapy. Flutamide (250 mg orally 3 times daily) was taken from day 1 until disease progression. Depot leuprolide (7.5 mg IM) was started on day 5 and repeated every 4 weeks indefinitely. The pharmacokinetically derived dosing schedule for suramin sought to maintain concentrations between 175 and 300 µg/mL. Patients also received daily doses of replacement hydrocortisone for suramin-induced adrenal insufficiency.

Results.—The mean age of the patient group was 59; 90% had bone metastases and 50% had soft-tissue metastases. Extent of disease was classified as severe in 82% and minimal in 18%. Three patients (6%) achieved a complete remission, which was maintained at 19, 37, and 42 months. Partial remissions that ranged in duration from 5 months to >61 months occurred in 30 (60%) patients, 10 of whom had not progressed at follow-up ranging from 10 to 61 months. Although the overall response rate was 69%, 36 (72%) of the 50 patients have progressed and 18 (36%) have died. Grade 3 to 4 toxicity, reported in 38% of patients, was predominantly hematologic and reversible in all cases.

Discussion.—Progressive disease develops in nearly all patients with metastatic prostate cancer. In this phase II trial of patients with a poor prognosis, the 3-agent therapy with suramin produced a high response rate and prolonged survival. A decline in prostate-specific antigen level to <0.5 ng/ml was associated with excellent 2-year survival of 92%.

▶ This is exactly the type of innovative study that is necessary for men with metastatic prostate cancer. The plethora of studies evaluating conventional vs. total androgen deprivation have defined fairly accurately the ability of this form of treatment to prolong survival. This study was undertaken to test the hypothesis that early inhibition of both androgen-dependent and androgen-independent prostate cancer cells may result in overall prolonged survival. To test this hypothesis, the authors enrolled men with high-risk stage D disease, as defined by the presence of poorly differentiated primary tumor. This pilot study of 50 men shows an overall response rate of 67% and an estimated median survival rate of 63% at 3 years (median survival has not yet been reached). These results are encouraging when one considers the poor prognosis of this group as a whole. However, one must balance the improved response and apparent improved survival in these patients against the 38% incidence of grade III to IV toxicity and also the expense of this therapy. Moreover, this trial must be placed in perspective, along with other innovative approaches measuring not just survival but also quality-of-life endpoints for patients with advanced prostate cancer. Specifically, this therapy should be tested against conventional forms of total androgen blockade, intermittent total androgen blockade, and oral anti-androgen therapies followed by conventional approaches.

G.L. Andriole, Jr., M.D.

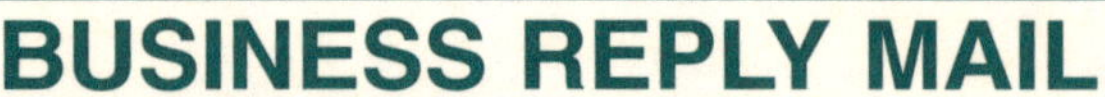

BUSINESS REPLY MAIL
FIRST-CLASS MAIL   PERMIT NO 135   ST LOUIS MO

POSTAGE WILL BE PAID BY ADDRESSEE

 Mosby

PAT NEWMAN
11830 WESTLINE INDUSTRIAL DRIVE
PO BOX 46908
ST. LOUIS   MO 63146-9934

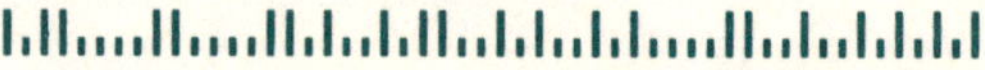

BUSINESS REPLY MAIL
FIRST-CLASS MAIL   PERMIT NO 135   ST LOUIS MO

POSTAGE WILL BE PAID BY ADDRESSEE

Mosby

PAT NEWMAN
11830 WESTLINE INDUSTRIAL DRIVE
PO BOX 46908
ST. LOUIS   MO 63146-9934

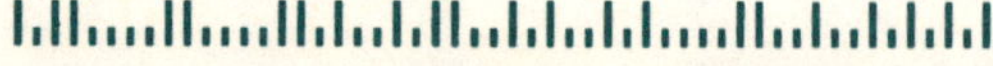

Want to speed up the process?

To order, you also may call 1-800-426-4545.

Mosby, Inc.
11830 Westline Industrial Drive
St. Louis, MO   63146 U.S.A.

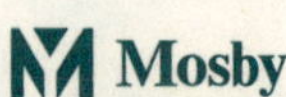 Mosby

Disease-Free and Overall Survival After Cryosurgical Monotherapy for Clinical Stages B and C Carcinoma of the Prostate: A 20-Year Followup
Porter MP, Ahaghotu CA, Loening SA, et al (Univ of Iowa, Iowa City)
J Urol 158:1466–1469, 1997   17–26

Introduction.—There is ongoing controversy regarding the use of cryosurgery for prostate cancer. The debate cannot be answered without long-term follow-up of cryosurgically treated patients. The long-term results of cryosurgical monotherapy for patients initially treated in the 1970s were reported.

Patients.—The single-center study included 66 patients receiving cryosurgical monotherapy for prostate cancer from 1973 to 1977. The patients' mean age was 67 years. There were 51 patients (mean age, 67 years) with clinically localized prostate cancer: stage B in 11 patients and stage C in 40. Eleven patients had well-differentiated tumors, 26 had moderately differentiated tumors, 11 had poorly differentiated tumors, and 3 had undetermined differentiation. Follow-up information was available for all patients but 2 at a mean follow-up of 94 months.

Outcomes.—Seventy-eight percent of patients had recurrence. There were 34 local and 6 unspecified recurrences. Adjuvant therapy was used to treat all recurrences. Forty-seven percent of patients died of prostate cancer, and 33% died of unspecified causes. The median overall progression-free survival was 34 months and the median overall survival was 75 months, according to Kaplan-Meier analysis. By grade, median progression-free survival was 34 months for patients with well-differentiated tumors, 36 months for those with moderately differentiated tumors, and 14 months for those with poorly differentiated tumors. The median progression-free survival was 57 months for patients with stage B disease and 30 months for those with stage C disease. The median overall survival was 114 months for well-differentiated tumors, 80 months for moderately differentiated tumors, 82 months for poorly differentiated tumors, 60 months for stage B disease, and 78.5 months for stage C disease.

Conclusion.—Long-term follow-up suggests that cryosurgery does not achieve effective local control of prostate cancer. Many patients die of prostate cancer, and most of these have local relapse at the time. Although duration of tumor response differs significantly with tumor stage and grade, overall survival does not.

▶ This long-term follow-up from the institution that launched cryosurgery in the early 1960s is eye opening. Forty of 51 patients died of prostate cancer if they had localized disease that was treated with cryosurgery monotherapy alone. Although these data cannot be compared with data on the contemporary use of cryosurgery (i.e., US-guided, using multiple freeze-thaw cycles, and treating tumors that are likely to be significantly smaller than those in this series), it is nonetheless discouraging that such a high proportion of patients died of prostate cancer and that most of them manifested local failure as a component of their disease progression.

G.L. Andriole, Jr., M.D.

The Efficacy and Complications of Salvage Cryotherapy of the Prostate
Pisters LL, von Eschenbach AC, Scott SM, et al (Univ of Texas, Houston)
J Urol 157:921–925, 1997   17–27

Background.—When local recurrence of prostate cancer develops after radiation therapy, tumor behavior is aggressive and outcome is poor. In some of these patients, the persistent disease appears to be localized only, with undetectable serum prostate-specific antigen (PSA) after salvage prostatectomy. Additional, aggressive local treatment might be beneficial in this subgroup. Cryotherapy was evaluated as salvage therapy for patients with local recurrence of prostate cancer after full-dose radiation therapy, systemic therapy, or both.

Methods.—The phase I/II trial included 150 patients who had locally recurrent prostate cancer after primary therapy with radiation, hormonal therapy, and/or systemic chemotherapy. All received salvage cryotherapy, consisting of a single freeze-thaw cycle in 71 patients and a double freeze-thaw cycle in 79 patients. The mean follow-ups were 17 and 10 months, respectively. The patients were followed up with PSA measurements every 3 months and sextant biopsy every 6 months. In addition to review of complications, quality of life was assessed by questionnaire.

Results.—Serum PSA became persistently undetectable in 31% of patients. The negative biopsy rate for patients treated by radiation therapy and then a double freeze-thaw cycle was 93%, compared with 71% for those who had a single freeze-thaw cycle. The double–freeze-thaw-cycle group also had a lower biochemical failure rate (i.e., an increase in serum PSA of 0.2 ng/mL above the nadir) at 44% vs. 65%, for the single freeze-thaw group. Seventy-three percent of patients experienced urinary incontinence, 67% had obstructive symptoms, and 72% had impotence. Severe perineal pain occurred in 8% of patients.

Conclusion.—For patients with locally recurrent prostate cancer, salvage cryotherapy provides a high rate of negative follow-up biopsies. Efficacy seems greater if a double freeze-thaw cycle is used rather than a single cycle. Salvage cryotherapy carries considerable long-term morbidity, as does salvage prostatectomy. Further study of cryotherapy for localized prostate cancer is needed.

▶ This report details results in 150 patients with locally recurrent prostate cancer after receiving radiation alone or in combination with other therapies. The net impact of salvage cryotherapy in this group of patients does not seem that impressive. Only 31% of patients had persistently undetectable serum PSA and between 18% and 36% of patients had persistent prostate cancer at posttreatment biopsy. Moreover, the sequalae of this therapy appear to be significant and included high rates of incontinence, obstruction, and impotence.

Based on these considerations, I find it hard to recommend salvage cryotherapy for patients with recurrence disease after radiation therapy. I think that it is probably more reasonable to consider salvage radical prostatectomy. Contemporary series have shown diminishing complications from this procedure, and 1 of the large cooperative cancer groups (Cancer and Leukemia Group B) has initiated a prospective study assessing the disease control capabilities and side effects of salvage radical prostatectomy. However, until the results of that study are available, salvage radical prostatectomy and salvage cryotherapy should probably be used sparingly for patients with persistent local disease after radiation therapy.

G.L. Andriole, Jr., M.D.

18 Outcomes/Quality of Life

Discrepancies Between Meta-analyses and Subsequent Large Randomized, Controlled Trials
LeLorier J, Grégoire G, Benhaddad A, et al (Hôtel-Dieu de Montréal Hosp; Univ of Montreal)
N Engl J Med 337:536–542, 1997
18–1

Background.—Although large, randomized, controlled clinical trials are considered definitive treatment efficacy evaluations, they are not always available. In the absence of such trials, clinicians are increasingly relying on meta-analysis to interpret data available from multiple small trials available from the literature. To understand the accuracy of meta-analysis projections, the results of a series of large randomized, controlled trials were compared to those of previously published relevant meta-analyses.

Study Design.—The *New England Journal of Medicine*, the *Lancet*, the *Annals of Internal Medicine*, and the *Journal of the American Medical Association* were searched for large randomized, controlled trials published from 1991 through 1994. Prior meta-analyses on these same topics were sought. The results of each trial were compared to those of the corresponding meta-analyses. Both principle and secondary outcomes were evaluated.

Findings.—The literature search identified 12 large randomized, controlled trials with 19 corresponding meta-analyses. Of the 40 primary and secondary outcomes analyzed, agreement bewteen these 2 methods was only fair. The positive predictive value of the meta-analyses was 68%, and the negative predictive value was 67%. In each case where findings disagreed, a significant treatment effect was determined by one method and no significant effect was found by the other method.

Conclusions.—The results of meta-analyses were not predictive of the results of large randomized, controlled clinical trials in about one third of cases. This implies that on the basis of meta-analysis alone, an ineffective treatment would have been advocated one third of the time.

▶ The field of meta-analyses represents a growth industry in the medical literature, as evidenced by the steadily increasing number of publications in this area in major U.S. and European journals. No area of medicine is complete until a rigorous meta-analysis is performed. Unfortunately, the field of meta-analysis is often closer to a science, with important methodologic considerations varying between these analyses (for example, inclusion and exclusion criteria for the relevant studies, variable quality of the studies, and review of individual patient-level data vs. study-based overview). Where discrepancies exist between the results of large randomized, controlled trials and meta-analyses, debate will follow about which study represents the "truth." This issue is especially relevant in metastatic prostate cancer where rigorous meta-analyses evaluating total androgen blockade and a large number of large randomized, controlled trials have produced conflicting results. While a significant proportion of both types of studies has found evidence supporting total androgen blockade, an almost equally large proportion of both types of studies has not been supportive. The end result is extreme confusion among clinicians, instead of the order that is the goal of the meta-analyses. Additional research in the area of meta-analyses of total androgen blockade is needed in order to explain why these discrepancies exist.

C.L. Bennett, M.D., Ph.D.

Use of Radical Prostatectomy Among Medicare Beneficiaries Before and After the Introduction of Prostate Specific Antigen Testing
Lu-Yao GL, Friedman M, Yao S-L (Johns Hopkins Oncology Ctr, Baltimore, Md)
J Urol 157:2219–2222, 1997   18–2

Background.—Nerve-sparing radical prostatectomy significantly increased the number of patients willing to undergo surgery for early stage prostate cancer. Improvements in early detection using prostate-specific antigen (PSA) further increased the incidence of this procedure. More recently, studies have demonstrated long-term survival in patients treated more conservatively. A national database was employed to evaluate the use of radical prostatectomy before and after the advent of PSA testing.

Study Design.—The hospitalization bills of all Medicare beneficiaries from 1984 through 1995 were examined to identify patients undergoing radical prostatectomies. Patients were excluded if they were younger than 65 years, outside the United States, were not enrolled in Medicare part A, or were enrolled in HMOs. Medicare enrollment files were used to define the at-risk population, and age-adjusted rates were standardized to the 1990 U.S. Medicare population.

Findings.—The rates of radical prostatectomy increased from 1984 to 1992 and then decreased. During the peak year, the age-adjusted rate of radical prostatectomy for white men aged 65 to 79 years was 461/100,000 and for black men was 294/100,000. Between 1992 and 1995, rates decreased, especially among whites and elderly men. The differences in the age-adjusted rates of radical prostatectomy between black and white men narrowed in more recent years.

Conclusions.—In the U.S. Medicare population, there was an increase in the use of radical prostatectomy for the treatment of early stage prostate cancer which peaked in 1992. After 1992, the use of radical prostatectomy decreased, especially among white and elderly men. Racial differences in the rate of use of radical prostatectomy has lessened in recent years.

▶ Health services research studies in prostate cancer are important to policy makers. One of the richest data sources is the Medicare data files, given the demographic characteristics of patients with prostate cancer. Lu-Yao *et al.* have been at the forefront of these outcomes studies, with important analyses of data from the Health Care Financing Administration.

Documenting the marked increase in the rate of radical prostatectomies through Medicare files is one example of these kinds of analyses. Of note is the peak of radical prostatectomies in 1992, immediately after PSA testing peaked. While racial differences in radical prostatectomies were apparent in 1992, these differences had narrowed by 1995. Finally, age-related variations in rates of radical prostatectomies are apparent in these analyses, with significantly higher rates among younger individuals (as expected). These studies represent an important area of research. Additional studies from other databases (such as the Veterans Administration and managed care organizations) will be important in the future.

C.L. Bennett, M.D., Ph.D.

References

1. Lu-Yao GL, Greenberg ER. Changes in prostate cancer incidence and treatment in USA. *Lancet* 343:251, 1994.
2. Lu-Yao GL, McLerran D, Wasson J, et al: An assessment of radical prostatectomy. Time trends, geographic variation, and outcomes. *JAMA* 269:2633, 1993.
3. Baron JA, Lu-Yao GL, Barrett JA, et al: Internal validation of Medicare claims data. *Epidemiology* 5:541, 1994.

Relative Importance of Sexuality and Quality of Life in Patients With Prostatic Symptoms: Results of an International Study
Da Silva FC, Marquis P, Deschaseaux P, et al (Hosp Desterro, Lisbon, Portugal; MAPI, Lyon, France; Pierre-Fabre Médicament, Castres, France; et al)
Eur Urol 31:272–280, 1997   18–3

Background.—Outcomes, including quality of life (QoL) and sexual functioning, are important in evaluating the effect of treatment for benign prostatic hyperplasia (BPH). There is no consensus on what should be assessed to determine the effect of treatment on QoL. A study was performed to determine what issues BPH patients felt were most important to their QoL.

Study Design.—A literature search of Medline, Excerpta Medica, Psychabstract, and OLGA was conducted for QoL surveys for BPH patients and for sexual functioning surveys. Ten BPH specific questionnaires and 18 sexual functioning questionnaires were identified. A French and English questionnaire was generated that included at least 1 question for every concept covered by the surveys derived from the literature search. These questionnaires were given to 117 prostatic patients in France and the United Kingdom who were over 50 years of age, had symptoms for at least 6 months, and had an International Prostate Symptom Score (I-PSS) of at least 7. French and United Kingdom data were compared using Cochran-Mantel-Haenzel statistics.

Findings.—This group of prostate patients reported that the most important issues were sleep, anxiety about the disease, mobility, leisure, daily activities, sexual activities, and satisfaction in sexual relationships. French patients considered the sexual aspects to be more important than English patients.

Conclusions.—This study confirms that quality of life, including sexual functioning, is important to BPH patients. It also demonstrates the value of cross-cultural comparisons.

► Assessment of quality of life is increasingly important in health care today. Development of standardized tools that allow for evaluation of health status in urology is imperative. The I-PSS is an important effort in this regard. This paper is important and allows for additional data about the utility of the I-PSS in various clinical settings.

The paper by Da Silva et al. builds on the concept of international validation of QoL instruments, including the I-PSS. Cross-cultural assessments are rarely done but with the widespread dissemination of quality of life instruments are becoming very important. Identification of specific aspects of quality of life, such as sexual function, that are likely to be important to broad populations of individuals is likely to be useful to physicians and policy makers. Of interest is the finding that sexual function was more important to French than English men with benign prostatic hypertrophy. Additional studies of QoL instruments in more countries are needed.

C.L. Bennett, M.D., Ph.D.

Quality of Life and Treatment Outcomes: Prostate Carcinoma Patients' Perspectives After Prostatectomy or Radiation Therapy
Shrader-Bogen CL, Kjellberg JL, McPherson CP, et al (HealthSystem Minnesota, Minneapolis; Univ of Minnesota, Minneapolis)
Cancer 79:1977–1986, 1997   18–4

Background.—Prostate cancer was diagnosed in 317,000 U.S. men in 1996. A majority of cases (57%) are diagnosed when the disease is still localized, and survival for this group is excellent (98%). Prostatectomy and radiotherapy are the standard treatments, yet both are associated with long-term side effects. How either treatment affects patient-reported quality of life after 5 years is the subject of this article.

Methods.—Two hundred seventy-four men with stage I or II adenocarcinoma of the prostate were questioned 1 to 5 years after their initial treatment. Prostatectomy had been performed in 132 men (48%), and radiotherapy was used in 142 men (52%). Each received a questionnaire that included demographic information, a Functional Assessment of Cancer Therapy-General (FACT-G) form (to evaluate overall quality of life), and a newly created Prostate Cancer Treatment Outcome Questionnaire (PCTO-Q) (to measure specific changes in bowel, urinary, and sexual functions).

Findings.—Patients who had undergone prostatectomy were significantly younger (average age 66.2) than patients who had undergone radiotherapy (average age 75.3); thus the 2 data sets were adjusted for age. The 2 groups did not differ significantly in any of the subscales of the FACT-G. As for the PCTO-Q, bowel function was significantly worse in patients who had received radiotherapy, particularly relating to diarrhea, urgency, and bleeding with bowel movement; the difference in reported quality of life scores between the 2 patient groups was not significant. Urinary symptoms were significantly worse in patients who had received a prostatectomy, particularly regarding leaking, leaking with coughing or sneezing, and nocturia. The difference in reported quality of life scores between the 2 patient groups was significant. Finally, sexual function was significantly worse in patients who had undergone a prostatectomy, particularly regarding the ability to achieve an erection. The difference in reported quality-of-life scores between the 2 patient groups was significant.

Conclusions.—The FACT-G, a more general measure of well-being, did not reveal significant quality-of-life differences between radiotherapy and prostatectomy. However, the more specific PCTO-Q did uncover significant differences between the 2 groups in bowel function (worse with radiotherapy), urinary symptoms (worse with prostatectomy), and sexual function (worse with prostatectomy). These results should be openly discussed when counseling patients about therapy options.

▶ In one of the larger studies of quality of life of men with prostate cancer, this report provides pilot information on 274 men with localized prostate cancer who were between 1 and 5 years out from radiation therapy or prostatectomy. A cancer specific questionnaire, the FACT-G, which has been extensively tested and validated in the general cancer population, and a newly developed prostate cancer tool (the PCTO-Q) were used. Scores in the FACT-G were similar between the 2 groups, while the PCTO-Q instrument identified more bowel dysfunction among the radiotherapy group and more urinary and sexual dysfunction problems among the prostatectomy group. The study results suggest that validation of prostate cancer specific instruments for both localized and metastatic disease patients is important and should be the focus of research in the future.

C.L. Bennett, M.D., Ph.D

Results of Hospital Cancer Registry Surveys by the American College of Surgeons: Outcomes of Prostate Cancer Treatment by Radical Prostatectomy

Mettlin CJ, Murphy GP, Sylvester J, et al (Roswell Park Cancer Inst, Buffalo, NY; Northwest Hosp, Seattle; American College of Surgeons, Chicago; et al)
Cancer 80:1875–1881, 1997   18–5

Introduction.—For the treatment of patients with prostate cancer, there has been an increased use of radical prostatectomy. Continuous monitoring and assessment on the long-term outcomes and complications of this procedure are necessary. Trends in radical prostatectomy use and outcomes from the perspective of cancer registries in which the procedure is performed are analyzed.

Methods.—In 1993, surveys were sent to hospital cancer registries requesting data on patients treated by radical prostatectomy on up to 5 patients treated in their institutions in 1990. There were 482 hospitals concerning 2,122 patients in response to this survey. Three years later, surveys were sent requesting data on treatment administered to the 1990 patients up to 5 years after surgery and data on new patients diagnosed in 1993. There were 265 hospitals who provided data on 1,304 patients in this survey. The probability of additional treatment after radical prostatectomy was determined with Kaplan-Meier survival curves.

Results.—For both sets of patients, similar surgical pathology outcomes were reported. For 1990, 27.5% of patients maintained erectile function adequate for intercourse after surgery, and for 1993, 29.7% of patients maintained erectile function. For 1990, 81.3% of patients reported complete control or only occasional urinary incontinence requiring no pads. For 1993, this was true for 79.8% of patients. For both groups of patients, the surgical mortality rates were less than 1%. There was a 10.5% 5-year cumulative probability of any additional treatment after radical prostatectomy. Greater probability of additional treatment was significantly associated with seminal vesicle involvement, positive surgical margins, lymph node involvement, capsular penetration, high Gleason score, and high prostate specific antigen.

Conclusion.—To reconcile the differences in outcomes reported from different data sources, continuing evaluation of the outcomes of prostate cancer treatments is needed.

▶ An additional unanswered question about early detection of prostate cancer relates to how the surgery relates to quality of life following surgical treatment. If the likelihood of maintenance of sexual functioning is low, then additional concerns over large-scale early detection programs are raised. In this study based on voluntary reporting from tumor registries, between 25% and 30% of men retained erectile function that would be satisfactory for intercourse, whereas 80% reported satisfactory urinary function. Comparison of these results with more recent studies is needed because many studies report higher rates of sexual function after nerve-sparing radical prostatectomy. As with most other studies, African-American men are underrepresented, accounting for between 5% and 10% of the patients. Additional studies in African-American men and in more recent time periods are needed.

C.L. Bennett, M.D., Ph.D.

Patient Satisfaction With Short Stays for Radical Prostatectomy
Litwin MS, Shpall AI, Dorey F (Univ of California, Los Angeles)
Urology 49:898–906, 1997

18–6

Introduction.—In a previous study, the authors reported that shortening of postoperative length of stay (LOS) after radical prostatectomy could achieve significant cost savings without increasing rates of complications or readmissions. There is concern, however, that patient satisfaction will be diminished with the increasingly shorter hospital stays. A questionnaire administered to 129 men sought to answer the question of whether shorter LOS lowers patient satisfaction.

Methods.—All patients had undergone radical retropubic prostatectomy for localized prostate cancer after a short-stay clinical care pathway was implemented. Their satisfaction with care was assessed by means of a previously validated, self-administered instrument. The 24-item survey included a global rating of overall satisfaction with care and questions related to hospital admission, daily care, level of patient information, nursing care, physician care, ancillary hospital staff, hospital atmosphere and building, discharge, and hospital billing. A separate instrument was used to collect sociodemographic and comorbidity data.

Results.—The survey response rate was 98%. Respondents had a mean age of 61.3; mean duration of time since surgery was 7.6 months. The majority of patients were white (90%) and employed full or part time (64%); 54% reported an annual income more than $75,000. Patient satisfaction was uniformly high, particularly in the area of physician care. Length of stay was 3 days for 97 patients, 2 days for 21, and at least 4 days for 11. Patient satisfaction did not vary by LOS, and 78% reported their LOS to be "just right." Health-related quality of life outcomes were also rated high, especially for physical and social function scores.

Discussion.—The introduction of a clinical care pathway to shorten LOS after prostatectomy did not lead to low levels of patient satisfaction. Reported levels of satisfaction in this group of relatively affluent patients did not appear to be correlated with LOS or with general or prostate-specific health-related quality-of-life scale scores.

▶ Satisfaction with care is important. Managed care organizations are rated, with some of the input based on patients' assessments of their satisfaction with the plan, medical facility, physician, and staff. Controversy exists over managed care plans initiating programs to shorten stays for radical mastectomies and radical prostatectomies. However, it is reassuring to find evi-

dence of patient satisfaction with short stays following radical prostatectomy, as reported by Litwin et al. Critical pathways may result in decreased
health care costs and increased patient satisfaction. Other centers have
found similar results.[1]

C.L. Bennett, M.D., Ph.D.

Reference

1. Palmer JS, Worwag EM, Conrad WG, et al: Same day surgery for radical retropubic
   prostatectomy: Is it an attainable goal? *Urology* 47:23–28, 1996.

**Caremap Management for Postoperative Prostatectomy Care at Home:
A Comparative Study**
Wilson DE, Jirsch DW, Mador DR, et al (Univ of Alberta, Edmonton, Canada)
Can J Surg 40:39–43, 1997   18–7

Objective.—The early discharge program providing community-based
home care for patients who underwent transurethral resection of the
prostate (TURP) was compared to traditional hospital care.

Methods.—The prospective comparative study involved 81 patients
who underwent TURP and were discharged on postoperative day 1 to a
community-based home care program provided by professional nurses and
117 TURP patients who remained in the hospital until postoperative day
2 or 3 and received standard hospital care. Readmission rate, reuse of
healthcare services, postoperative complications, and patient satisfaction
were determined in a structured telephone interview conducted 2 weeks
after discharge.

Results.—Of the 117 remaining in the hospital and receiving standard
care, 32 were hospitalized for 4 or more days as a result of complications.
Of the 85 patients discharged on day 2 or 3, 64 were contacted by
telephone 2 weeks later. Of the 81 early discharge patients, 63 were
contacted by telephone. There were no differences between groups with
respect to pain, reuse of health services, readmission, or complications.
Both groups were equally satisfied with care.

Conclusion.—There were no differences between early discharge and
standard care TURP patients with respect to pain, reuse of hospital services, readmission, complications, or patient satisfaction with care.

▶ Cost containment considerations have affected all aspects of medical
care, with the largest effects being seen among hospitalized individuals.
Efforts to decrease costs of care while maintaining or improving quality of
care are important. One such area is among men undergoing prostatectomy
for which programs that allow for early transfer to the home setting have
been implemented. Success of these programs has been documented in
many medical practice settings in the United States and Canada. However,
these efforts require coordination between the medical providers, home
care, nursing staff, and the patient pre- and postoperatively. This study from

Alberta, Canada, showed that among men undergoing a transurethral resection of the prostate, a 1-day hospitalization could be achieved without compromising patient satisfaction or clinical outcomes. Factors for success in this program are identified: local development of the care map, multidisciplinary input into the program, continuing education for all providers, and objective assessment of the program with respect to clinical and economic parameters.

C.L. Bennett, M.D., Ph.D.

Surgical Care and Outcome for Patients in Their Nineties
Burns-Cox N, Campbell WB, van Nimmen BAJ, et al (Royal Devon and Exeter Hosp, England)
Br J Surg 84:496–498, 1997   18–8

Background.—A growing number of very elderly patients are seen in hospitals. There are few data on the surgical outcomes of patients aged 90 and older. A 2-year experience with surgical patients in this age group is presented.

Patients.—The experience included 129 patients aged 90 or older who were hospitalized under the care of 5 general surgeons and 2 urologists. The patients were 88 women and 41 men, median age 92. The patients were admitted a total of 141 times, including 96 emergency and 45 elective admissions. Forty percent of admissions were for GI conditions, 16% were for undiagnosed abdominal pain, 16% were for hernia, 13% were for arterial disease, and 7% were for urologic problems.

Outcomes.—Sixty-six percent of admissions led to surgery, including 82% of elective admissions and 58% of emergency admissions. Hospital mortality was 12%—10% after elective surgery and 14% after emergency surgery. None of 9 surgical patients in American Society of Anesthesiologists grade 1 died. Mortality was 4% for patients in grade 2, 20% for those in grade 3, and 60% for those in grade 4. Survivors stayed in the hospital for a median of 6 days. Sixty-eight percent of patients who were admitted from home were discharged there.

Conclusions.—This study documents reasonably low mortality among very elderly patients admitted for surgery. Mortality is higher after emergency admission. Some patients in this age group admitted for "surgical" conditions may be better treated without surgery. Such decisions should include input from consultants, nursing staff, and the patient's family.

▶ As people live longer, studies of care of the elderly will increase in frequency. This study of surgical care and outcome for patients in their nineties is of general interest to surgeons. How old is too old comes up most frequently for elderly patients with hernias, gastrointestinal disorders such as acute cholecystitis, or bowel problems. In this study, only 7% of the admissions were for urologic conditions. Of note, 12% of the patients died postoperatively with a 10% rate for elective procedures. While the authors conclude that there is a reasonable expectation of survival for the nonagenarians, it is also reasonable to view the results as suggesting that there is enough mortality in the very old that one should be hesitant to recommend elective surgery in this group. At some point, being too old for surgery is likely to be a realistic statement. Ninety appears to be close to that point, at least as far as elective surgery is concerned.

C.L. Bennett, M.D., Ph.D.

Predictors of General Quality of Life in Patients With Benign Prostate Hyperplasia or Prostate Cancer

Krongrad A, Granville LJ, Burke MA, et al (Univ of Miami, Fla; Univ of Texas, Dallas; Univ of Illinois, Chicago)
J Urol 157:534–538, 1997   18–9

Objective.—There is a scarcity of information about quality of life issues and predictors of quality of life in patients with prostate disease. Most studies examine quality of life as it relates to disease-specific variables rather than to the emotional component. The role of emotional quality of life was evaluated using a neural network model to create predictive tools for assessing quality of life.

Methods.—Fifty veterans with either benign prostate hyperplasia or prostate cancer completed the 17-item Rand Mental Health Index at 1 and 6 months. These scores and clinical data were analyzed statistically using the feed-forward, back propagation neural networks, Baye's classifiers linear and quadratic discriminant function analysis, and stepwise logistic regression analysis.

Results.—The 1-month quality of life neural network model had a classification accuracy of 89%, compared with 49% for both linear and quadratic discriminant function analysis. At 6 months, the quality of life neural network model had an overall accuracy of 90%, compared with 57% and 43%, respectively, for linear and quadratic discriminant function analysis. Logical regression analysis was better able than the neural network model to identify significant inputs.

Conclusion.—Models of general quality of life for patients with prostate disease should include emotional quality of life measures to provide accurate predictions.

▶ Comparisons of quality of life of cancer patients are often made to persons in the general population or among individuals with the same diagnosis. Studies of men with benign and malignant prostate cancer provide an opportunity to evaluate health status in a group of men with similar symptoms and differing prognoses. In a pilot study of 50 veterans with benign prostate hyperplasia or prostate cancer, assessments were made at 1 month and 6 months time, using the 17-item version of the RAND Mental Health Index. As with other studies, the effort is limited by the small sample size. However, it does provide additional support for including health status

assessments for persons with similar symptoms, regardless of the underlying etiology.

C.L. Bennett, M.D., Ph.D.

Health-related Quality of Life Among Patients With Metastatic Prostate Cancer
Albertsen PC, Aaronson NK, Muller MJ, et al (Univ of Connecticut, Farming-
ton; Antoni Van Leeuwenhoek Hosp, Amsterdam; New England Med Ctr, Boston)
Urology 49:207–217, 1997   18–10

Objective.—Because of the increase in the incidence of prostate cancer, quality of life of survivors with advanced prostate cancer is a growing issue. Results are presented of a study quantifying and comparing the health-related quality of life (HRQL) of patients with advanced prostate cancer who had received a luteinizing hormone-releasing hormone agonist plus flutamide with the HRQL of age-matched normal controls.

Methods.—In a multicenter cross-sectional study, men with stage D2 prostate cancer receiving combination therapy self-administered the European Organization for Research and Treatment of Cancer Core Quality of Life Questionnaire-C30 and the Medical Outcomes Study Short Form Health Survey (SF-36). Patients were divided into 2 groups: those in remission (n = 60) and those with progression (n = 55). Responses were compared statistically.

Results.—Patients with progressive disease were more likely to have weight loss, extensive disease, a poorer performance rank, and more pain. Patients in remission reported a significantly better quality of life, a higher level of physical and social function and mental health, less fatigue, less weight loss, less appetite loss, and less pain than those with disease progression. Reports of urinary symptoms, sexual function, sexual satis-faction, hot flashes, diarrhea, and constipation were similar between groups although men in remission tended to rate them more highly. The HRQL responses for men in remission were similar to those reported for the general population of age-matched controls.

Conclusion.—The HRQL responses of men with advanced prostate cancer in remission were similar to those responses of age-related controls, whereas HRQL responses of men with advanced and progressive prostate cancer were significantly worse in all areas except for treatment-related problems.

▶ Prostate cancer treatments for localized and metastatic disease are characterized by considerations of both quantity and quality of life. One important area of debate of prostate cancer treatment is maximal androgen
blockade, where controversy exists over clinical benefit and quality of life.
General health status assessments with the Medical Outcomes SF-36 suggested that overall quality of life is similar between men in the general

population and those with metastatic prostate cancer in remission and receiving maximal androgen blockade therapy, whereas both groups reported better health status than did men with progressive metastatic prostate cancer who were receiving maximal androgen blockade. However, with respect to cancer-specific considerations, the stable and progressive prostate cancer groups did not differ significantly, as measured by a validated instrument, the European Organization for Research and Treatment of Cancer Quality of Life Questionnaire-C30. The study is limited by being a cross-sectional study of 113 patients (that is, only one interview for each prostate cancer patient). As with other quality-of-life reports, it is most important as a pilot effort. In addition, with the U.S. Medicare program moving toward incorporation of health status as an important measure of patient outcome, the study provides additional evidence of the feasibility of this effort.

C.L. Bennett, M.D., Ph.D.

Health Related Quality of Life Outcomes in Patients Treated for Metastatic Kidney Cancer: A Pilot Study
Litwin MS, Fine JT, Dorey F, et al (Univ of California, Los Angeles)
J Urol 157:1608–1612, 1997   18–11

Objective.—Quality-of-life issues are particularly important for patients treated for advanced cancer. Therapies for metastatic renal cell carcinoma do not significantly improve survival. The health-related quality of life in patients with kidney cancer surviving nephrectomy and tumor infiltrating lymphocytes plus interleukin-2 therapy were compared with those of the general population or those of patients having chronic diseases or other malignancies.

Methods.—Twenty of 25 patients, 20 men with metastatic kidney cancer treated with nephrectomy, tumor infiltrating lymphocytes, and interleukin-2 returned the RAND 36-Item Health Survey 1.0 (SF-36) measuring health-related quality of life and the Cancer Rehabilitation Evaluation System-Short Form measuring cancer-targeted quality of life. Responses were compared with those of patients with other types of cancer, with those of patients with diabetes, hypertension, arthritis, or congestive heart failure, and with responses from the general population. Medical comorbidity, sociodemographic, and tumor response data were collected.

Results.—Responses to therapy were complete for 20% of patients and partial for 25%. Thirty percent of patients had stable disease, 15% experienced progression, and 10% were not evaluable. Patients with metastatic kidney cancer surviving nephrectomy and therapy had health-related quality-of-life scores significantly higher than those of patients with heart failure, significantly lower than those of the general population, similar to or worse than those of patients with hypertension and diabetes, and similar to or better than those of patients with other cancers. Kidney cancer patients with more comorbid conditions tended to have lower scores.

Conclusion.—Kidney cancer patients surviving nephrectomy and subsequent therapies had higher quality of life scores than did patients with other cancers and heart failure but lower or similar quality-of-life scores than did patients with hypertension and diabetes. Health-related quality of life scores for kidney cancer patients were worse than for those of the general population. Additional larger studies need to be conducted before the results can be generalized.

▶ Health-related quality-of-life evaluations are becoming an integral aspect of cancer care. While many studies have addressed health status assessments for breast and prostate cancer, fewer studies have investigated these issues for less common malignancies. Health status includes aspects of general life issues, cancer-related concerns, and considerations specific to the particular type of cancer.

This paper on health-related quality of life for renal cancer provides some of the first assessments for persons with renal cell cancer, of which there are 25,000 new cases annually. While only 20 patients provided responses to the questions, the data are important in terms of being a pilot effort for a rarer disease. General health status issues were evaluated with a generic tool, the RAND 36-Item Health Survey (also known as the Medical Outcomes Short-Form 36), which has been evaluated in multiple studies of persons with and without cancer. The small number of patients, all of whom were being treated with tumor infiltrating lymphocytes and interleukin-2, reported worse overall quality of life than did the general population in 6 of 8 scales. Cancer-related quality-of-life assessments (using the Cancer and Rehabilitation Evaluation System-Short Form) were comparable to persons with other cancers in most dimensions. Although the study suggested that quality of life for renal cell patients receiving immunotherapy is better than for many other patient groups, caution is required. Any study that is based on 20 renal cancer patients, with only 3 persons with progressive disease with therapy, is unlikely to be broadly representative of the total population. Other studies with more patients are needed.

C.L. Bennett, M.D., Ph.D.

Which Patients Will Benefit From Psychosocial Intervention After Cystectomy for Bladder Cancer?

Månsson Å, Colleen S, Hermerén G, et al (Univ Hosp, Lund, Sweden)
Br J Urol 80:50–57, 1997   18–12

Background.—Patients with invasive bladder cancer vary in their ability to cope with diagnosis, treatment, and associated quality-of-life changes. Previous studies have indicated that both physical and psychosocial functioning were negatively affected by cystectomy. A psychosocial intervention program was created to improve adjustment of bladder cancer patients. The effects of this psychosocial program on the adjustment of bladder cancer patients was examined in a randomized clinical trial.

Methods.—The study population consisted of 40 men and 10 women, aged 46 to 84, with invasive bladder cancer, who did not receive preoperative chemotherapy. Prior to surgery, these patients were interviewed on their general outlook on life, and their psychological defensive strategies were assessed by the Meta-Contrast Technique. Half of these patients were randomized to receive a postoperative counseling program. Of the 50 patients, 17 received an ileal urinary conduit, 17 a continent reservoir with abdominal stoma, and 16 an orthotopic neobladder. Three months after surgery, the outlook on life was again ascertained and the standardized Sickness Impact Profile (SIP) questionnaire was administered.

Results.—There was no significant difference between the SIP results of these 2 groups of patients. Intervention benefited patients with continent cutaneous diversion, with lower SIP psychosocial scores. Meta-Contrast Technique analysis identified 3 groups of patients: those characterized by isolation and repression, repression and stereotypy, or sensitivity and stereotypy. Three clusters of philosophical outlook were identified. In patients characterized by a belief in a supernatural power and philosophical interest, those who participated in the counseling sessions had lower SIP scores than did those who did not participate.

Conclusions.—Invasive bladder cancer patients with pessimistic attitudes and an interest in philosophical questions, who use stereotypy and repression as defensive strategies, may benefit from post-surgical counseling.

▶ Quality-of-life studies of cancer patients are increasing in frequency, with little information on how they can be used to improve patient care. While a small number of studies have shown improved patient outcomes when they are involved in psychosocial interventions for breast cancer and melanoma, widespread use of these programs has yet to occur. These interventions are unlikely to be useful across the board. This study suggests that, among bladder cancer patients, those with certain attributes (pessimistic disposition, general interest in philosophical questions, and likely to use defensive strategies of stereotypy and repression) are more likely to benefit from psychosocial interventions than are others. Although these results are from a small study, they provide support for further evaluation in bladder cancer patients, many of whom face important questions related to quality of life.

C.L. Bennett, M.D., Ph.D.

19 Infertility

Endocrine Evaluation of Infertile Men
Sigman M, Jarow JP (Brown Univ, Providence, RI; Johns Hopkins Outpatient Ctr, Baltimore, Md)
Urology 50:659–664, 1997   19–1

Introduction.—Screening for treatable endocrinopathies is the purpose of endocrinologic testing of infertile men. The intact function of the hypothalamic-pituitary-gonadal axis is necessary for male reproductive and sexual function. Severe abnormalities of spermatogenesis and resultant oligospermia or azoospermia are typically associated with inadequate levels of gonadotropins and testosterone. The incidence of endocrinopathies in the infertile population is quite low, despite the fact that the prevalence of endocrine abnormalities among infertile men is higher than in the general adult male population. Men having a fertility evaluation frequently have routine endocrine testing. Limiting testing to only those patients with severe abnormalities on semen analysis is another approach. There is still no consensus as to who should be tested. The incidence of endocrinologic abnormalities among men having infertility evaluations was determined, and criteria to identify those men most likely to benefit from endocrine screening were identified.

Methods.—There were 1,035 men who were retrospectively reviewed. To determine whether endocrinologic screening could be limited to a specific subpopulation, results of endocrine testing were compared with medical history and physical and laboratory findings.

Results.—Upon repetitive testing, only 99 of 1,035 patients (9.6%) had abnormal endocrine studies. An isolated elevation of serum follicle-stimulating hormone levels was seen in the majority of these patients. A clinically significant endocrinopathy that would have had an effect on disease management was seen in only 1.7% of these men. For the detection of clinically significant endocrinopathy, screening with serum testosterone and follicle-stimulating hormone levels alone was just as effective as screening with a complete hormonal panel of testosterone, follicle-stimulating hormone, luteinizing hormone, and prolactin. If hormonal screening was limited to only those patients with sperm density of less than 10×10^6/mL, only 1 man with clinically significant endocrinopathy would not have been identified.

Conclusion.—A rare cause of male infertility is endocrinopathies. The vast majority of clinically significant endocrinopathies can be detected by endocrine screening with serum testosterone and follicle stimulating hormone levels alone of men with sperm counts of less than 10 million/mL.

▶ I agree with the authors that most infertile men are hormonally intact, especially those men with obvious diagnosis such as varicoceles. We have encountered 2 cases of asymptomatic hyperprolactinemia with normal testosterone levels, although such cases are rare. We have also observed that oligospermic men with low normal follicle-stimulating hormone levels tend to respond to clomiphene citrate better than those with high normal values. It is possible that some of these men have subtle pituitary deficiency that is not otherwise apparent. Ross reported a 8.4% incidence of adrenal dysfunction as evidenced by elevated dehydroepiandrosterone (DHEA) sulfate/17 hydroxyprogesterone levels.[1] These men are asymptomatic and manifest no other abnormalities. Seminal improvement is possible after low-dose prednisone therapy. I obtain follicle-stimulating hormone, testosterone, and DHEA-S in most patients.

J. Yuan, M.D.

Reference

1. Ross LS: Routine hormonal screening of infertile men: Is it worthwhile? *J Urol* 126:756–758, 1981.

Effects of Subinguinal Varicocele Ligation on Sperm Concentration, Motility and Kruger Morphology
Seftel AD, Rutchik SD, Chen H, et al (Case Western Reserve Univ, Cleveland, Ohio)
J Urol 158:1800–1803, 1997
19–2

Background.—There is ongoing debate over the effects of varicocelectomy on sperm morphology. In recent years, the Kruger strict criteria for morphologic characterization of sperm have become the new gold standard. However, these criteria have not been used to describe the effects of varicocelectomy on sperm morphology. This retrospective study examined the effects of varicocelectomy on Kruger morphology, sperm count, and motility.

Methods.—The study included 30 patients undergoing subinguinal varicocelectomy, including 25 bilateral and 5 unilateral cases. Sperm density, motility, and morphology were assessed before and after varicocele repair. Preoperative levels of follicle-stimulating hormone, luteinizing hormone, and testosterone were compared with those of fertile sperm donors.

Results.—For men with clinical bilateral varicoceles, varicocelectomy was followed by significant improvements in sperm density and motility. However, there were no accompanying changes in strict morphology. Men with subclinical varicocele or unilateral clinical varicocele showed no change in morphology, concentration, or motility. Measured hormone levels were not significantly different between the preoperative varicocele patients and the fertile controls. Successful term pregnancies were achieved for 12 patients: 6 through natural-cycle intercourse, 5 through in vitro fertilization with embryo transfer, and 1 through intracytoplasmic sperm injection.

Conclusions.—According to strict Kruger morphologic criteria, there is no change in sperm morphology after varicocelectomy. However, sperm motility and concentration do change significantly. Infertility in men with varicocele does not appear to be related to hormonal difference. Even though varicocelectomy does not affect Kruger morphology, varicocele repair is necessary because of the importance of sperm motility to fertilization and pregnancy.

Response of Routine Semen Analysis and Critical Assessment of Sperm Morphology by Kruger Classification to Therapeutic Varicocelectomy
Vazquez-Levin MH, Friedmann P, Goldberg SI, et al (Beth Israel Med Ctr, New York)
J Urol 158:1804–1807, 1997   19–3

Background.—The effect of surgical correction of varicoceles on the ability to father children has been reported. The efficacy of varicocelectomy before assisted reproductive procedures is less well established. The effect of surgical correction of varicoceles evidenced by sperm morphologic characteristics using the Kruger classification was determined.

Methods and Findings.—Thirty-three subfertile men undergoing semen assessment before and after varicocelectomy were studied. Sperm concentration and count were improved significantly 3 to 4 and 6 to 8 months after varicocelectomy. According to Kruger classification, morphologic assessment showed an overall significant increase in the percentage of normal A forms 3 to 4 and 6 to 8 months postoperatively. Forty-six percent of the patients with abnormal sperm morphology before surgery and more than 4% A forms achieved normal levels 3 months after surgery. At 6 months postoperatively, only 6 patients maintained normal values. Three of the initial 14 nonresponders achieved normal values. Sperm morphology improved in 3 patients with severe teratozoospermia. Varicocelectomy did not affect sperm morphology in the 4 patients with normal morphology before surgery.

Conclusions.—Surgical correction of varicocele results in significantly improved sperm morphology, according to Kruger classification. Both concentration and count were improved as early as 3 months after surgery.

► Varicocele causes impaired fertility, and its repair leads to improved seminal parameters and pregnancy rate. It is the preferred treatment when subfertility and varicoceles coexist. Varicocele may result in a variety of seminal defects ranging from reduced count and overall and/or sustained motility to isolated functional defects. The question is, should varicoceles be repaired for abnormal morphology but in the presence of normal count, motility, and hamster egg test or some other functional assays? No definitive study exists to answer this question. Given that morphology does correlate with conventional IVF outcome and the wide range of impairment imposed by the presence of varicoceles, my current approach is to proceed with artery-sparing microscopic repair.

J. Yuan, M.D.

Patient Noncompliance After Vasectomy

Maatman TJ, Aldrin L, Carothers GG (Michigan Urological Clinic, Grand Rapids)
Fertil Steril 68:552–555, 1997   19–4

Introduction.—A popular and safe method of birth control in the United States is bilateral vasectomy. After vasectomy, semen analyses are traditionally performed to determine the presence or absence of sperm in the ejaculate. Patients must follow instructions after a vasectomy to determine the success of the operation. In men having bilateral vasectomy, the postoperative instruction compliance rate was reported.

Methods.—To determine the rate of compliance with postvasectomy follow-up instructions, the records of men having vasectomy were reviewed. Until a man has 2 consecutive negative semen analyses 1 month apart, it is policy to have him continue to use some form of birth control. To screen for the rare man who recanalizes, a yearly semen analysis, after achieving sterility, is recommended. At this private practice, verbal instructions on 1 occasion and written follow-up instructions on 3 occasions are given to the patient after vasectomy.

Results.—After vasectomy, 644 men (34%) never returned, thus no semen analyses were available for examination. A single semen analysis was performed on 619 men (33%) who returned. A second negative semen analysis was performed on 629 men (33%) who returned. Postvasectomy follow-up instructions were followed by only 60 men (3%); these men returned for a yearly semen analysis. Despite the fact that 8 pregnancies occurred, none of the patients in this group pursued litigation.

Conclusion.—There is a poor rate of compliance in following instructions for determining sterility after vasectomy. Despite the low rate of recanalization, yearly semen analysis is still recommended.

▶ The authors reported a well-known phenomenon: patient noncompliance and lack of follow-up after vasectomy. The 1% early failure rate is consistent with that in the literature. Proper documentation, with a detailed consent form listing all the pros and cons as well as patient responsibility, is the only way we physicians can protect ourselves from litigious patients.

J. Yuan, M.D.

Fertility Options After Vasectomy: A Cost-effectiveness Analysis
Pavlovich CP, Schlegel PN (New York Hosp-Cornell Med Ctr; The Population
Council, New York)
Fertil Steril 67:133–141, 1997   19–5

Background.—Two percent to 6% of men undergoing vasectomy subsequently seek a reversal to restore fertility. A cost-effectiveness analysis (cost per delivery) was performed using 2 different initial approaches to postvasectomy infertility.

Methods.—Data on men treated in 1994 at U.S. centers which had experience in vasectomy reversal or sperm retrieval and intracytoplasmic sperm injection (ICSI) were included in the model of expected costs and outcomes. All had female partners aged 39 years or younger. Treatment charges, complication rates, and pregnancy and delivery rates associated with initial microsurgical vasectomy reversal were compared with those associated with retrieved epididymal or testicular sperm.

Findings.—The cost per delivery with initial vasectomy reversal was $25,475. The delivery rate was 47%. The cost per delivery after sperm retrieval and ICSI was $72,521. Mean costs for percutaneous or testicular sperm retrieval and for surgical epididymal sperm retrieval were $73,146 and $71,896, respectively. After 1 cycle of sperm retrieval and ICSI, the delivery rate was 33%.

Conclusion.—Microsurgical vasectomy reversal is the most cost-effective approach to the treatment of postvasectomy infertility. This approach also has the best chance of resulting in the delivery of a child after a single intervention.

▶ This excellent article gives a state-of-the-art review of vasectomy reversal and in vitro fertilization (IVF) outcome and examines the overall cost of each approach. The cost of IVF is indirect and is not appreciated by the infertile couples. Men are now being referred to urologists for sperm retrieval for IVF without ever being formally consulted for vasectomy reversal or, worse, sperm retrievals are being performed directly by the gynecologists.

Many couples are quite concerned at the 30% IVF dropout rate and the prospect of an up to 45% chance of multiple gestation in conjunction with IVF. These concerns are especially true of men with vasectomies because these patients are often self-paying, have children from a previous marriage, and are looking to have an additional child—rather than having children at all cost—as in the case with some primarily infertile couples. We need to share this information with our gynecologist colleagues and patients so that our patients can be properly served.

J. Yuan, M.D.

Vasoepididymostomy for Vasectomy Reversal: A Critical Assessment in the Era of Intracytoplasmic Sperm Injection

Kolettis PN, Thomas AJ Jr (Cleveland Clinic Found, Ohio)
J Urol 158:467–470, 1997

19–6

Background.—Vasoepididymostomy has been successful in vasectomy reversal, yet it is a technically challenging procedure. Other approaches, such as microsurgical epididymal sperm aspiration with intracytoplasmic sperm injection, might be more cost effective and successful. These authors compared the costs and success rates of these 2 methods to see whether a clearly superior method could be identified.

Methods.—Medical records were reviewed for 55 men who underwent microsurgical vasoepididymostomy for vasectomy reversal. Patients were followed after surgery to assess patency, contraception and delivery rates, complications, and costs associated with the procedure and with delivery. The cost per newborn was also calculated. These findings were compared with those reported in the literature after microsurgical epididymal sperm aspiration with intracytoplasmic sperm injection.

Findings.—No major complications occurred in the group undergoing vasoepididymostomy. Patency, pregnancy, and live delivery rates in the vasoepididymostomy group were 85%, 44% (24 pregnancies), and 36% (17 live births), respectively. Pregnancy and delivery rates reported for microsurgical epididymal sperm aspiration with intracytoplasmic sperm injection averaged 56% and 29%, respectively. Total costs per newborn associated with the procedures were $31,099 for vasoepididymostomy and $51,024 for microsurgical epididymal sperm aspiration with intracytoplasmic sperm injection.

Conclusion.—Even though it is tempting to generalize the successes of intracytoplasmic sperm injection to all cases of male infertility, this study showed that microsurgical vasoepididymostomy was at least as successful as, and substantially less expensive than, microsurgical epididymal sperm aspiration with intracytoplasmic sperm injection. It would seem that this latter method should be used only when surgical reconstruction is not an option.

▶ The advent of in vitro fertilization/intracytoplasmic sperm injection (ICSI) has led some to suggest that treatment for male factor infertility is irrelevant and unnecessary. This retrospective cost-effectiveness analysis comparing cost per live delivery between vasectomy reversal and ICSI clearly favors surgical reconstruction as the procedure of choice in men with epididymal obstruction. The overall pregnancy rate following vasectomy reversal is about 30%, provided it is performed by those familiar with microsurgical reconstruction.

J. Yuan, M.D.

Effect of Level of Anastomosis and Quality of Intraepididymal Sperm on the Outcome of End-to-Side Epididymovasostomy
Jarow JP, Oates RD, Buch JP, et al (Bowman Gray School of Medicine, Winston-Salem, NC; Boston Univ; North Texas Male Infertility, Dallas; et al)
Urology 49:590–595, 1997   19–7

Background.—The outcomes of epididymovasostomy are believed to be better if the procedure is done at the most distal site of the epididymis, where whole sperm (regardless of their motility status) are present in the lumen. The effects of the level of epididymal anastomosis and the quality of sperm on surgical outcomes were investigated.

Methods.—One hundred thirty-one azoospermic men, with a mean age of 39 years, underwent an end-to-side epididymovasostomy. The mean obstruction interval was 18 years. The cause of obstruction was vasectomy in 48%, infection in 19%, congenital anomaly in 20%, and unknown in 13%. The overall rate of patency was 67%; the pregnancy rate was 27%. Subgroups of patients with an anastomosis to the same level of the epididymis on all functional sides included caput (56 patients), corpus (28), and cauda (13).

Findings.—Motile sperm were more often present in the caput and corpus than in the cauda epididymis (54%, 61%, and 25%, respectively). These subgroups did not differ significantly in patency rates. The postoperative total motile sperm count and pregnancy rate for the corpus epididymis group were significantly better than for the caput group but no different from that of the cauda group. The patency and pregnancy rates for anastomoses done at levels showing motile sperm were not significantly better than at sites with nonmotile sperm. However, the postoperative total motile sperm count was better.

Conclusion.—The outcomes of epididymovasostomy to the corpus and cauda epididymis are roughly equivalent and better than to the caput. Thus, moving more proximally from the cauda to the corpus in the search for motile sperm for cryopreservation during an end-to-side epididymovasostomy may be reasonable. By contrast, moving from the corpus to the caput epididymis adversely affects outcomes.

▶ This is a multi-institution report on epididymovasostomy outcome in a large group of men. It confirms previous observations that anastomosis to the epididymal caput is associated with a lower pregnancy rate.[1] Intracytoplasmic sperm injection in conjunction with percutaneous sperm aspiration or testicular sperm extraction have lessened the need for direct epididymal sperm retrieval at the time of reconstruction. However, one should not hesitate to proceed with epididymal caput exploration and anastomosis if sperm is not found more distally, as the absence of epididymal sperm at the level of anastomosis will likely result in failure.

J. Yuan, M.D.

Reference

1. Niederberger C, Ross LS: Microsurgical epididymovasostomy: Predictors of success. *J Urol* 149:1364–1367, 1993.

Fibrin-Glue Assisted Vasoepididymostomy: A Comparison to Standard End-to-Side Microsurgical Vasoepididymostomy in the Rat Model
Shekarriz BM, Thomas AJ Jr, Sabanegh E, et al (Cleveland Clinic Found, Ohio)
J Urol 158:1602–1605, 1997   19–8

Purpose.—Animal models of vasovasostomy have shown very good patency rates with fibrin glue. If fibrin glue were used instead of microsutures, it might simplify the microsurgical technique of vasoepididymostomy. A vasoepididymostomy technique using fibrin glue was studied in rats.

Methods.—Twenty-four male Sprague-Dawley rats underwent bilateral vasoepididymostomy by a conventional microsurgical technique on 1 side and a fibrin-assisted glue technique on the other. The animals were killed for examination after 30 days. To determine anastomotic patency, the vasal fluid was inspected for sperm, and methylene blue dye was injected into the vas deferens. The effects of each technique on granuloma formation were assessed as well.

Results.—Patency rates were 79% for fibrin glue anastomoses versus 63% for suture anastomoses. The 2 groups were similar in their incidence of sperm granuloma formation in patent anastomoses: 50% versus 67%, respectively. Anastomoses were created much more quickly using fibrin glue.

Conclusions.—The use of fibrin glue may greatly simplify the procedure of vasoepididymostomy. The patency rates achieved in this model are similar to those obtained with microsutured anastomoses. If the fibrin-glue technique can be introduced into clinical practice, it may offer good outcomes at a significantly reduced cost.

▶ A number of methods have been used to facilitate vasal and epididymal reconstruction. These include fibrin glue, CO_2 laser welding, intra-vasal stenting, and the latest, laser-activated tissue soldering. These modified approaches appear to have comparable patency rates to that of the suture-only conventional technique. Regardless of the modifications, accurate luminal approximation with sutures is still required initially. This procedure may be less time-consuming but not necessarily easier, because it is the inner-layer anastomosis for vasovasostomy/vasoepididymostomy (VV/VE) which presents the technical challenge.

The triangulated technique is an ingenious approach to performing VE. It allows for the placement of sutures into a still somewhat-distended epididymal tubule and partially intussucepts the tubule into the vasal lumen. Early patency rate is impressive, and I anxiously await the pregnancy rate and the long-term results.

J. Yuan, M.D.

Distribution of Spermatogenesis in the Testicles of Azoospermic Men: The Presence or Absence of Spermatids in the Testes of Men With Germinal Failure

Silber SJ, Nagy Z, Devroey P, et al (St Luke's Hosp, St Louis; Vrije Universiteit Brussel, Belgium)
Hum Reprod 12:2422–2428, 1997

19–9

Introduction.—Testicular sperm extraction and intracytoplasmic sperm injection (TESE-ICI) has become a practical treatment for men with azoospermia, whether caused by "incomplete" maturation or "incomplete" Sertoli cell only. The histologic findings in patients with nonobstructive azoospermia undergoing this procedure are highly variable. Testicular histologic studies are often performed at the same time as TESE, and have not been quantitatively analyzed for the presence of mature spermatids. The ability of preprocedural diagnostic testicle biopsy to predict the success of TESE-ICI in patients with nonobstructive azoospermia caused by testicular failure was evaluated. The study also examined the minimal threshold of testicular sperm production necessary for spermatozoa to reach the ejaculate.

Methods.—Testicular biopsy was performed before TESE-ICI in 45 patients with nonobstructive azoospermia caused by testicular failure. After quantitative analysis, the biopsy findings were compared with those of men with normal spermatogenesis. The relationship to the results of TESE-ICI was assessed as well.

Distribution of spermatogenesis in the testis

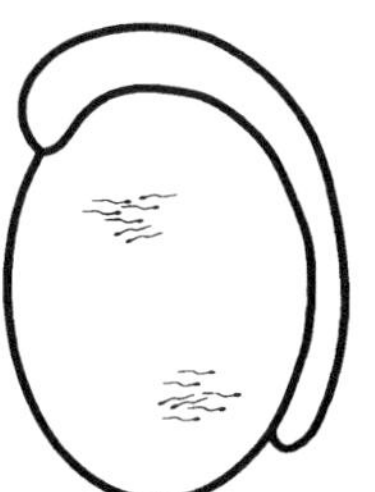

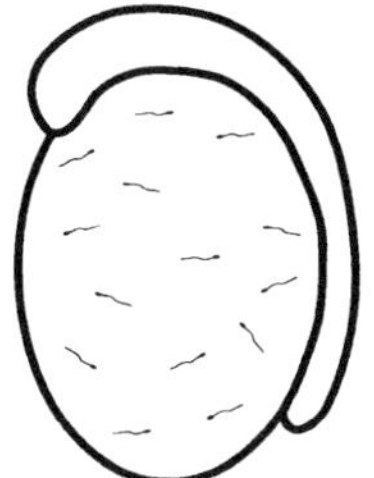

FIGURE 5.—The reliability of prior diagnostic biopsy suggests a homogeneous distribution of spermatogenesis in nonobstructive azoospermia, and not a patchy distribution. (Courtesy of Silber SJ, Nagy Z, Devroey P, et al: Distribution of spermatogenesis in the testicles of azoospermic men: The presence or absence of spermatids in the testes of men with germinal failure. *Hum Reprod* 12:2422–2428, 1997. Copyright European Society for Human Reproduction and Embryology, by permission of Oxford University Press.)

Results.—The mean number of mature spermatids per seminiferous tubule was 0 to 6 in men with nonobstructive azoospermia caused by germinal failure, compared with 17 to 35 in those with normal spermatogenesis but obstructive azoospermia. The results in the former group were similar, regardless of the type of testicular failure. Twenty-six men had mature spermatids found in their preprocedural testis biopsy; in 22 of these, spermatozoa were successfully obtained for ICI. For any spermatozoa to reach the ejaculate, at least 4 to 6 mature spermatids had to be present in the testis biopsy, the results indicated.

Conclusions.—In men with nonobstructive azoospermia, diagnostic testicular biopsy can predict the likelihood of success with TESE-ICI. As incomplete testicular failure may involve sparse spermatogenesis throughout the testicle, massive sampling from many different areas of the testes may not be needed for TESE-ICI to be successful (Fig 5). This study identifies a threshold of spermatogenesis that is necessary for any spermatozoa to reach the ejaculate.

▶ In vitro fertilization with intracytoplasmic sperm injection (IVF/ICSI) has revolutionized the treatment in men with severely impaired spermatogenesis, including those with Sertoli-only or maturation arrest. In up to 60% of these men, sperm may be extracted for IVF/ICSI. The inability to find sperm at the time of egg retrieval, leading to IVF cancellation, exacts tremendous emotional and financial toll on the patients. Testicular tissue cryopreservation without initial sperm extraction and individual sperm storage within prepared zona pellucida are attempts to prevent such disappointments. Controversy continues as to whether patchy spermatogenesis exists outside 1 to 2 generously obtained and thoroughly examined testicular biopsy samples showing no evidence of any mature sperm. Our approach is to proceed with diagnostic testis biopsy with concurrent TESE with attempted cryopreservation. If positive, we will then proceed with re-biopsy/TESE and IVF/ICSI following a 6-month waiting period.

J. Yuan, M.D.

Physiological Consequences of Testicular Sperm Extraction
Schlegel PN, Su L-M (New York Hosp-Cornell Med Ctr; Ctr for Biomedical Research, New York)
Hum Reprod 12:1688–1692, 1997   19–10

Introduction.—Retrieval of spermatozoa from the testes of men with non-obstructive azoospermia may provide an opportunity for fertility despite limited sperm production. In conjunction with intracytoplasmic sperm injection, testicular sperm extraction has been used as a therapeutic procedure for obstructive and non-obstructive azoospermia. Little is known about the physiologic consequences of this new technique on testicular function. Men who had multiple testicular sperm extraction procedures were studied to determine the physiologic effects of this technique on subsequent testicular function.

Methods.—Sixty-four men who had testicular sperm extraction for nonobstructive azoospermia were studied. Physical examinations were performed along with serial scrotal sonography, histologic analyses, and evaluation of the success of repeated sperm retrieval attempts.

Results.—Ultrasonographic abnormalities in the testis suggesting resolving inflammation or hematoma at the biopsy site were seen in 82% of the men at 3 months after testicular sperm extraction. These acute inflammatory changes typically resolved after 6 months and left linear scars or calcifications. Documented impaired testicular blood was evident in 2 patients. One patient had complete devascularization of the testis after testicular sperm extraction with multiple biopsies. There was a greater chance for spermatozoa to be retrieved in a repeat testicular sperm extraction done more than 6 months after the procedure (80%) than 1 done within 6 months (25%) of the initial procedure. For up to 6 months after testicular sperm extraction, transient adverse physiologic effects are common.

Conclusion.—After testicular sperm extraction procedures with multiple biopsies, permanent devascularization of the testis can occur. By using an open biopsy technique with optical magnification to directly identify testicular vessels, the risk of this complication may be minimized.

▶ Despite efforts at predicting the outcome of testicular sperm extraction (TESE) in men with nonobstructive azoospermia, sperm may not be retrieved as much as 60% of the time. The overall yield is related to the degree of spermatogenesis, amount of tissue examined, and, to a large extent, the persistence of the embryologist. Less invasive techniques, such as aspiration, are less successful when spermatogenesis is only scantly present. Refinement in our ability to cryopreserve previously extracted sperm is 1 possible way to avoid repeated TESE; I am adopting the authors' recommendation of waiting at least 6 months before another attempt at TESE.

J. Yuan, M.D.

The Effect of Female Age and Ovarian Reserve on Pregnancy Rate in Male Infertility: Treatment of Azoospermia With Sperm Retrieval and Intracytoplasmic Sperm Injection
Silber SJ, Nagy Z, Devroey P, et al (St Luke's Hosp, St Louis; Dutch-Speaking Free Univ, Brussels, Belgium)
Hum Reprod 12:2693–2700, 1997   19–11

Background.—In patients with male infertility undergoing assisted reproduction procedures, factors other than spermatozoa may be the major determinant of success. The effect of the partner's age and ovarian reserve on the success rates of assisted reproduction performed for azoospermia was studied.

TABLE 3.—Obstructive Azoospermia: Effect of Age of Wife

Age of wife (years)	No. of cycles (% of total)	No. of eggs at MII	No. of 2PN oocytes (% of MII eggs)	Normal cleaved embryos (% of 2 PN)	No. delivered pregnancies per cycle (% of cycles)	Implantation rate % (per embryo)
<30	50 (27)	735	392 (53)	302 (77)	22 (44)[a]	22[b]
30–36	87 (47)	1111	610 (55)	413 (68)	30 (34)[a]	19[c]
37–39	24 (13)	207	113 (55)	90 (80)	3 (12)[a]	4[d]
40+	25 (13)	281	147 (52)	101 (69)	1 (4)[a]	7[e]
Totals	186 (100)	2334	1262 (54)	906 (72)	56 (30)	16.2

[a]$P < 0.001$ between all four groups; [b,d]$P < 0.001$; [c,e]$P, < 0.001$; [c,d,e]$P < 0.001$.

MII = metaphase II; 2PN = two-pronuclear.

(Courtesy of Silber SJ, Nagy Z, Devroey P, et al: The effect of female age and ovarian reserve on pregnancy rate in male infertility: Treatment of azoospermia with sperm retrieval and intracytoplasmic sperm injection. *Hum Reprod* 12:2693–2700, 1997, by permission of Oxford University Press.)

Methods.—Two hundred forty-nine consecutive couples with male infertility caused by azoospermia underwent microsurgical epididymal sperm aspiration (MESA) or testicular sperm extraction (TESE) with intracytoplasmic sperm injection (ICSI). One hundred eighty-six men had irreparable obstructive azoospermia. Sixty-three had nonobstructive azoospermia caused by testicular failure.

Findings.—Neither fertilization nor pregnancy was affected by the pathology, source, quantity, or quality of the spermatozoa. Maternal age and ovarian reserve did not affect fertilization or embryo cleavage but dramatically influenced embryo implantation, pregnancy rates, and delivery rates. Women in their 20s had a 46% live delivery rate per cycle, compared with 34% for women aged 30 to 36 years and 13% for those aged 37 to 39 years. Women aged 40 years or older had a live delivery rate per cycle of only 4%. Number of eggs retrieved affected pregnancy and delivery rates to a lesser degree than maternal age. Sufficient spermatozoa could be retrieved to perform ICSI, with normal fertilization and embryo cleavage, from virtually all men with obstructive azoospermia and 62% of men with nonobstructive azoospermia caused by germinal failure (Table 3).

Conclusions.—The success of MESA-ICSI and TESE-ICSI for male factor infertility is limited by the partner's age and possibly ovarian reserve. Live delivery rates of 42% per cycle are readily achieved when the woman is younger than 37 years and when 9 or more eggs are retrieved.

▶ The only meaningful outcome for all fertility treatment is the delivery of healthy infants or the live birth rate; other considerations are cost and complication rate. Statistics such as fertilization rate etc. are practically meaningless to the infertile couples. This report confirms the observation by Oehninger et al.[1] in that female age is the most important predictor of outcome. Other reports have suggested that IVF/ICSI birth rate are lower in patients with nonobstructive azoospermia using extracted testicular sperm. The average difference is about 15% to 20% lower.[2] When counseling couples prior to IVF, expected delivery rate should be based on the female age and possibly the etiology of the male factor rather than the cumulative average encompassing all cases.

J. Yuan, M.D.

References

1. Oehninger S, Veeck L, Lanzendorf S, et al: Intracytoplasmic sperm injection: Achievement of high pregnancy rates in couples with severe male factor infertility is dependent primarily upon female and not male factors. *Fertil Steril* 64:977–981, 1995.
2. Mansour RT, Kamal A, Fahmy I, et al: Intracytoplasmic sperm injection in obstructive and non-obstructive azoospermia. *Hum Reprod* 12:1974–1979, 1997.

Reconstitution of Spermatogenesis From Frozen Spermatogonial Stem Cells

Avarbock MR, Brinster CJ, Brinster RL (Univ of Pennsylvania, Philadelphia)
Nature Med 2:693–696, 1996   19–12

Introduction.—Few efforts have been documented of cryopreservation of male germline stem cells. Considering the difficulty associated with freezing mature spermatozoa, successful cryopreservation of spermatogonial stem cells by routine procedures is surprising. The most valuable use of cryopreservation may be for germ lines of valuable experimental males in research, agriculture animals that die before puberty or are too old to breed, and males from exotic or endangered species.

Methods.—Testis cells were collected from prepubertal or adult mice carrying a *lacZ* transgene that allows round spermatids and cells in later steps of spermiogenesis to be stained blue when incubated. This was done to determine whether male germ cells could be cryopreserved in suspension. The donor testis cells were collected, frozen, and stored. They were thawed and transplanted into the seminiferous tubules of recipient mice. Blue staining helped in readily identifying the areas of the recipient testes populated by cryopreserved donor cells.

Results.—Male germline stem cells were successfully cryopreserved. Spermatogenesis was generated from the donor testis cells frozen from 4 to 156 days at $-196°C$. Rat spermatogenesis was subsequently generated when the stem cells were transplanted to the testis of an immunodeficient mouse.

Conclusion.—The preserved male germ lines may be considered biologically immortal because transplanted testis stem cells will ultimately undergo replication and meiotic recombination during spermatogenesis. Clones of the original male may be established at any time after spermatogonial transplantation to multiple recipients with cryopreservation of the germ line.

▶ The authors have shown that stem cells can be harvested, cryopreserved, and later used to repopulate a germ-cell depleted testis. The same authors have also reported cross-species stem-cell transplant from rat to mouse.[1] Aside from the vast potential in veterinarian medicine and agriculture, it is conceivable that in conjunction with other advances, such as germ cell culture and gene therapy, male infertility because of defective spermatogenesis may possibly be treated through extensions of such techniques in the future.

J. Yuan, M.D.

Reference

1. Clouthier DE, Avarbock MR, Maika SD, et al: Rat spermatogenesis in mouse testis. *Nature* 381:418–421, 1996.

Simultaneous Injection of Round Spermatid Nuclei From Mice and Hamster Oscillogen Can Initiate the Normal Development of Mouse Embryos
Sasagawa I, Tomaru M, Adachi Y, et al (Yamagata Univ, Japan)
J Urol 158:2006–2008, 1997   19–13

Background.—Research has shown that mature mouse oocytes injected with spermatid nuclei fail to become activated. Additional stimulation is needed to trigger oocyte activation, leading to embryo development. The current study determined whether simultaneous injection of mouse round spermatids and hamster oscillogen can fertilize oocytes and contribute to normal embryo development.

Methods.—Mouse oocytes were injected simultaneously with mouse round spermatid nuclei and a preparation of oocyte-activating protein from hamster spermatozoa. Findings were compared with those of injection of testicular spermatozoa.

Findings.—The incidence of normal fertilization and embryo development after simultaneous injection of round spermatid nuclei and hamster oscillogen did not differ significantly from that after testicular spermatozoa injection. The rate of development of 2-cell embryos to term also did not differ greatly between the 2 oocyte groups.

Conclusions.—These findings suggest that oscillogen should be included with the injection of round spermatid nuclei to effectively activate oocytes and embryo development. Additional studies should be done with purified rather than a crude preparation of oscillogen.

▶ Factors other than the physical introduction of sperm nuclear content into an oocyte are required for normal embryo development. Concerns regarding the use of spermatid for direct oocyte injection center on the cell cycle imbalance and the lack of oocyte activation, which result in reduced embryo development. Following reports of successful laboratory attempts using round spermatid for injection (ROSNI), several human births have likewise been achieved. The overall success is low (less than 10%) and should be considered as investigational;[1] we do not offer ROSNI at this time for reasons cited above.

J. Yuan, M.D.

Reference

1. Fishel S, Aslam I, Tesarik J: Spermatid conception: A stage too early or a time too soon? *Hum Reprod* 11:1371–1375, 1996.

Assisted Ejaculation and In-Vitro Fertilization in the Treatment of Infertile Spinal Cord–Injured Men: The Role of Intracytoplasmic Sperm Injection

Hulting C, Rosenlund B, Levi R, et al (Karolinska Inst, Stockholm; Huddinge Univ, Sweden)
Hum Reprod 12:499–502, 1997   19–14

Introduction.—Men with spinal cord injuries have as strong an instinct to father children as men without injuries. Assisted ejaculation by means of vibratory or electrical stimulation is usually needed for men with spinal cord injuries. The outcome of assisted ejaculation in combination with in-vitro fertilization and intracytoplasmic sperm injection was analyzed. The results of treatment when only in-vitro fertilization was available was compared with results when micromanipulation could also be used.

Methods.—Couples in which the man had spinal cord injuries seeking treatment for their infertility were included in the study if they had a stable relationship, motile spermatozoa in a diagnostic sample, and no contraindications in the woman. Electro-ejaculation or vibratory stimulation were used to retrieve spermatozoa. Standard in-vitro fertilization was performed if the sperm quality was sufficient. If the semen quality was extremely poor, intracytoplasmic sperm injection was performed.

Results.—There were 25 couples in 52 cycles who had 81 ovum retrievals and 47 embryo transfers. Sperm counts ranged from 0.01×10^6 to 978×10^6. The fertilization rate was 30% before the introduction of intracytoplasmic sperm injection. The fertilization rate increased to 88% with this new technique. The sperm count, level of injury, or fertilization technique was not associated with the pregnancy rate. There were 16 clinical pregnancies and 11 deliveries with a cumulative pregnancy rate per couple of 56%.

Conclusion.—Similar pregnancy results occurred with severe male-factor infertility and severe male-factor infertility combined with tubal-factor infertility. When home insemination is ineffective, patients with male-factor infertility because of spinal cord injury should be offered in-vitro fertilization or intracytoplasmic sperm injection. High-order multiple pregnancy in these couples can be avoided with these techniques because the number of embryos transferred can be limited to 2 or 3. For maximizing the probability of success, availability of intracytoplasmic sperm injection is important.

▶ Assisted ejaculations, either electro-ejaculation or penile vibratory stimulation, are highly effective in producing sperm; however, pregnancy rate after insemination had been low. In the insensate patients in whom repeated electro-ejaculations can be performed in the office and in those responding to penile vibratory stimulation, a trial of insemination is worthwhile, assuming the motile sperm count is acceptable. We are leaning toward in-vitro fertilization and intracytoplasmic sperm injection as the primary treatment in sensate patients in whom general anesthesia is required for each electro-ejaculation attempt and in those with extremely poor sperm motility.

J. Yuan, M.D.

Men Homozygous for an Inactivating Mutation of the Follicle-Stimulating Hormone (FSH) Receptor Gene Present Variable Suppression of Spermatogenesis and Fertility

Tapanainen JS, Aittomäki K, Min J, et al (Oulu Univ, Finland; Univ of Helsinki; Univ of Turku, Finland)
Nature Genet 15:205–206, 1997

19–15

Objective.—The pituitary gonadotropins luteinizing hormone and follicle-stimulating hormone (FSH) regulate gonadal function. Luteinizing hormone governs gonadal steroidogenesis, whereas FSH is critical for folliculogenesis in females and spermatogenesis in males. A new inactivating point mutation in the FSH receptor (FSHR) gene—which, in homozygous females, causes recessively inherited hypergonadotropic ovarian failure—is reported.

Findings.—The 566C→T mutation was found in 22 of 75 Finnish females with hypergonadotropic ovarian dysgenesis. These subjects, who came from 13 families, were tested along with 15 of 25 brothers. The mutation was found in exon 7 of the FSHR gene, where the extracellular domain of the receptor molecule is encoded, and predicted an alanine to valine substitution. In functional tests, the mutant FSHR showed obviously reduced ligand binding and signal transduction. Without functional FSH, affected females were infertile because of the failure of ovarian follicles to mature. Males homozygous for the inactivating FSHR mutation had spermatogenic failure to a varying extent, but did not have azoospermia or absolute infertility.

Conclusions.—An inactivating point mutation of the FSHR gene associated with hypergonadotropic ovarian failure in females is reported. However, the same mutation in males does not produce complete azoospermia. The mutation appears to cause a partial, rather than a complete, blockade of FSH action. The findings suggest that FSH may play a more important role in fertility among females than males.

▶ This article examines the effect of FSH receptor point mutation, which causes ovarian failures in affected females, in 5 men. Despite all the men having some degree of FSH elevation and measurable reduction in FSH receptor activity in vitro, the clinical findings vary with regard to fertility status, sperm count and testicular size. Other researchers have reported biologically inactive FSH or luteinizing hormone as a potential cause of hypogonadism. It is quite possible that some cases of hypergonadotropic hypogonadism may be due to functional disturbances along the hypothalamus-pituitary-gonadal axis, as described in this article, and that they may be diagnosed as we refine our understanding in male reproductive biology.

J. Yuan, M.D.

Azoospermic Men With Deletion of the *DAZ* Gene Cluster Are Capable of Completing Spermatogenesis: Fertilization, Normal Embryonic Development and Pregnancy Occur When Retrieved Testicular Spermatozoa Are Used for Intracytoplasmic Sperm Injection
Mulhall JP, Reijo R, Alagappan R, et al (Boston Univ; Massachusetts Inst of Technology; Cambridge; Reproductive Science Ctr, Waltham, Mass)
Hum Reprod 12:503–508, 1997   19–16

Background.—Some men with nonobstructive azoospermia have fully formed spermatozoa that can be used to achieve pregnancy by intracytoplasmic sperm injection (ICSI). Recent research suggests that the *DAZ* gene cluster is a strong candidate for one of the elusive azoopsermia factors (*AZFs*) located on the long arm of the Y chromosome. In 13% of azoospermic men and a small proportion of severely oligozoospermic men, the *DAZ* gene cluster is deleted. Vertical transmission of *AZF* region deletions from father to son may also occur. The current study explored whether azoospermic men with *AZF/DAZ* region deletions can complete minimal spermatogenesis and whether any spermatozoa may participate in fertilization, embryo development, and pregnancy.

Methods and Findings.—Eighty-three patients underwent *AZF/DAZ* region microdeletion analysis. All had small, soft testes; normal epididymides and vasa deferentia; and increased serum follicle-stimulating hormone, indicating nonobstructive azoospermia. Three of the 6 men found to have *AZF/DAZ* deletions were also found to have spermatozoa in the harvested testicular tissue. These spermatozoa were used for ICSI. Fertilization occurred in 36% of injected oocytes, which compared favorably with testicular spermatozoa obtained from nonobstructive azoospermic men without *AZF/DAZ* gene deletions. One fertilization resulted in a twin conception; it was the first term pregnancy reported using spermatozoa from an azoospermic man with *AZF/DAZ* deletions.

Conclusion.—Men with nonobstructive azoospermia and *AZF/DAZ* deletions may harbor spermatozoa in their testicular parenchyma that may be retrieved for use in ICSI to achieve pregnancy. Although the male offspring of such men may be infertile or sterile, it seems unlikely that other somatic abnormalities would occur in these children.

▶ Recent advances in assisted reproduction and molecular biology have enabled us to enter into previously uncharted territory in human genetics and reproduction. *DAZ*/Y-chromosomal microdeletions and other genetic factors not yet described are likely to be the responsible factors in many men currently being given a diagnosis of idiopathic oligospermia and nonobstructive azoospermia. Although *DAZ* deletion is not a contraindication for in vitro fertilization/ICSI, the current consensus for managing these men is genetic testing and consultation before ICSI, with preimplantation embryo biopsy-genetic testing in selected cases, such as Klinefelter's syndrome.

J. Yuan, M.D.

Microdeletions in the Y Chromosome of Infertile Men

Pryor JL, Kent-First M, Muallem A, et al (Univ of Minnesota, Minneapolis; Promega Corp, Madison, Wis; Univ of Wisconsin, Madison)
N Engl J Med 336:534–539, 1997   19–17

Background.—Small deletions in the long arm of the Y chromosome are present in some infertile men with azoospermia or severe oligospermia. How predictable are these microdeletions? And do similar microdeletions occur in fertile men? This study examined the prevalence of these microdeletions to determine if specific phenotypes could be associated with specific deletions.

Methods.—The study included samples from 200 men with infertility and 200 banked samples from men who were fertile. A detailed questionnaire and thorough physical examination identified the cause of infertility (including idiopathic infertility). Genomic DNA was analyzed by polymerase chain reaction at least 3 times per sample, and Southern blot hybridization was used to confirm the polymerase chain reaction results.

Findings.—Microdeletions of the Y chromosome were found in 14 infertile men (7%) and in 4 fertile men (2%). In 12 of the 14 infertile men, the microdeletion involved deletion interval 6 or included some portion of it. In the other 2 infertile men, a deletion in the proximal p arm and a deletion in the proximal portion of deletion interval 5 were involved. However, neither the location nor the size of the deletion correlated with the patient's sperm count. Nine patients had azoospermia or severe oligospermia, 4 had oligospermia, and 1 had normospermia. Fathers of 6 of the infertile men with Y chromosome deletions also were examined (paternity was established by DNA analysis). In 2, the father's microdeletion was identical to that of his son, but the other 4 fathers had no microdeletions.

Conclusions.—No relationship was found between the location or extent of a microdeletion and the severity of spermatogenic failure. Furthermore, because even fertile men had microdeletions, a microdeletion by itself does not indicate infertility.

▶ Of men with nonobstructive azoospermia, 10% to 15% have various deletions in their Y chromsomes, including the AZF/DAZ gene in the distal long arm. Additional factors, including those that may be present on the autosomes, are being examined for their roles in spermatogenesis. Vertical transmission from father to son of Y-linked microdeletion has been reported. These men should be tested and even if they are found to be AZF intact, they should be made aware that our current understanding in human reproductive genetics is incomplete, and other causative factors may be present and possibly inherited when infertility is overcome with IVF/ICSI.

J. Yuan, M.D.

Submicroscopic Deletions in the Y Chromosome of Infertile Men

Girardi SK, Mielnik A, Schlegel PN (New York Hosp-Cornell Med Ctr; Ctr for Biomedical Research, New York)
Hum Reprod 12:1635–1641, 1997

19–18

Introduction.—The etiology of male-factor infertility is still poorly understood. Previous studies have found macroscopic deletions of the distal long arm of the Y chromosome in infertile men. Homology of RNA-binding protein was associated with a family of genes from this deleted region. The entire euchromatic region of the long arm of the Y chromosome was screened in infertile men to determine the regions and frequency of deletions.

Methods.—In 160 infertile men, the frequency of Y-chromosome deletions was evaluated using a series of 36 sequence-tagged sites, emphasizing intervals 5 and 6 of the long arm of the Y chromosome. To minimize potential overestimation of the frequency of deletion, peripheral leukocyte DNA was extracted and amplified with 2 parallel techniques. The presence of deletions, relative to a patient's sperm concentration, testis volume, and hormonal parameters, was evaluated.

Results.—A 7% prevalence of submicroscopic Y-chromosome deletions was found in men with sperm concentrations less than 5×10^6/mL. In 7% of azoospermic men, deletions were detected. In 10% of men with sperm concentrations less than 1×10^6/mL, deletions were detected, as they were in 8% of men with sperm concentrations greater than 1×10^6 but less than 5×10^6/mL. Y-chromosome deletions before polymerase chain reaction–based testing for the presence of sequence-tagged sites were not identified with other clinical parameters. Distinct regions of Y-chromosome deletions were detected, ~3.6 Mb in length in the AZFb region and 1.4 Mb in length in the AZFc region. In the AZFa region, there were no deletions detected.

Conclusion.—There is a high risk of Y-chromosome deletions among men with severe male infertility. Before treatment with assisted reproduction, testing for these genetic abnormalities is indicated.

▶ The Cornell group likewise confirms the presence of Y-chromosome microdeletion in men with severe male-factor infertility. They also noted that 1 man's sperm count deteriorated from severe oligospermia to azoospermia during a 30-month follow-up. Similar deterioration has also been seen in the Klinefelter's syndrome and in my own practice. Should we consider cryopreservation in men with severe oligospermia early on to prevent the uncertainty of testicular sperm extraction later on?

J. Yuan, M.D.

20 Penis and Urethra

Treatment Results and Prognostic Factors in 101 Men Treated for Squamous Carcinoma of the Penis
Sarin R, Norman AR, Steel GG, et al (Inst of Cancer Research, Sutton, Surrey, England)
Int J Radiat Oncol Biol Phys 38:713–722, 1997   20–1

Objective.—Cancer of the penis is a rare condition. Treatment is directed at preserving the organ and function while maximizing survival. The outcome of different treatments and prognostic factors for locoregional control and survival were evaluated retrospectively.

Methods.—Records of 101 men, aged 24–91 years, treated for invasive squamous carcinoma (n = 99) or verrucous carcinoma (n = 2) of the penis at Royal Marsden Hospital between 1960 and 1990 were reviewed. Median age at diagnosis was 64 years. The tumor was confined to subepithelial connective tissue in 79 patients and was node negative in 82. Histologic grades were G1 in 36 patients, G2 in 18, G3 in 28, and unknown in 19. Patients were treated with external beam radiation therapy (EBRT) (n = 53), interstitial radiation therapy (n = 12), wide excision (n = 2), wide excision plus EBRT (n = 5), wide excision plus interstitial radiation therapy (n = 1), partial penectomy (n = 17), partial penectomy plus EBRT (n = 1), or total penectomy (n = 10). Patients with G3 or T2/3/4 tumors were significantly more likely to have positive nodes than patients with lower grade tumors. A total of 59 patients received EBRT of 60 Gy at 2 Gy/fraction for 46 days. Patients were followed up for an average of 5.2 years. Overall survival, cause-specific survival, local progression-free survival, and local disease-free survival were determined.

Results.—During the follow-up period, 56 patients died, 31 of their disease and 2 of unknown causes for a 5- and 10-year overall survival of 56.5% and 39% and a 5- and 10-year cause-specific survival of 66% and 57%, respectively. The pattern of initial failure was recurrent or residual disease in 36 patients. Residual or recurrent inguinal or pelvic nodes were found in 37 patients. Distant metastases developed in 14 patients. Multivariate analysis identified poorly differentiated tumors, ulcerative or ulceroproliferative tumors, tumors extending beyond the glans, node-positive disease, and age 60 years or older as independent, significant adverse prognostic factors for cause-specific survival. The biological effective EBRT dose was significant in predicting local failure with but not without applying the time factor in 44 assessable patients with T1 tumors. After local failure, 26 of 36 patients were salvaged with radiation therapy or surgery. Local control was accomplished in 74 of 77 patients with T1 tumors, 7 of 12 with T2, 3 of 3 with T3, and 3 of 5 with T4. Treatment complications of EBRT included urethral stricture (n = 7) and penectomy for radiation necrosis (n = 1) and severe urethral damage (n = 1) in 56 patients. Three surgically treated patients had urethral stricture.

Conclusion.—There is a high risk of loco-regional recurrence of penile cancer after radiotherapy, although surgical or additional radiation therapy can salvage most patients. Although this study is small, patients receiving radiotherapy had significantly higher local failure rates.

▶ This manuscript presents fairly long-term follow-up (median of 5.2. years) of patients with penile cancer who, for the most part, were initially treated with either EBRT or interstitial therapy. One of the most impressive aspects of this series is the relatively high local failure rates for patients with T1 penile cancers treated with irradiation therapy (17 out of 44 or 39%). Moreover, this series, in conjunction with 4 others reviewed in this manuscript, discloses overall local failure rates after radiation therapy ranging between 15% and 43%, urethral stricture rates ranging between 14% and 41%, and necessity for penectomy because of radiation-induced complications from 2.9% to 15.7%. Although the authors could not demonstrate that local failure was associated with death from penile cancer, there certainly was a trend in this direction, and it probably would have been observed if more patients had been evaluated.

I take these data to suggest that patients with low volume penile cancer may be best treated surgically, although radiation therapy remains an option for patients who are particularly interested in the potential for penile preservation.

G.L. Andriole, Jr., M.D.

Carcinoma of the Penis: Appraisal of a Modified Tumour-staging System
Heyns CF, van Vollenhoven P, Steenkamp JW, et al (Univ of Stellenbosch, Cape Town, South Africa)
Br J Urol 80:307–312, 1997   20–2

Objective.—Lymph node involvement in patients with penile cancer carries a poor prognosis. However, lymph node dissection can result in significant morbidity. Moreover, 20% of patients with negative nodes have occult metastases, and half of clinically palpable nodes have no metastases on histologic examination. Variables predictive of lymph node metastases in patients with squamous carcinoma of the penis were investigated.

Methods.—Histologic or cytologic records of the inguinal lymph nodes of 35 patients aged 34–88 years with penile carcinoma treated between

November 1983 and April 1995 were reviewed. Tumors were staged using a modified clinical TNM staging system.

Results.—Preoperatively, 26 (74%) patients had palpable nodes. Inguinal lymph node cytologic findings in 12 patients were positive in 8, negative in 3, and insufficient in 1. At surgery, a penectomy was performed in 34 patients, a partial amputation in 20, and a radical penectomy in 17. Histologically, 17 tumors were grade 1, 13 were grade 2, and 5 were grade 3. Lymphadenectomy was performed in 31 patients at an average of 75 days after penectomy. Complications after lymphadenectomy were wound sepsis in 12 patients, wound dehiscence in 7, lymphocele in 6, lymph leak in 4, wound abscess in 3, necrosis of wound edges in 2, hematoma in 1, and pneumonia in 1. Six patients required reoperation. Lymph node metastases were found in no patients with T1 tumors, 5 of 19 with T2 tumors, and 2 of 2 with T4 tumors. Lymph node metastases were found in 2 of 8 patients without clinically palpable nodes, in 3 of 14 with clinically suspected infection, and in 11 of 12 with clinically suspected malignancy. Lymph node metastases were found in 5 of 17 patients with grade 1 tumors, 9 of 13 with grade 2 tumors, and 3 of 5 with grade 3 tumors. Using the modified histologic T-staging system, lymph node metastases were found in 1 of 9 patients with T1 tumors, 8 of 16 with T2 tumors, 5 of 5 with T3 tumors, and 3 of 5 with T4 tumors.

Conclusion.—Findings of lymph node metastases in about 25% of patients without clinically palpable nodes and about 20% of those with palpable nodes thought to be infected agree with other studies. According to the modified histologic T-staging system, lymphadenectomy can be avoided in patients with T1 tumors. In all other patients bilateral lymphadenectomy is recommended 6–8 weeks after penectomy.

▶ This carefully reported study evaluated a modified T-staging system that combines histologic tumor differentiation and extent of pathologic invasion to predict the presence of lymph node metastases. This staging system was originally proposed by McDougal.[1]

In the current series, lymph node metastases were present in one quarter of those who had palpably benign lymph nodes and in 20% of those whose palpable lymph nodes normalized after antibiotic therapy. However, no patient with a T1 lesion with palpably normal nodes had metastases, whereas 16% with T1 lesions with palpable lymph nodes had metastases. The rate of metastases was successively higher as the modified T stage advanced, reaching a peak of 88% for patients with T4 lesions associated with palpably abnormal inguinal lymph nodes.

This study validates the earlier study by McDougal and supports the role of modified lymphadenectomy for patients with palpably benign tumors whose primary tumors are of advanced T stage or are poorly differentiated histologically.

G.L. Andriole, Jr., M.D.

Reference

1. McDougal WS: Carcinoma of the penis: Improved survival by early regional lymphadenectomy based on the histological grade and depth of invasion of the primary lesion. *J Urol* 154:1364–1366, 1995.

Long-term Follow-up of Men Undergoing Modified Inguinal Lymphadenectomy for Carcinoma of the Penis

Colberg JW, Andriole GL, Catalona WJ (Washington Univ, St Louis)
Br J Urol 79:54–57, 1997

20–3

Introduction.—Total lymphadenectomy has been recommended for patients with carcinoma of the penis and clinically negative lymph nodes, but the procedure carries a risk of significant morbidity and would be of no

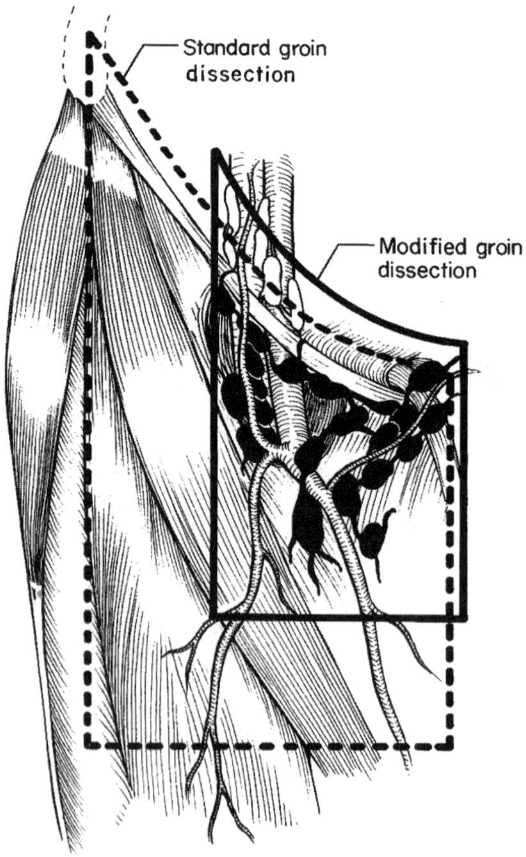

FIGURE 1.—Comparison of the limits of dissection of modified groin dissection with standard groin dissection. (Courtesy of Colberg JW, Andriole GL, Catalona WJ: Long-term follow-up of men undergoing modified inguinal lymphadenectomy for carcinoma of the penis. *Br J Urol* 79:54–57, 1997.)

benefit in about 80% of cases. An alternative option involves a modification of the standard inguinal lymphadenectomy, which removes more nodes than sentinel biopsy. Nine men who underwent the modified procedure were followed up for long-term outcome.

Methods.—All 9 patients had histologically confirmed squamous cell carcinoma of the penis. Lymph nodes were clinically normal in 7 patients and slightly enlarged in 2. Chest x-ray and CT findings were negative for metastases. A modified inguinal lymph node dissection (Fig 1) was performed in all cases. Specimens from 3 patients showed lymph node metastases, and these patients underwent extended inguinal dissection and pelvic lymphadenectomy. Mean follow-up was 67.5 months.

Results.—Two of the 3 patients with histologically involved lymph nodes had T3 squamous carcinoma. In all 3 cases, however, extended inguinal and pelvic node dissections did not reveal cancer. Early postoperative complications included skin-flap necrosis, which healed without complication. Although all patients experienced mild lower extremity edema and 4 required support stockings, none had debilitating lymphedema. All patients were alive at the latest follow-up with no evidence of recurrent disease. A patient with nodal metastases was treated with platinum-based adjunctive chemotherapy.

Discussion.—Because of the pattern of lymphatic drainage of the penis, complete groin dissection is a radical approach for most patients with carcinoma of the penis and clinically negative nodes. The modified inguinal lymphadenectomy excises the most likely sites for nodal metastases, provides staging information similar to that obtained from the standard procedure, and yields good long-term results.

▶ Lymph node dissection is the most effective means of eradicating minimal metastatic disease in patients with invasive carcinoma of the penis. The difficulties with recommending standard inguinal node dissection for every patient with invasive penile cancer are that only a minority harbor micrometastatic disease, and operation may cause substantial morbidity. As an alternative, Cabanas has suggested a sentinel node biopsy, but long-term results have disclosed a significant proportion of falsely negative sentinel node biopsies. In 1988, a modified inguinal lymphadenectomy was described using boundaries shown in the accompanying figure. This operation appears to effectively discover and eradicate early stage micrometastatic disease without inducing significant morbidity. In this article, long-term follow-up (median 67.5 months) discloses that no patient has had recurrent disease develop in the inguinal region. These results, coupled with the acceptable morbidity of this operation, suggests that it should be recommended for patients with invasive penile carcinoma.

G.L. Andriole, Jr., M.D.

Reconstruction of Deformities Resulting From Penile Enlargement Surgery

Alter GJ (Univ of California, Los Angeles)
J Urol 158:2153–2157, 1997

20–4

Introduction.—Although penile enlargement surgery has become more common, there are no standardized techniques. This report describes a series of patients who presented for reconstruction of penile deformities secondary to penile enlargement surgery.

Methods.—Between 1994 and 1996, the author operated on 19 patients to reconstruct complications of penile augmentation. Complaints related to suspensory ligament release with a large V-Y advancement flap included scars, hairless concavity in the suprapubic region, loss of penile length, deformity at the base that created a proximal penile hump, low hanging penis, scrotal "dog ears," and loss of sensitivity. Complications related to autologous fat injections included fat disappearance, lumps and nodules, shaft distortion, excess penile skin, and inadequate rigidity. Other complaints included impotence, incontinence, and pain.

Results.—The 19 men in this study underwent 24 operations. Of the 17 patients with V-Y scar revisions, 12 had partial or complete reversal of the V-Y advancement flap with removal of scrotal dog ears, 2 had scar revisions only, and 3 had scar revisions and dorsal hump thinning. Fourteen men had removal of fat nodules. Complications included a hematoma requiring drainage, slight wound separation in 2 patients, and an infection that resolved with antibiotics. One patient required further surgery for an inadequate reversal of the V-Y advancement flap. Penile appearance and function were improved in all cases.

Conclusions.—Penile augmentation procedures are not standardized, and complications are not uncommon. Correcting these complications is difficult and may require more than 1 procedure.

▶ This is another large series that reveals potential complications of penile enhancement surgery. It is unknown how many men undergo this type of surgery, but it seems that the patient dissatisfaction rate must be relatively high. The concerns relate to asymmetric fat injection, scarring, and even impotence and persistent penile pain. The author describes how to undo the damage. These enhancement operations should clearly not be performed in infants and children, and I doubt that there is a role in the adult for what is purely a cosmetic operation.

D.E. Coplen, M.D.

Use of Multiple UroLume Endourethral Prostheses in Complex Bulbar Urethral Strictures

Tillem SM, Press SM, Badlani GH (Long Island Jewish Med Ctr, New Hyde Park, NY)
J Urol 157:1665–1668, 1997

20–5

Introduction.—Patients who received the UroLume Wallstent (American Medical Systems, Minnetonka, Minnesota) showed marked improvement in urine flow rates and symptom scores after 2 years of follow-up. The multicenter study reported, however, that 41 of 175 patients (23%) required placement of multiple stents, either initially or for repeat treatment. Patients with multiple stents were evaluated to determine if their results were as good and as durable as the results for the entire study group.

Patients and Methods.—Patients were enrolled in a prospective trial of the UroLume endourethral prosthesis for treatment of recurrent bulbar urethral strictures. Twenty-five patients required multiple stents as part of the primary procedure and 16 for repeat treatment. Strictures were generally longer in patients who required more than 1 stent (mean 3.6 cm) than in those who received a single stent (mean 2.3 cm). All patients with multiple stents had failed previous therapy and most had undergone multiple urethral dilations and internal urethrotomies.

Results.—The number of multiple stents required ranged from 2 (78%) to 4 (7%). Repeat treatment rates were 14.3% for the entire study group vs. 43.9% for the multiple stent group. Just as in the study group overall, patients who required multiple stents exhibited marked improvement in peak urine flow rates and symptom scores. More than half of patients in each group reported pain 6 weeks after the procedure, but only 1 patient in each group described pain as "marked" at 1 year. Hematuria was more common in the multiple stent group at 1 year (24% vs. 9%). Incontinence, described as mild in most patients, tended to improve with time and did not differ between single and multiple stent groups.

Conclusion.—In the North American UroLume Wallstent trial, multiple stents were required initially for strictures longer than 2.5 cm and for multiple, separate strictures. Secondary insertion was necessitated by recurrent stricture adjacent to the stent, hyperplastic tissue growth within the stent, and gaps between previously adjacent stents. Patients with multiple stents had higher rates of repeat treatment, but their outcome in terms of urine flow and symptom scores was equivalent to that of the study group overall.

▶ The urethral stent in complex urethral strictures is moderately successful. Hyperplastic tissue (presumably recurrent fibrosis) occurs in up to 20% of patients with multiple stents and 7% of all patients. Recurrent stricture adjacent to the stent occurs nearly 10% of the time. Whether this was related to insufficient initial stent length or peri-stent irritation is unclear. The most distressing outcome is the incidence of urinary incontinence in 24% of patients after stent placement. A formal urethroplasty is preferential in most patients, and this device should be limited to complex failures or debilitated patients who cannot withstand an open urethroplasty.

D.E. Coplen, M.D.

Role of Preoperative Sonourethrography in Bulbar Urethral Reconstruction

Morey AF, McAninch JW (Univ of California, San Francisco; San Francisco Gen Hosp, Calif)
J Urol 158:1376–1379, 1997   20–6

Background.—Sonourethrography is useful for evaluation of bulbar urethral strictures. The role of preoperative sonourethrography in prospective procedure selection for bulbar urethral reconstruction was investigated in 67 male patients.

Methods.—All patients had bulbar urethral strictures of ≤25 mm or less on preoperative radiographic retrograde urethrography and were considered good candidates for resection and end-to-end anastomosis. Sonourethrography was performed just prior to incision. These 2 measurements were compared, and the sonographic measurement was used to guide selection of the urethroplasty technique.

Results.—Sonographic measurements of bulbar urethral strictures were longer than retrograde urethrography measurements in a significant number of cases. Of the 67 patients, the 26 patients with short strictures on retrograde urethrography were treated successfully by resection and end-

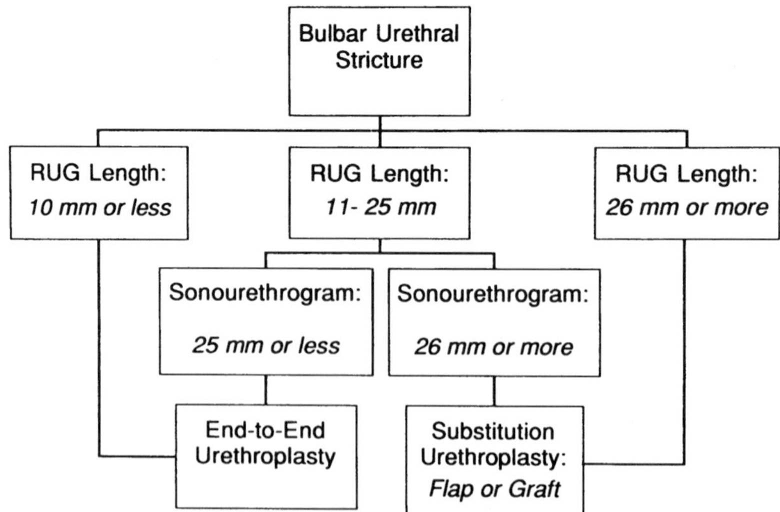

FIGURE 6.—Algorithm of role of preoperative sonourethrography in reconstruction of bulbar urethral strictures. *Abbreviation: RUB,* retrograde urethrography. (Courtesy of Morey AF, McAninch JW: Role of preoperative sonourethrography in bulbar urethral reconstruction *J Urol* 158:1376–1379, 1997.)

to-end anastomosis. Sonographic assessment did not change the management of these patients. Ultrasonic measurements did affect the reconstructive technique selected in 15 of 41 patients with strictures of intermediate length (11–25 mm).

Conclusions.—Sonourethrography is more accurate than retrograde urethrography for assessing the length of bulbar urethral strictures. This increased accuracy becomes important in the prospective selection of urethral reconstruction technique in patients with intermediate length strictures. These authors propose that sonourethrography be prospectively performed in patients with intermediate length strictures on retrograde urethrography. Excisional therapy should be used for those <25 mm on sonography, and substitution urethroplasty should be performed for longer strictures (Fig 6).

▶ The authors have extensive experience with urethral sonography in stricture disease. They now use sonography only in the evaluation of select bulbar urethral strictures. Sonography was performed intraoperatively, but no correlation was made between sonographic stricture length and actual length at the time of surgery. When the stricture length was >25 mm as determined with sonography, then substitution urethroplasty was performed regardless of the intraoperative findings. Intraoperative measurement of the stricture length might be as informative. The authors follow the algorithm in Figure 6, but no surgical outcomes are reported.

D.E. Coplen, M.D.

21 Erectile Dysfunction

The International Index of Erectile Function (IIEF): A Multidimensional Scale for Assessment of Erectile Dysfunction
Rosen RC, Riley A, Wagner G, et al (Univ of Medicine and Dentistry of New Jersey, Piscataway; Springfield Univ Hosp, London; Univ of Copenhagen; et al)
Urology 49:822–830, 1997
21–1

Background.—A National Institutes of Health (NIH) Consensus Development Conference has defined erectile dysfunction as the inability to achieve or maintain an erection adequate for satisfactory sexual performance. A brief, reliable measure of erectile function was designed to be cross-culturally valid and psychometrically sound.

Methods.—Relevant domains of sexual function in various cultures were identified, and an initial questionnaire was developed for administration to patients with erectile dysfunction. The final 15-item questionnaire—the International Index of Erectile Function (IIEF)—was tested for its sensitivity, specificity, reliability, and construct validity (Appendix).

Findings.—In a principal components analysis, 5 factors with eigenvalues exceeding 1.0 were identified: erectile function, orgasmic function, sexual desire, intercourse satisfaction, and overall satisfaction. Test-retest repeatability correlation coefficients for the scores in these domains were very significant. Construct validity was adequate. All 5 domains showed a

---

APPENDIX—Individual Items of International Index of Erectile Function Questionnaire and Response Options (US Version)

Question*	Response Options
Q1: How often were you able to get an erection during sexual activity?	0 = No sexual activity 1 = Almost never/never
Q2: When you had erections with sexual stimulation, how often were your erections hard enough for penetration?	2 = A few times (much less than half the time) 3 = Sometimes (about half the time) 4 = Most times (much more than half the time) 5 = Almost always/always
Q3: When you attempted sexual intercourse, how often were you able to penetrate (enter) your partner?	0 = Did not attempt intercourse 1 = Almost never/never 2 = A few times (much less than half the time)
Q4: During sexual intercourse, <u>how often</u> were you able to maintain your erection after you had penetrated (entered) your partner?	3 = Sometimes (about half the time) 4 = Most times (much more than half the time) 5 = Almost always/always

(Continued)

APPENDIX (cont.)

Question*	Response Options
Q5: During sexual intercourse, <u>how difficult</u> was it to maintain your erection to completion of intercourse?	0 = Did not attempt intercourse 1 = Extremely difficult 2 = Very difficult 3 = Difficult 4 = Slightly difficult 5 = Not difficult
Q6: How many times have you attempted sexual-intercourse?	0 = No attempts 1 = One to two attempts 2 = Three to four attempts 3 = Five to six attempts 4 = Seven to ten attempts 5 = Eleven+ attempts
Q7: When you attempted sexual intercourse, how often was it satisfactory for you?	0 = Did not attempt intercourse 1 = Almost never/never 2 = A few times (much less than half the time) 3 = Sometimes (about half the time) 4 = Most times (much more than half the time) 5 = Almost always/always
Q8: How much have you enjoyed sexual inter-course?	0 = No intercourse 1 = No enjoyment 2 = Not very enjoyable 3 = Fairly enjoyable 4 = Highly enjoyable 5 = Very highly enjoyable
Q9: When you had sexual stimulation <u>or</u> inter-course, how often did you ejaculate? Q10: When you had sexual stimulation <u>or</u> inter-course, how often did you have the feeling of orgasm or climax?	0 = No sexual stimulation/intercourse 1 = Almost never/never 2 = A few times (much less than half the time) 3 = Sometimes (about half the time) 4 = Most times (much more than half the time) 5 = Almost always/always
Q11: How often have you felt sexual desire?	1 = Almost never/never 2 = A few times (much less than half the time) 3 = Sometimes (about half the time) 4 = Most times (much more than half the time) 5 = Almost always/always
Q12: How would you rate your level of sexual desire?	1 = Very low/none at all 2 = Low 3 = Moderate 4 = High 5 = Very high
Q13: How satisfied have you been with your over-all <u>sex life</u>? Q14: How satisfied have you been with your <u>sexual relationship</u> with your partner?	1 = Very dissatisfied 2 = Moderately dissatisfied 3 = About equally satisfied and dissatisfied 4 = Moderately satisfied 5 = Very satisfied
Q15: How do you rate your <u>confidence</u> that you could get and keep an erection?	1 = Very low 2 = Low 3 = Moderate 4 = High 5 = Very high

All questions are preceded by the phrase "Over the past 4 weeks."

(Courtesy of Rosen RC, Riley A, Wagner G, et al: The International Index of Erectile Function (IIEF): A multidimensional scale for assessment of erectile dysfunction. *Urology* 49:822–830. Copyright 1997, with permission from Elsevier Science.)

high degree of sensitivity and specificity to the effects of treatment. Significant changes between baseline and posttreatment scores were noted in all 5 domains in treatment responders but not in the nonresponders.

Conclusions.—The IIEF addresses the relevant domains of male sexual function and is psychometrically sound. The questionnaire is self-administered and available in 10 languages. It is sensitive and specific enough to detect treatment-related changes in men with erectile dysfunction.

▶ The IIEF is an excellent attempt to quantify erectile function (for example, symptom score) addressing several aspects of sexual function. With a brief 15 items, this scale appears to satisfy both clinical and research needs of simplicity, reliability, and specificity and would be a valuable adjunct to any multidisciplinary approach to the treatment of erectile dysfunction.

D.P. O'Brien, M.D.

Modified Nesbit Procedure for the Treatment of Peyronie's Disease: A Comparative Outcome Analysis
Licht MR, Lewis RW (Cleveland Clinic Florida, Ft Lauderdale; Med College of Georgia, Augusta)
J Urol 158:460–463, 1997   21–2

Introduction.—Peyronie's disease causes a bending deformity of the penile shaft. Surgical correction is needed when the deformity makes normal sexual function impossible. Among the various surgical techniques, the Nesbit procedure removes an ellipse of tunica albuginea opposite the plaque to straighten the penis. A surgical modification of the Nesbit procedure was compared with 2 other techniques: the standard Nesbit procedure and plaque excision with synthetic patch-graft repair.

Methods.—Two groups (28 patients each) had previously undergone a standard Nesbit procedure or plaque excision with a polyethylene-terephthalate mesh–reinforced silicone-sheet patch graft. Thirty patients were treated with the modified Nesbit procedure (Figure), in which a vertical incision in the tunica albuginea is closed in a horizontal fashion. Permanent suture knots are buried beneath the tunica in a running looped manner, providing a watertight closure with no exposed suture material.

Results.—The 3 treatment groups were similar in mean age, mean plaque size, percentage of impotence, previous therapy, and history of trauma. Mean follow-up time was almost 2 years in the standard Nesbit and patch-graft groups and 12 months in the modified Nesbit group. Compared with the standard Nesbit and patch-graft groups, more patients in the modified Nesbit group had penile curvature completely eliminated (79%, 61%, and 93%, respectively). Overall patient satisfaction was 83% with the modified Nesbit procedure, 79% with the standard Nesbit procedure, and 30% with the patch-graft technique. Postoperative impotence (de novo loss of erection after surgery) occurred in 1 patient after the standard Nesbit procedure and in 4 after patch graft, but in none of the modified Nesbit group. Thirteen of 14 patients who were impotent pre-

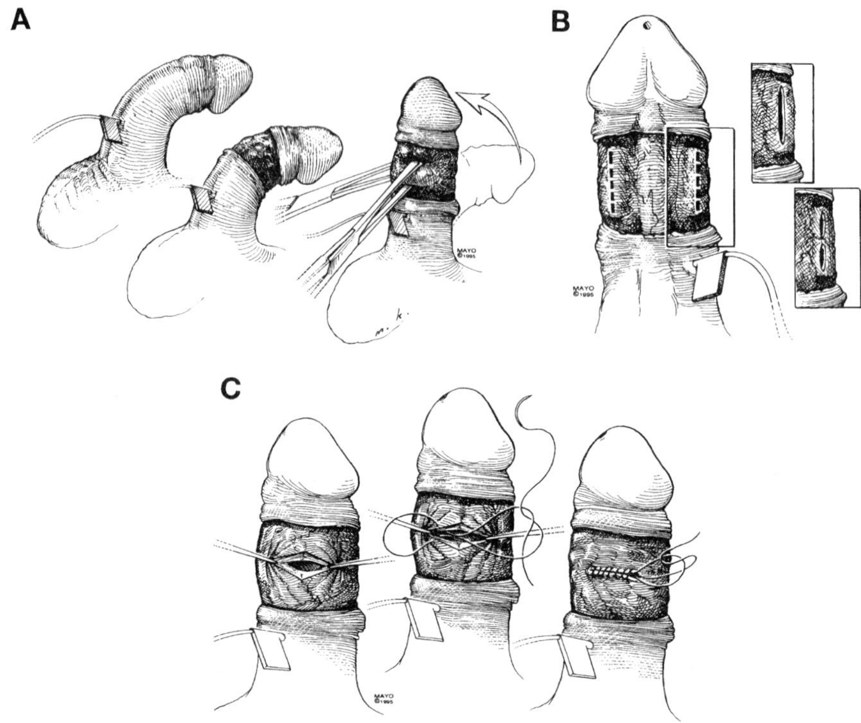

FIGURE.—A, Allis clamps are used to grasp and gather tunica albuginea opposite the point of maximum penile curvature during artificial erection. **B,** 1 longitudinal or multiple smaller incisions are made between indentations left by Allis clamp. **C,** incisions are closed horizontally using running permanent suture with knots buried at both ends. (Courtesy of Licht MR, Lewis RW: Modified Nesbit procedure for the treatment of Peyronie's disease: A comparative outcome analysis. *J Urol* 158:460–463, 1997. By permission of Mayo Foundation.)

operatively remained impotent; 1 in the modified Nesbit group reported return of erectile function.

Conclusion.—The modified Nesbit procedure was more successful than the other 2 procedures in achieving penile straightening and yielded a higher rate of patient satisfaction. Differences in outcomes between the standard and modified Nesbit procedures were not always significant, but patch grafting was significantly less successful in eliminating curvature and providing patient satisfaction. The Nesbit procedure is relatively easy to perform and requires a minimum of postoperative care and recovery.

▶ This is an excellent and practical article describing a nice modification to the Nesbit procedure. I have used a similar modification[1] (including permanent buried sutures) without the incision for several years with similar success. These procedures all cause some shortening and work better on a penis with good initial length. Correction of lateral curvatures is also more successful in preventing real or perceived shortening of the penis by the patient than is correction of dorsal curvatures, particularly if the curve is severe. A shorter penis or one with a severe curve is best treated with plaque excision and grafting or penile prostheses in patients with concomitant impotence.

D.P. O'Brien, M.D.

Reference

1. Walton KN: A modified Nesbit procedure for Peyronie's disease. Presented at the Societie' de Internationale Urologie, Vienna, July 1985.

MUSE Therapy: Preliminary Clinical Observations
Werthman P, Rajfer J (Univ of California, Los Angeles)
Urology 50:809–811, 1997

21–3

Background.—Treatment of erectile dysfunction relies on intracavernosal injection of vasodilating agents. An alternative form of pharmacotherapy has recently been introduced: a transurethral delivery system (MUSE) for alprostadil (prostaglandin E_1). Preliminary clinical observations were reported.

Methods.—One hundred consecutive patients with erectile dysfunction underwent MUSE treatment. Doses ranged from 125 to 1,000 µg. Erections were observed in a clinical setting. All men had had intracavernosal injections of combination pharmacotherapy in the past.

Findings.—Only 7% of the men treated with MUSE had well-sustained, rigid erections. Thirty percent had full erections with partial rigidity. The remaining 63% of the men did not have erections that they thought were sufficient for penetration. Twenty-four percent of the men had penile pain, perineal pain, or both. Three percent had a syncopal episode, and another 3% had urethral bleeding. One patient had priapism that needed to be drained. Intracavernosal injections resulted in sustained rigid erections in 49%, full erections with partial rigidity in 40%, and an inadequate response in 11%.

Conclusions.—Intracavernosal injections are more effective than MUSE administration of alprostadil in producing a rigid, sustained erection suitable for intercourse in most men with erectile dysfunction. The authors have developed a practical clinical algorithm for selecting patients for MUSE therapy, in which all men with erectile dysfunction are required to undergo an initial diagnostic injection of intracavernosal medication.

▶ As noted in this article, the majority of patients using MUSE therapy do not have rigid erections. In this series, 37% of patients had erections adequate for penetration. A larger percentage of patients using intracavernosal injection therapy have erections adequate for penetration. Office titration and sufficient home trials are necessary for full evaluation of MUSE therapy, which may not be as effective as some initial studies have shown.

D.P. O'Brien, M.D.

Long-term Follow-up of Patients Receiving Injection Therapy for Erectile Dysfunction

Sundaram CP, Thomas W, Pryor LE, et al (Univ of Minnesota, Minneapolis; Sackler School of Medicine, Tel Aviv, Israel)
Urology 49:932–935, 1997   21–4

Background.—Vasoactive intracavernosal pharmacotherapy (VIP) is widely used by men with erectile dysfunction. Medications such as papaverine, phentolamine, and prostaglandin E_1 are injected singly or in combination, causing relaxation of the cavernous and arteriolar smooth muscle, filling of the penile sinusoids with blood, and restriction of venous outflow. Patients who were started on VIP between 1984 and 1989 were studied 5 years later to determine long-term complications and dropout rates.

Methods.—Between November 1984 and July 1989, 186 men entered the VIP self-injection program at the University of Minnesota; 108 were available for follow-up, and 100 completed a questionnaire about their VIP experience. The hospital records of these 100 men were reviewed. Those who discontinued VIP were compared with those who continued therapy.

Results.—Seventy-seven respondents had used a combination of papaverine and phentolamine. The median total number of injections per patient was 100. During their time on VIP, respondents had a median of 4 injections per month. Nearly half of the patients increased the dosage of the vasoactive agent from the initial titration. Side effects were common (41%) but relatively minor. Sixty-eight patients discontinued self-injection therapy, 38 within a year of starting injections. Those who discontinued VIP were older than those who did not (mean age, 51.3 years vs. 44.8 years). The incidence of side effects was similar in these 2 groups. Frequently cited factors leading to discontinuation of injection therapy were the desire for a permanent modality (29.4%), lack of a partner (26.5%), and poor response (23.5%).

Conclusions.—The initial dropout rate is high among men who start injection therapy for erectile dysfunction, but those who continue for 2 years tend to continue long-term therapy. Side effects continue to be relatively minor during long-term follow-up. Regular follow-up of patients is important, especially during the first year of VIP use and for men older than 50 years.

▶ This is one of the longest follow-up studies reported on patients using injection therapy for erectile dysfunction. The most important data showing diminished dropout after 2 years of therapy indicate the continued need for close patient observation either for reassurance to continue the injections or to promote some other form of therapy before irreversible penile changes occur. It is also important to note the low rate of long-term complications (e.g., penile fibrosis).

D.P. O'Brien, M.D.

Predictors of Success and Risk Factors for Attrition in the Use of Intracavernous Injection
Gupta R, Kirschen J, Barrow RC II, et al (New York Hosp)
J Urol 157:1681–1686, 1997   21–5

Introduction.—Although intracavernous pharmacologic therapy is a safe and effective option for most patients with erectile dysfunction, reported attrition rates range from 11% to 80%. A large group of patients enrolled in an erectile dysfunction unit was studied for potential predictors of attrition, length of time from initiation of injections to their discontinuation, and alternative therapies chosen.

Methods.—Data were available on 1,089 patients enrolled in a program for pharmacologically assisted erection between 1988 and 1996. All completed a sexual function questionnaire, were given a detailed history and physical examination, and had psychological inhibition ruled out as a cause of the dysfunction. Patients were invited to take part in a home injection trial if a good response was obtained after the first injection of papaverine (30 mg) plus phentolamine (0.5 mg) or low-dose prostaglandin E_1 (5–10 µg). An attempt was made to contact those who discontinued injection therapy after entering the maintenance phase of the program.

Results.—Approximately two thirds (62.4%) of patients remained active participants for a mean of 26.2 months, 37.7% discontinued therapy, and 20.8% did not complete follow-up. The active and inactive groups did not differ in mean age (61.5 vs. 62.8 years), mean duration of erection (48.6 vs. 48.1 minutes), or mean injection frequency (5.8 vs. 4.9 times per month), but more patients in the inactive group had vascular dysfunction as a cause of impotence. Half of those who ceased therapy did so early in the course of treatment, after receiving the first 20 injections. The mean period of participation for patients who eventually discontinued therapy did not differ significantly according to medication (18.5 months for papaverine plus phentolamine vs. 15.4 months for prostaglandin E_1), but significantly more patients discontinued papaverine plus phentolamine than remained on this regimen. Patients who dropped out in the first month often cited inconvenience, pain, and ineffectiveness as causes; lack of efficacy continued to be a predominant reason. Data on follow-up treatment were available for 150 patients, 52% of whom received a penile prosthesis.

Conclusion.—Most patients who discontinue intracavernous injection therapy do so in the first 2 months. Lack of treatment efficacy and vascular dysfunction are risk factors for attrition, and most who discontinue injections seek alternative therapies. Clinicians should counsel patients at high risk for treatment failure about other options.

▶ This is a valuable study of the reasons for attrition of patients from an injection therapy protocol for erectile dysfunction. This study points out the need for attentive follow-up for this group of patients. This type of intensive detail not only diminishes attrition but also promotes patient acceptance of other modalities of therapy (e.g., prosthetics rather than abandoning treatment altogether).

D.P. O'Brien, M.D.

Comparative Study of Papaverine Plus Phentolamine Versus Prostaglandin E1 in Erectile Dysfunction

Bechara A, Casabé A, Chéliz G, et al (Hosp Durand, Buenos Aires, Argentina)
J Urol 157:2132–2134, 1997   21–6

Introduction.—A number of vasoactive drugs have been used successfully in the diagnosis and treatment of sexual erectile dysfunction. Papaverine plus phentolamine is far more effective than papaverine alone, and the addition of these 2 agents to prostaglandin E_1 has a reported efficacy of 85%. Responses and short-term adverse effects of papaverine plus phentolamine vs. prostaglandin E_1 were studied in patients undergoing erection testing.

Methods.—Sixty patients aged 22–78 years (mean, 58 years) participated. None had neurologic impairment or had undergone a previous test of pharmacologically induced erection. The patients were randomly assigned to 6 groups to be tested 1 week apart with the 2 active solutions and placebo. Weekly injections contained 30 mg of papaverine hydrochloride and 0.5 mg of phentolamine mesylate in a 1-mL solution, 30 μg of prostaglandin E1 in a 1-mL solution, or a 1-mL isotonic sodium chloride solution. Erectile responses were classified on a scale from E0 (without tumefaction) to E5 (complete rigidity). Positive responses (E4 and E5) allowed penetration.

Results.—Response rates were 54% for papaverine plus phentolamine and 50% for prostaglandin E_1; no patient responded to placebo. The 2 active solutions did not differ significantly in their ability to achieve an erectile response that allowed penetration. Prolonged erection occurred in 15% of patients given prostaglandin E_1 and in 18% given papaverine plus phentolamine; pain was reported in 35% and 15%, respectively, of these 2 groups.

Discussion.—Although prostaglandin E_1 and the combination of papaverine and phentolamine did not differ significantly in the rate of positive responses or of prolonged erection, prostaglandin E_1 injections were reported to be significantly more painful. Because prostaglandin E_1 causes more pain and costs considerably more per dose, papaverine plus phentolamine appears to be the drug of choice for erection testing and for self-injection treatment.

▶ This is a nice randomized study with placebo control that, in the same population, combined several observations of the injection reaction, the most valuable of which is the determination that a papaverine-phentolamine mixture may be the most suitable combination for a test of pharmacologically induced erection.

D.P. O'Brien, M.D.

The Impact of Aging on Penile Hemodynamics in Normal Responders to Pharmacological Injection: A Doppler Sonographic Study
Chung WS, Park YY, Kwon SW (Ewha Woman's Univ, Seoul, Korea)
J Urol 157:2129–2131, 1997   21–7

Introduction.—Elderly men with impotence often have stenosis or occlusions in the vascular system responsible for erection; however, erectile function can also be affected by the natural aging process. Sixty-four patients with erectile dysfunction were studied for age-related changes in penile arterial flow during pharmacologically induced erection.

Methods.—The patients ranged in age from 17 to 74 years and were classified into 4 groups according to age: younger than 30 years (n = 12), 30–39 years (n = 22), 40–49 years (n = 15), and 50 years or older (n = 15). All responded well to intracavernous injection of prostaglandin E_1 (10 µg), with sustained nonbuckling rigidity of the penis lasting longer than 1 hour. After the injection, real-time color duplex US of the cavernous arteries was performed, and flow parameters, including peak systolic and end-diastolic flow velocities, were recorded 3 times. The flow parameters of the cavernous arteries were compared among the 4 age groups.

Results.—All patients had a maximum peak systolic velocity of greater than 30 cm per second and a minimum end-diastolic velocity of less than 3 cm per second. The average maximum peak systolic velocity was statistically different, however, in the various age groups. Peak systolic velocity decreased with age, with the greatest decrease observed between patients in the third and fourth decades. When peak systolic velocity was compared for each measurement according to the sampling time by age group, all average peak systolic velocities were similar regardless of the sampling time in men in their 20s and 30s. Patients 40 years and older demonstrated a significant increase in peak systolic velocity at the second and third measurements compared with the first measurement.

Conclusion.—Cavernous arterial flow during pharmacologically induced erections clearly decreases with age, with the greatest decrease occurring between the third and fourth decades. After age 50, maximum peak systolic velocity is reached later after intracorporeal injection than in younger patients. These changes should be considered when penile vascular inflow is evaluated in elderly patients.

▶ This study is an interesting addition to the rapidly increasing knowledge base regarding aging and the physiologic changes related to erection. Although modified by use of the pharmacologic agent, the data suggest a decrease in cavernous arterial flow and diminution of tissue response with aging. Further study of these tissues at the molecular level will be necessary to document the changes and to modify them in the future.

D.P. O'Brien, M.D.

Long-term Mechanical Reliability of AMS 700 Series Inflatable Penile Prostheses: Comparison of CX/CXM and Ultrex Cylinders

Daitch JA, Angermeier KW, Lakin MM, et al (Cleveland Clinic Found, Ohio)
J Urol 158:1400–1402, 1997   21–8

Background.—Recently, the incidence of revisions needed in patients with the length- and girth-expanding AMS 700 Ultrex inflatable penile prosthesis has been increasing. The long-term mechanical reliability of the AMS Ultrex inflatable penile prosthesis was compared with that of the girth-expanding AMS 700 CX and CXM inflatable penile prostheses in men with organic erectile dysfunction.

Methods.—Accurate follow-up data were obtained on 111 of 142 (78.2%) men with CX or CXM prostheses implanted between 1986 and 1995 and on 152 of 179 (84.9%) men implanted with Ultrex prostheses between 1989 and 1995. The end points compared were mechanical failure caused by any malfunctioning component, device failure caused by any cylinder complication, and cylinder aneurysms or leaks.

Findings.—Mechanical failures occurred in 9% of the CX/CXM group and in 17.1% of the Ultrex group. The incidences of cylinder complications were 4.5% and 8.6%, respectively. Cylinder aneurysms or leaks occurred in 2.7% of the CX/CXM and in 5.9% of the Ultrex devices. Kaplan-Meier estimates showed that mechanical survival (for all 3 end points) was significantly lower in the Ultrex group than in the CX/CXM group.

Conclusions.—Though Ultrex cylinders provide length and girth expansion, these prostheses have a greater mechanical failure rate than CX/CXM devices in a shorter length of follow-up. Patients with Ultrex cylinders should be monitored closely for problems.

▶ This is a companion study to Abstract 21–9 on the Mentor unit. I have had similar aneurysm and leak results with the Ultrex components and now use the CX/CXM system exclusively. Long-term results and reliability are excellent with either the Mentor or AMS products.

D.P. O'Brien, M.D.

Safety and Efficacy Outcome of Mentor Alpha-1 Inflatable Penile Prosthesis Implantation for Impotence Treatment

Goldstein I, Newman L, Baum N, et al (Boston Univ)
J Urol 157:833–839, 1997   21–9

Introduction.—Recent years have seen important changes in the design of the multicomponent inflatable penile prosthesis. Many studies have evaluated the success rates of specific penile prostheses; however, most have been single-center studies of approximately 100 patients. This broad-ranging, multicenter retrospective study evaluated the safety and efficacy of the Alpha-1 inflatable penile prosthesis (Mentor Corp., Santa Barbara, Calif) for treatment of impotence.

Methods.—The 2-phase study included medical record and questionnaire data from consecutive eligible patients of 7 physician-investigators. Only physicians experienced with penile prosthetic implantation were invited to participate in the study. The overall study population included 434 patients; 234 patients responded to the outcomes questionnaire. Ninety-one percent of the patients underwent implantation of the Alpha-1 prosthesis.

Results.—There were no deaths among 434 patients receiving Alpha-1 implants. Ninety-one percent of the patients were completely free of morbidity. Ninety-three percent of the prostheses remained free from replacement or revision surgery during the study period; 404 patients still had their original implant in place. In 7 patients, infection necessitated explantation of the prosthesis. In 5 patients, device malfunctions such as auto-inflation and fluid loss required implant removal. Five patients required surgical revision for pump replacement; in 4 of these, implantation was via a scrotal approach. The longest follow-up was 3.6 years, and 40% of the patients were followed up for at least 2 years.

Eighty-nine percent of the questionnaire respondents reported that the prosthesis met their expectations for impotence therapy. The results were as expected in 28% of the patients, better than expected in 31%, and much better than expected in 30%. Satisfaction rates were ≥80% for erectile ability, confidence with intercourse, and device function.

Conclusions.—Follow-up study of the patients with Alpha-1 penile implants shows zero mortality. Morbidity risk is 9%, risk of explantation or surgical revision is 7%, and mechanical failure risk is 2.5%. At 3-year follow-up, 85% of the devices are functioning and 75% of the patients have required no surgical intervention. Patient satisfaction is high. Contrary to conventional wisdom, the safety and efficacy of the Alpha-1 penile implant is comparable to that of noninflatable rod-type prostheses.

▶ Although this paper has some flaws, which the authors state, it does show clearly that, in experienced hands, the inflatable prosthesis can be implanted with a complication rate approaching that of rigid or semirigid rod surgery. Patient satisfaction was high in responders. I have found that the level of preoperative teaching is directly related to patient expectations and satisfaction postoperatively.

D.P. O'Brien, M.D.

Outpatient Inflatable Penile Prosthesis Insertion
Garber BB (Graduate Hosp, Philadelphia)
Urology 49:600–603, 1997   21–10

Background.—Inflatable penile prosthesis (IPP) implantation has been traditionally done on an inpatient basis. However, refinements in operative technique permit IPP insertion on an ambulatory basis, without the routine use of IV antibiotics, drains, urethral catheters, prosthesis inflation, and compression dressings. The initial outcomes of an ambulatory, outpatient, multiple-component IPP insertion protocol were reported.

Methods.—Ninety-five men with organic impotence were included. The operative technique involved a 2.5-cm-high vertical midline scrotal incision, exposed by a LoneStar retractor. Prosthetic components were prepared and soaked in an antibiotic irrigant solution consisting of polymyxin B sulfate (500,000 U), bacitracin (50,000 U), and gentamicin (80 mg/L of normal saline). Mean follow-up was 1 year.

Outcomes.—The prosthetic infection rate was 1%, which is comparable to that reported from inpatient implantation protocols. The most common complication was urinary retention, occurring in 4% of the patients. This complication was managed easily with temporary catheterization.

Conclusions.—Multiple-component IPP insertion can be adapted easily to an outpatient setting. Early results suggest that outpatient IPP insertion is safe and effective in men with organic impotence.

▶ This study shows gratifying results in 95 patients who had multiple-component IPPs, either Mentor or AMS types, placed in an ambulatory outpatient setting. An excellent infection rate (1%) was obtained, and the most frequent complication was urinary retention (4%). Certainly this form of cost management deserves consideration by all experienced implanters.

D.P. O'Brien, M.D.

Immediate Sexual Rehabilitation by Simultaneous Placement of Penile Prosthesis in Patients Undergoing Radical Prostatectomy: Initial Results in 50 Patients

Khoudary KP, DeWolf WC, Bruning CO III, et al (Harvard Med School, Boston)
Urology 50:395–399, 1997
21–11

Background.—Most men experience some degree of erectile dysfunction after radical prostatectomy, despite attempts at nerve sparing. In addition, nerve-sparing surgery may be contraindicated in some men. The outcomes of simultaneous placement of a penile prosthesis and radical prostatectomy were reported.

Methods.—Between 1993 and 1996, 50 men underwent a combined procedure of non–nerve-sparing radical retropubic prostatectomy and penile prosthesis placement. The records of these men were reviewed retrospectively. Findings were compared with those of 72 men undergoing radical prostatectomy alone during the same time. The 2 groups were comparable preoperatively.

Findings.—Prosthesis insertion required a mean of 82 minutes of operative time. Mean time to sexual intercourse was 12.7 weeks. At an average follow-up of 1.7 years, there have been no infections. Eight percent of the

TABLE 2.—Postoperative Complications

Complication	Rad Px (n = 72)	Comb (n = 50)
Prosthesis infection	N/A	0
Bladder neck contracture	10	5
Abscess	2	0
Biochemical failure	2	1
Rectal perforation	1	0
Bladder neck calculus	0	1
Incontinence—sphincter	0	1
Revision of prosthesis	N/A	4*
Postoperative hypotension	0	1

*All occurred in the first 25 patients.

Abbreviations: Rad Px, radical prostatectomy; *Comb,* combined procedure; *NIA,* not applicable.

(Courtesy of Khoudary KP, DeWolf WC, Bruning CO III, et al: Immediate sexual rehabilitation by simultaneous placement of penile prosthesis in patients undergoing radical prostatectomy: Initial results in 50 patients. *Urology* 50:395–399. Copyright 1997, with permission from Elsevier Science.)

men needed revision of the inflatable penile prosthesis. The 2 treatment groups did not differ significantly in estimated blood loss, length of hospitalization, or analgesic use (Table 2).

Conclusions.—The placement of a penile prosthesis during radical prostatectomy enables early return to sexual function, with no apparent increase in morbidity. Additional research is needed to determine the impact of such surgery on psychosocial adjustment and quality of life.

▶ This is an excellent presentation of the efficacy of simultaneous placement of a penile prosthesis at the time of radical prostatectomy in promoting rapid return to sexual function postoperatively. The lack of morbidity is a testament to the need for attention to detail as is mandatory in any prosthetic endeavor. This also obviates the difficult reservoir placement following extensive pelvic surgery and could be considered for utilization in patients undergoing cystoprostatectomy .

D.P. O'Brien, M.D.

Recovery of Spontaneous Erectile Function After Nerve-sparing Radical Retropubic Prostatectomy With and Without Early Intracavernous Injections of Alprostadil: Results of a Prospective, Randomized Trial

Montorsi F, Guazzoni G, Strambi LF, et al (Univ of Milan, Italy)
J Urol 158:1408–1410, 1997

21–12

Background.—Recovery of normal erections after a nerve-sparing radical prostatectomy requires several months. This prolonged interval, characterized by the absence of frequent and rigid erections, may be associated with cavernous hypoxia and subsequent damage to the cavernous tissue, resulting in erectile dysfunction. The effects of early postoperative intracavernous injections of alprostadil on cavernous hypoxia and tissue damage were investigated.

Methods.—Thirty men with clinically localized prostate cancer underwent nerve-sparing radical retropubic prostatectomy and were then assigned randomly to alprostadil injections 3 times a week for 12 weeks (group 1) or observation with no erectogenic treatment (group 2). Patients were assessed at 6 months.

Findings.—Eighty percent of the patients in group 1 completed treatment. Sixty-seven percent of these 12 patients reported the recovery of spontaneous erection adequate for satisfactory sexual intercourse, compared with 20% in group 2. This difference was significant. All but 1 man reporting normal postoperative erections in group 1 also had normal erections during nocturnal testing. Color Doppler sonography demonstrated normal penile hemodynamics in all group 1 patients. In this group, failures resulted from cavernous veno-occlusive dysfunction (17%) and cavernous nerve injury (17%). Group 2 patients with normal erections had normal nocturnal testing and penile hemodynamics. Failures in this group resulted from cavernous veno-occlusive dysfunction (53%), cavernous arterial insufficiency (13%), or cavernous nerve injury (20%). Complications in group 1 included a penile nodule in 2 men (13%) and prolonged penile erection in 1 (6%). None of the patients in group 2 had complications.

Conclusions.—Early postoperative injections of alprostadil significantly increase the recovery rate of spontaneous erections after nerve-sparing radical retropubic prostatectomy. Programmed vasoactive injections may improve cavernous oxygenation, thereby limiting the development of hypoxia-induced tissue damage. This treatment may produce complications, which must be explained clearly to patients.

▶ This article has small numbers but a large message that early return to erectile function by injection therapy may preserve, promote earlier return of spontaneous erections, or both by limiting the development of hypoxia-induced cavernosal tissue damage. We have used both injection therapy and MUSE therapy in the early postoperative period following radical prostatectomy with good success. The psychological benefit of this approach is obvious, but the physiologic benefits need further experimental documentation.

D.P. O'Brien, M.D.

Apoptosis in the Rat Penis After Penile Denervation
Klein LT, Miller MI, Buttyan R, et al (Columbia Univ, New York)
J Urol 158:626–630, 1997   21–13

Objective.—Patients undergoing radical prostatectomy are at risk for erectile dysfunction. Although the risk for this complication has been lessened by nerve-sparing radical prostatectomy, at least 30% of patients will be impotent. Some patients complain of decreased penile size after the operation. This has led the authors to hypothesize that injury to the cavernous nerves may lead to programmed cell death within the penis. This process, also called apoptosis, is a basic biological process that governs tissue size and form. Early molecular events after penile denervation were studied in rats, including the occurrence of penile apoptosis.

Methods.—Bilateral cavernous neurotomy or a sham operation was performed in male Sprague-Dawley rats. Penile amputation was performed at 1 to 10 days postoperatively. Penile extracts were prepared for analysis of messenger RNA.

Results.—The denervated rat penes showed distinct internucleosomal degradation of DNA, providing evidence of apoptosis. In situ end-labeling techniques showed apoptotic bodies in the cavernous tissue after denervation. Denervation also induced expression of sulfated glycoprotein-2 (SGP-2), a gene product reportedly elevated in apoptotic tissues. The level of SGP-2 increased slightly in the later days after sham operation, but not to the levels seen after denervation. Thus, apoptosis appeared to be an early event after denervation.

Conclusions.—This rat model of penile denervation suggests that apoptosis of the penis occurs after injury to the cavernous nerves. Apoptosis may play a role in the loss of penile mass in patients undergoing prostatectomy. The findings offer new insights into our understanding of the molecular events underlying erectile dysfunction.

▶ This excellent study attempts to evaluate the molecular basis for erectile dysfunction or decrease in penile size following the denervation that obtains after radical prostatectomy. The study also adds fodder to the speculation that treatment of impotence after prostatectomy should begin in the early postoperative period to prevent further deterioration of the mechanisms of erection.

D.P. O'Brien, M.D.

Age Decreases Nitric Oxide Synthase-containing Nerve Fibers in the Rat Penis

Carrier S, Nagaraju P, Morgan DM, et al (Univ of California, San Francisco)
J Urol 157:1088–1092, 1997   21–14

Background.—Although erectile dysfunction is common in elderly men, it should not be considered a normal consequence of aging. Intracavernous smooth-muscle relaxation, the most important step in the mechanism of erection, appears to involve vasoactive intestinal polypeptide (VIP) and nitric oxide (NO). A rat model was used to clarify the effect of aging on the number and distribution of VIP- and (NO) synthase (NOS)–containing nerve fibers within the corpus cavernosum and dorsal nerve. The erectile response to apomorphine, electrostimulation of the cavernous nerve, and intracorporeal papaverine injection was also investigated.

Methods.—Twenty-three adult male Sprague-Dawley rats were used. Eight were 2.5 months old (young group), 8 were 8.5 months old (intermediate group), and 7 were 24 months old (old group). All were kept on a 12-hour light/dark cycle. The rats were observed for the number of erections after injection of apomorphine. During a surgical procedure, the pelvic nerves and the cavernous nerves were identified and exposed. Intracavernous pressures and blood pressures were measured and recorded. The cavernous nerve was electrostimulated on each side, and after a 15-minute rest period, a 900–µg dose of papaverine hydrochloride was administered intracavernously. A mid-shaft penile segment was taken for staining of the cavernous tissue and dorsal nerve.

Results.—The 3 age groups differed significantly in the number of observed erections and yawns in the 30-minute observation period. Young rats had the greatest number of erections in the apomorphine study (mean, 3.6), significantly more than the old group (mean, 1.0). Old rats had significantly fewer NOS-containing nerve fibers than did young and intermediate-aged rats (mean, 63.3; 135.1; and 127.8, respectively). During electrostimulation, the latency period before a rise in intracavernous pressure increased with age (6.77 vs. 2.3 seconds in young rats). The maximal intracavernous pressure after papaverine injection showed an age-dependent decrease, but pressures were lower than those achieved with electrostimulation.

Discussion.—Aging in rats was associated with a reduction in neurotransmitters, increasing the threshold to stimuli and diminishing responsiveness. The reduction in NOS-containing nerve fibers appears to have a central role in the age-related decreased response of the erectile mechanism.

▶ This quality study adds to the growing physiologic data of the aging phenomenon of erections at the cellular and molecular level. As noted by the authors, the erectile mechanism itself appears to remain intact, so that treatment of the erectile dysfunction of aging in the future will be directed at modifying the physiologic changes of the neuromuscular response.

D.P. O'Brien, M.D.

22 Testis Tumor

International Germ Cell Consensus Classification: A Prognostic Factor-based Staging System for Metastatic Germ Cell Cancers
Mead GM, for the International Germ Cell Cancer Collaborative Group (Royal South Hants Hosp, Southampton, England)
J Clin Oncol 15:594–603, 1997   22–1

Background.—The incidence of seminomatous and nonseminomatous germ cell tumors (GCTs), the most frequent cancers of young men, is increasing rapidly. Mortality from metastatic GCTs was high until the introduction of cisplatin-containing chemotherapy; now, overall cure rates of GCTs are better than 80%. A simple prognostic factor-based staging classification system for metastatic GCTs was developed for use in clinical practice and collaborative trials.

Methods.—The study included clinical data on 5,202 patients with nonseminomatous GCTs (NSGCTs) and 660 patients with seminomas, all treated with cisplatin-containing chemotherapy. The patients were treated by collaborative groups from 10 countries; the median follow-up was 5 years. Multivariate analyses were performed to identify prognostic factors for progression and survival. The multivariate models were then validated in an independent data set of more recently treated patients.

Results.—Independent adverse factors for patients with NSGCTs were the mediastinal primary site, α-fetoprotein level, human chorionic gonadotropin level, lactate dehydrogenase (LDH) level, and presence of nonpulmonary visceral metastases. The latter was the main adverse prognostic factor for patients with seminoma. A model constructed from these factors identified 3 risk groups, each of which was classified as nonseminoma or seminoma (Fig 4). Sixty percent of patients were in the good prognosis group, which had a 5-year survival of 91%. Twenty-six percent were in the intermediate prognosis group, which had a 5-year survival of 79%. The remaining 14% of patients, all of whom had NSGCTs, were in the poor prognosis group, which had a 5-year survival of 48%.

Conclusions.—A clinically based prognostic classification system for GCTs is reported. This system has been agreed to by all major clinical trial groups currently active worldwide. Use of the classification in clinical practice and research will facilitate international communication regarding the assessment and treatment of GCTs.

GOOD PROGNOSIS	
NON-SEMINOMA	**SEMINOMA**
Testis/retroperitoneal primary *and* No non-pulmonary visceral metastases *and* Good markers - all of *AFP < 1000 ng/ml and hCG < 5000 iu/l (1000 ng/ml) and LDH < 1.5 x upper limit of normal* **56% of non-seminomas 5 year PFS 89% 5 year Survival 92%**	Any primary site *and* No non-pulmonary visceral metastases *and* Normal AFP, any hCG, any LDH **90% of seminomas 5 year PFS 82% 5 year Survival 86%**
INTERMEDIATE PROGNOSIS	
NON-SEMINOMA	**SEMINOMA**
Testis/retroperitoneal primary *and* No non-pulmonary visceral metastases *and* **Intermediate markers - any of:** *AFP ≥ 1000 and ≤ 10,000 ng/mL or hCG ≥ 5000 iu/l and ≤ 50,000 iu/l or LDH ≥ 1.5 x N and ≤ 10 x N* **28% of non-seminomas 5 year PFS 75% 5 year Survival 80%**	Any primary site *and* **Non-pulmonary visceral metastases** *and* Normal AFP, any hCG, any LDH **10% of seminomas 5 year PFS 67% 5 year Survival 72%**
POOR PROGNOSIS	
NON-SEMINOMA	**SEMINOMA**
Mediastinal primary *or* **Non-pulmonary visceral metastases** *or* **Poor markers - any of:** *AFP > 10,000 ng/ml or hCG > 50,000 iu/l (10000 ng/ml) or LDH > 10 x upper limit of normal* **16% of non-seminomas 5 year PFS 41% 5 year Survival 48%**	**No patients classified as poor prognosis**

FIGURE 4.—Definition of the germ cell consensus classification. *Abbreviations: AFP*, alpha-fetoprotein; *hCG*, human chorionic gonadotrophin; *LDH*, lactate dehydrogenase; *PFS*, progression-free survival. (Courtesy of Mead GM, for the International Germ Cell Cancer Collaborative Group. *J Clin Oncol* 15:594–603, 1997.)

▶ This manuscript presents a remarkable collaboration of groups from 10 countries who provided information on patients with metastatic GCTs treated with cisplatin-containing chemotherapy. The results of this collaboration are shown in Table 4 of the original article. When I look over this table, 3 things jump out to me. The first is that a major adverse factor was the presence of a mediastinal primary site in patients with nonseminomatous GCTs. A second concerns the presence of nonpulmonary visceral metastasis usually to the liver, bone, and brain but also occasionally including the bowel or the adrenal gland. Finally, serum LDH has now been confirmed as an important prognostic factor for all GCTs. Although the assay conditions have not been standardized, it is noteworthy that almost half of the patients with very high LDH levels (greater than 10 times normal) had high-risk tumors, and overall survival was poorer for these patients even when an elevated LDH level was the only poor risk factor.

G.L. Andriole, Jr., M.D.

Decision Analysis for Avoiding Postchemotherapy Surgery in Patients With Disseminated Nonseminomatous Germ Cell Tumors
Debono DJ, Heilman DK, Einhorn LH, et al (Indiana Univ, Indianapolis)
J Clin Oncol 15:1455–1464, 1997   22–2

Objective.—Nonseminomatous germ cell tumor (NSGCT) is a curable malignancy. However, there is debate over the role of postchemotherapy surgery and the identification of patients most likely to have residual fibrosis or necrosis, in whom postchemotherapy surgery might be averted. The authors' department has been following a policy of observation for all patients with NSGCT with serologic and radiographic complete remission (CR) after chemotherapy. The results of this policy at 7-year follow-up were reviewed.

Methods.—The retrospective study included 295 consecutive patients undergoing primary chemotherapy for disseminated NSGCTs. After primary chemotherapy, the patients were classified according to their response and the presence or absence of teratoma in the primary tumor. Group A included 78 patients with CR; group B, 50 patients with unresectable tumor; group C, 90 patients with serologic CR, a teratoma-positive primary tumor, and resectable partial remission (PR); group D, 50 patients with serologic CR, teratoma-negative primary tumor, and <90% radiographic PR; and group E, 27 patients with serologic CR, teratoma-negative primary tumor, and ≥90% radiographic PR. Routine postchemotherapy management was observation for patients in groups A, B, and E, whereas those in groups C and D underwent routine postchemotherapy surgical resection. The long-term results of these 2 approaches were analyzed to validate the policy of selective observation.

Results.—The percentage of patients who were continuously without evidence of disease was 92% in group A, 40% in group B, 87% in group C, 86% in group D, and 74% in group E. Overall and progression-free survival were similar for patients in group A (those in CR who were observed) and the patients in groups C and D (who underwent surgery). For patients in group A, the bulk of retroperitoneal disease at presentation had no significant effect on the results of treatment.

Conclusions.—For patients with NSGCT who have serologic and radiologic evidence of CR after primary chemotherapy, postchemotherapy retroperitoneal lymph node dissection is not necessary. For patients with serologic CR, ≥90% radiographic remission, and teratoma-negative tumor, the optimal approach to treatment is less clear; these patients are at increased risk for relapse if managed with observation. The authors make recommendations for postchemotherapy surgery in patients with disseminated NSGCTs. All such patients need lifelong follow-up, because of the risk of late relapse.

▶ This large retrospective study from Indiana University was undertaken to determine the role of postchemotherapy surgery in patients with NSGCTs. The large experience at this center allowed the authors to evaluate patients on the basis of their serologic and radiologic response as well as according to whether teratomatous elements were present in the primary tumor. The authors carefully analyzed their patients with follow-up as long as 10 years. The authors make the following recommendations regarding postchemotherapy management of patients with NSGCTs:

1. Postchemotherapy retroperitoneal lymph node dissection is recommended for all patients with teratoma-positive primary tumors who are left with resectable residual disease if they have had a serologic response.

2. Postchemotherapy surgery is recommended for patients with teratoma-negative primary tumor with a complete serologic response but who achieve <90% radiographic remission.

3. Patients who achieve serologic and radiographic CR, irrespective of initial tumor bulk, should be followed up without surgery.

4. Patients with a teratoma-negative primary tumor who achieve serologic CR and >90% radiographic regression after chemotherapy may undergo either resection or observation.

5. Lifelong follow-up is recommended for all such patients, as late relapse of disease occurs in 2% to 3%.

G.L. Andriole, Jr., M.D.

The Incidence of Seminoma and Expression of Cell Adhesion Molecule CD44 in Cryptorchid Boys and Infertile Men

Hadžiselimović F, Herzog B, Emmons LR (Univ Children's Hosp, Basel, Switzerland; Inst of Andrology, Liestal, Switzerland)
J Urol 157:1895–1897, 1997

22–3

Introduction.—The risk of seminoma is significantly increased in infertile male patients and in those with undescended testes. A large population of infertile men and cryptorchid boys was reviewed for the incidence of seminoma. The expression of CD44 adhesion molecules in carcinoma in situ and primordial germ cells was also analyzed.

Methods.—The study material consisted of 5,231 biopsies from 3,867 patients: 1,121 men with oligo-asthenoteratospermia syndrome, 218 men with azoospermia, and 2,528 boys with cryptorchidism. Light microscopy, fluorometry, electron microscopy, and immunohistochemistry were used to analyze testicular tissue embedded in Epon. Biopsies of all patients suspected of having carcinoma in situ were examined using an anti–CD44 monoclonal antibody for cell adhesion molecule CD44.

Results.—Six (0.5%) of 1,121 patients with oligo-asthenoteratospermia syndrome were found to have abnormal germ cells, characterized by a large nucleus with a well-differentiated large nucleolus and extensive accumulation of glycogen within the cytoplasm. Such atypical germ cells were not found in the azoospermia group. Seminoma in situ was present in 4 (0.2%) of 2,403 patients with cryptorchidism. Inclusion of those with persistent primordial germ cells increased the rate of atypical germ cells to 0.45% in the cryptorchid boys. Anti–CD44 monoclonal antibodies were bound specifically to all carcinoma in situ and to atypical spermatogonia in cryptorchid testes. The CD44 antigen was found to be internalized in the cytoplasm during later stages of maturation and metastasis.

Discussion.—Infertile men and boys with cryptorchid testes have a similar risk for seminoma, but their risk of cancer is much greater than that of the general population. Testicular biopsy during orchiopexy can help identify those at risk for development of seminoma. The finding that CD44 expression is associated with seminoma cells suggests that anti–CD44 molecule antibody can be used for early identification of this neoplasm.

▶ This large study examined over 5,000 biopsies from approximately 4,000 patients with either cryptorchidism, severe oligo-asthenoteratospermia, or azoospermia. Men with infertility and boys with cryptorchid testes have approximately the same risk for seminoma development, which is 4 to 5 times higher than the risk of testicular tumor in the general population. In this study, carcinoma in situ was discovered in 0.27% of the patients and primordial germ cells (a putative progenitor to seminoma cells) were found in an additional 0.30%. It is interesting that all seminomas and all patients with primordial germ cells expressed the CD44 adhesion molecules, suggesting that this marker may be an early indicator for malignant development. This study highlights the importance of considering the presence of malignancy in patients with severe oligospermia and older boys with undescended testes.

G.L. Andriole, Jr., M.D.

Prognostic Factors for Relapse in Stage I Testicular Seminoma Treated With Surveillance

Warde P, Gospodarowicz MK, Banerjee D, et al (Univ of Toronto; Princess Margaret Hosp, Toronto)
J Urol 157:1705–1710, 1997   22–4

Background.—There is a growing trend toward postorchiectomy surveillance for patients with stage I seminoma, with further treatment reserved for patients with occult metastases and relapse. This raises the need to identify patients at high risk for occult metastases and relapse who should receive adjuvant therapy postoperatively. Prognostic factors for relapse were analyzed in patients with stage I seminoma being managed by surveillance.

Methods.—The study included 34 patients (median age, 34 years) who were placed on surveillance after orchiectomy for clinical stage I seminoma. A wide range of potential prognostic variables were analyzed by the Cox proportional hazards model, including age, tumor size, mitotic count, S phase fraction, ploidy, presence of small-vessel invasion, syncytiotrophoblasts and tumor-infiltrating lymphocytes, and expression of β-human chorionic gonadotropin and low–molecular weight keratin on immunohistochemical analyses.

Findings.—Thirty-one patients had disease relapse during a median follow-up of 6 years. The actuarial 5-year relapse-free rate was 85%, survival was 97%, and cause-specific survival was 99.5%. Five-year freedom from relapse was 88% for patients with tumors smaller than 6 cm in greatest dimension, vs. 67% for those with larger tumors; 79% for patients aged 34 years or younger vs. 91% for older patients; and 86% for those with no small-vessel invasion vs. 69% for those with invasion. Age and tumor size were significant predictors of relapse on multivariate analysis, and small-vessel invasion was close to significance. For patients with none of these 3 risk factors, the risk of relapse was only 6%.

Conclusions.—For patients with stage I testicular seminoma managed by postorchiectomy surveillance, the key prognostic factors are age, primary tumor size, and small-vessel invasion. These prognostic factors will help in selecting the most appropriate therapy for individual patients. Other histopathologic factors, including DNA ploidy status, do not appear to be significant. However, additional follow-up and assessment of biological factors are indicated.

▶ This Canadian series corroborates experience from Europe showing that patients undergoing observation for stage I seminoma have only a 15% relapse rate during the first 5 years of follow-up. When these patients relapse, they are nearly always cured by chemotherapy or radiation therapy. In this study, young age and large tumor size (diameter, >6 cm) were predictive of relapse; therefore, such patients may not be the ideal candidates to undergo surveillance.

The potential benefits of surveillance include better fertility and diminished risk of a later, radiation-induced second malignancy. However, surveillance is expensive and requires diligent follow-up on the part of both the patient and the physician. I believe the majority of patients with early stage seminoma should receive radiation therapy, as it is effective, of relatively low morbidity, and obviates the need for intensive and repetitive radiographic follow-up.

G.L. Andriole, Jr., M.D.

MIB-1 Immunohistochemistry in Clinical Stage I Nonseminomatous Testicular Germ Cell Tumors Predicts Patients at Low Risk for Metastasis

Albers P, Bierhoff E, Neu D, et al (Bonn Univ, Germany)
Cancer 79:1710–1716, 1997

22–5

Introduction.—Clinical staging of low-stage nonseminomatous germ cell tumors (NSGCTs) is inaccurate in 30% of patients, leading to the use of histopathologic risk factors in making treatment decisions. Previous studies have linked low tumor proliferation rates to a low risk of occult metastatic disease. MIB-1 (Ki-67 receptor) was used to confirm the immunohistochemical assessment of tumor proliferation in patients with NSGCTs.

Methods.—The investigators analyzed orchiectomy specimens from 78 patients with clinical stage I NSGCTs. Pathologic stage was confirmed as stage I in 50 patients and stage II in 28. Retroperitoneal lymph node dissection was performed in all patients. Histopathologic reevaluation and MIB-1 immunostaging of the surgical specimens were performed to prove the reliability of immunohistochemical assessment.

Results.—The pathologic stage I specimens had 51.5% MIB-1–positive tumor cells, compared with 75% in the pathologic stage II specimens. At a cutoff point of 70%, 69% of cases were correctly classified. Sensitivity was 86%, specificity 60%, negative predictive value 88%, and positive predictive value 55%. The MIB-1 findings were the best predictor of low-risk status for metastases, better than such traditional risk factors as percentage of embryonal carcinoma and vascular invasion.

Conclusions.—Staining for MIB-1 can identify patients with clinical stage I NSGCTs who are at low risk for metastases. The technique offers a simple and reproducible means of improving risk classification for patients with this difficult-to-stage tumor. Identifying tumors with high proliferative activity does not identify high-risk patients, however. The mechanisms of tumor spread by highly proliferative testicular tumors are under study.

▶ This paper describes a prognostic marker in primary NSGCTs that may help guide selection of patients suitable for observation. The Ki-67 receptor, which is expressed by proliferating cells in late G1, S, G2, and M phases, may be labeled using the MIB-1 antibody. In this study, stratification of patients whose primary tumor contained fewer than 70% positive-staining cells was the best predictor of a low risk for metastases, even when compared with traditional factors such as percentage of embryonal carcinoma and presence of vascular invasion. MIB-1 staining was able to predict a low risk for occult metastases with an accuracy of 88%. Most of the patients who were misclassified were those who harbored pure teratoma, and the authors suggest that patients with pure teratoma be evaluated using traditional parameters to assess risk of occult metastases.

G.L. Andriole, Jr., M.D.

Cisplatin-based Chemotherapy Changes the Incidence of Bilateral Testicular Cancer

van Basten J-PA, Hoekstra HJ, van Driel MF, et al (Univ Hosp, Groningen, The Netherlands)
Ann Surg Oncol 4:342–348, 1997

22–6

Introduction.—Cisplatin-based chemotherapy has increased the survival rate of patients with testicular cancer, but the risk for a contralateral testicular tumor may be increased. The records of 365 consecutive patients were reviewed to establish the risk for development of contralateral tumors in testicular cancer patients and to investigate the effect of initial treatment on the second malignancy.

Methods.—All patients had a histologically verified nonseminomatous testicular germ-cell tumor (NSTGCT) that was treated at the study institution between 1980 and 1995. Treatment consisted of 4 courses of cisplatin, vinblastine, or etoposide and bleomycin. Patients with stage I NSTGCT were treated with orchidectomy alone followed by frequent checkups and screenings. The incidence rate of contralateral tumor was related to previous therapy, and observed and expected incidence rates compared.

Results.—The mean age of the patient group at diagnosis was 29 years. Cisplatin-based chemotherapy was administered to 225 men, and 140 had postorchidectomy surveillance. A contralateral tumor developed in 11 patients after a median follow-up of 84.5 months. Contralateral testicular tumors were more common in the surveillance group (5%) than in the chemotherapy-treated group (1.8%). The 2 groups did not differ in the time interval between the first and contralateral testicular tumor. Compared to Dutch men of similar age, the crude relative risk (RR) for a contralateral tumor to develop in nonseminoma patients was 60.9. Compared to patients undergoing orchidectomy and surveillance, the RR was 3 times lower in patients treated with chemotherapy.

Discussion.—The incidence of a contralateral testicular tumor was 3% in Dutch men who were treated for a nonseminoma testicular tumor; this

TABLE 6.—Incidence of Contralateral Tumor in Nonseminoma Patients in Relation to Treatment Given for First Primary Testicular Tumor

| | | Patients with bilateral testicular cancer/total nonseminoma patients | | Treatment prior to occurrence of contralateral tumor | | | |
| | | | | Surveil* | | Chemo† | |
Year	Reference	n	%	n	%	n	%
1991	Nicolai (16)	6/823	(0.7)	4/377	(1.1)	2/446	(0.5)
1993	Bokemeyer (15)	9/355	(2.7)	9/219	(4.1)	0/136	(0)
1995	Present series	11/365	(3.0)	7/140	(5.0)	4/225	(1.8)
Total		26/1,543	(1.7)	20/736	(2.7)	6/807	(0.7)

*Surveil: patients treated with orchidectomy alone (and surveillance) or retroperitoneal lymph node dissection (without additional treatment).
†Chemo: cisplatin-based chemotherapy.
(Courtesy of van Basten J-PA, Hoekstra HJ, van Driel MF, et al: Cisplatin-based chemotherapy changes the incidence of bilateral testicular cancer. *Ann Surg Oncol* 4:342–348, 1997. Copyright © the Society of Surgical Oncology, Inc.)

is 60 times greater than the expected incidence rate of a testicular GCT in a general population of Dutch men. Initial treatment was related to the incidence of a contralateral tumor (Table 6) in only 2 previous series, which also supports the hypothesis that cisplatin-based chemotherapy eliminates carcinoma in situ in the contralateral testis.

▶ This provocative article suggests that use of platinum-based chemotherapy lowers the occurrence of a contralateral testicular tumor. The results of this series and 2 earlier series in the literature are shown in Table 6.

This effect of cisplatin-based chemotherapy on occult carcinoma in situ or on a nascent contralateral testicular tumor is surprising, because earlier data suggested that men with bulky testicular tumors who receive platinum-based chemotherapy prior to orchiectomy often have viable residual tumor elements in the testis, despite eradication of tumor elsewhere (e.g., retroperitoneum or lungs). The inability of chemotherapy to ablate tumors in the testis has often been ascribed to the "blood testis barrier." However, this rather large series and other accumulating epidemiologic evidence do suggest some effect of chemotherapy on intratesticular neoplasms. These results raise the possibility that patients with a solitary testis may undergo enucleation of the index tumor and subsequently receive cisplatin-based chemotherapy to reduce the occurrence of another tumor in the remnant gonad. Such an approach, if feasible, may preserve the quality of life of such men in that lifelong testicular replacement therapy will not be necessary and the psychological implications of bilateral orchiectomy would be averted.

G.L. Andriole, Jr., M.D.

Sexuality and Fertility in Long-term Survivors of Testicular Cancer

Arai Y, Kawakita M, Okada Y, et al (Kyoto Univ, Japan)
J Clin Oncol 15:1444–1448, 1997   22–7

Background.—Once a highly lethal disease, testicular cancer now can be cured with multimodal therapy. More young men are surviving to cope with long-term reproductive and sexual effects of therapy. Postorchiectomy surveillance is increasing, so sexual function and fertility should be studied for surveillance as well as other forms of therapy.

Methods.—Patients with testicular cancer (n = 85) who were treated after orchiectomy by chemotherapy with retroperitoneal lymph node dissection, chemotherapy only, infradiaphragmatic radiotherapy, or surveillance were questioned regarding sexual function, marital status, and fertility.

Results.—From 20% to 30% in each group reported slight to severe sexual drive impairment. Reduction in erectile potential was (nonsignificantly) highest for radiotherapy, perhaps because of age. This group also often reported reduced orgasm intensity. As expected, a significant greater decline in semen volume at ejaculation was reported by men who had chemotherapy plus lymph node dissection; 74% reported dry ejaculation. Premature ejaculation was most common with radiotherapy (40%), with many patients noting decreased semen volume. Sexual satisfaction remained unchanged in most patients in all groups. About a third reported feeling less attractive from orchiectomy, especially in the surveillance group. Although 20 of the men in both chemotherapy groups (59%) wanted to father children, only 3 (9%) did so after treatment, whereas 4 (44%) in the surveillance group have done so.

Conclusions.—Quality of life in patients with testicular cancer can be improved by reducing sexual dysfunction and infertility, which are major, persistent side effects of treatment. The patients may also need sexual and marital counseling. Surveillance does not necessarily yield fewer sexual problems, and more extensive studies are needed on quality of life.

▶ This study dispels the notion that men undergoing surveillance for germ cell testicular tumors have normal sexual function. Whether the relatively high occurrence of sexual dysfunction observed in this series is the result of physiologic or psychological factors is not known, but it appears to be persistent over the long term. These data should be considered when discussing surveillance vs. early therapy for patients with germ cell tumors of the testis.

G.L. Andriole, Jr., M.D.

Risk of Second Malignant Neoplasms Among Long-term Survivors of Testicular Cancer

Travis LB, Curtis RE, Storm H, et al (Natl Cancer Inst, Bethesda, Md; Danish Cancer Society, Copenhagen; Karolinska Univ, Stockholm; et al)
J Natl Cancer Inst 89:1429–1439, 1997   22–8

Introduction.—One of the major breakthroughs in cancer treatment was the introduction of the heavy metal compound cisplatin into therapy protocols for testicular tumors. With a 5-year relative survival rate of more tha 90%, testicular cancer is now largely curable, and radiotherapy fields to treat testicular cancer have decreased in size in recent decades with use of lower doses. Possible late effects may be seen in men who were treated with earlier, more aggressive approaches. Long-term risks of second cancers among survivors have not been quantified. The site-specific risk of second malignant neoplasms among 1-year survivors of testicular cancer was quantified, as well as among 20-year survivors.

Methods.—There were 28,843 men identified in tumor registries and, of these, 3,300 men had survived more than 20 years. A search of registry files was conducted to find new invasive cancers.

Results.—In 1,406 men, second cancers were reported, with statistically significant excesses noted for acute nonlymphocytic leukemia; acute lymphoblastic leukemia; non-Hodgkin's lymphoma; and cancers of the stomach, rectum, colon, prostate, pancreas, bladder, kidney, connective tissue, and thyroid. After seminomas or nonseminomatous tumors, the overall

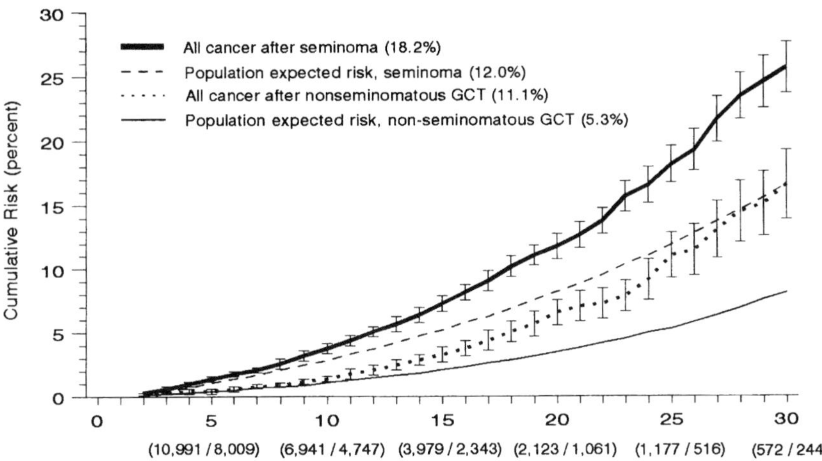

FIGURE 1.—Cumulative risk of second malignant neoplasms among 28,010 one-year survivors of testicular germ cell tumors (*GCT*). Percentages in parentheses indicate the actuarial risk at 25 years. Within the figure, 95% confidence intervals for point estimates are shown by *short vertical lines*. (Courtesy of Travis LB, Curtis RE, Storm H, et al: Risk of second malignant neoplasms among long-term survivors of testicular cancer. *J Natl Cancer Inst* 89:1429–1439, 1997. By permission of Oxford University Press.)

risk was similar (Fig 1). After the diagnosis of testicular cancer, the risk of solid tumors increased with time, yielding an observed-expected ratio of 1.54 among 20-year survivors. Radiotherapy and chemotherapy were associated with secondary leukemia. Radiotherapy was associated with excess cancers of the stomach, bladder, and possibly the pancreas.

Conclusion.—For more than 2 decades after initial diagnosis, men with testicular cancer continue to be at significantly elevated risk of second malignant neoplasms, including secondary leukemia; sarcoma; and cancers of the lung, gastrointestinal tract, and other urogenital sites. Although the precise roles of treatment, natural history, diagnostic surveillance, and other influences are yet to be clarified, patterns of excess second cancers suggest that many factors may be involved.

▶ This meticulously performed study shows that young men in North America and Europe surviving testicular cancer have a 1.43-fold increased incidence of cancers, most notably leukemias, lymphomas, and melanomas. The probability of experiencing a second neoplasm was most notable for men followed for more than 20 years, as shown in Figure 1. This information coupled with the overall increasing incidence of testis cancer (2% to 3% per year) will make it important for all physicians treating patients with testicular cancer to carefully monitor these patients for their entire life. The exact factors that contribute to the excess occurrence of neoplasms—such as diagnostic imaging, radiation therapy, or chemotherapy—will need to be investigated over the next several years.

G.L. Andriole, Jr., M.D.

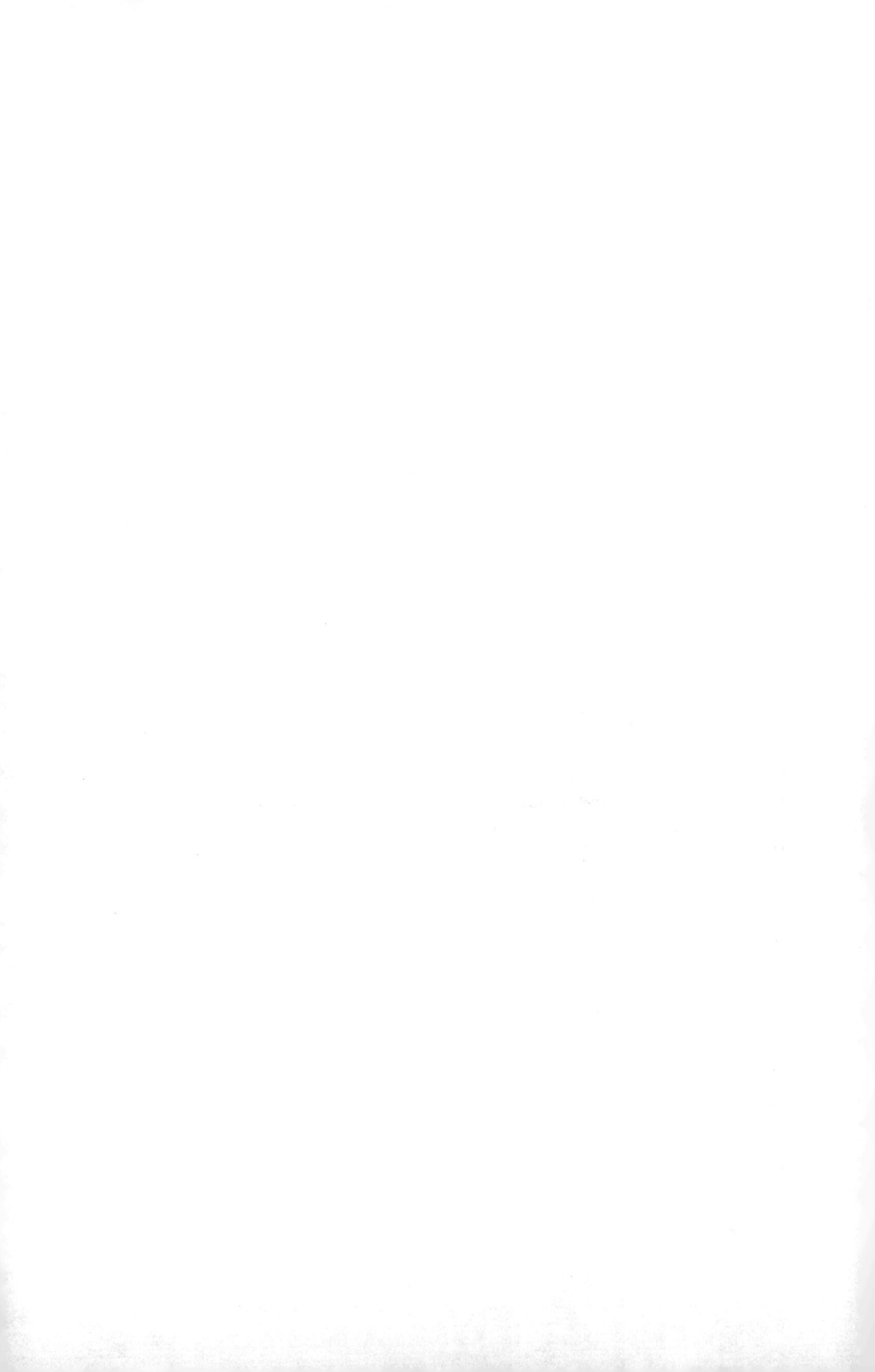

23 Pediatric Infections/ Reflux

Pediatric Vesicoureteral Reflux Guidelines Panel Summary Report on the Management of Primary Vesicoureteral Reflux in Children
Elder JS, Peters CA, Arant BS Jr, et al (American Urological Assoc, Baltimore, Md)
J Urol 157:1846–1851, 1997   23–1

Background.—Treatment for children with vesicoureteral reflux seeks to prevent renal injury, symptomatic pyelonephritis, and other complications. Reflux often resolves on its own, so antibiotics can be given to prevent infections until that occurs. In selected patients, surgery is performed to reduce the chances of renal injury and other complications. However, even experts disagree about the best treatment approach. The Pediatric Vesicoureteral Reflux Guidelines Panel of the American Urological Association offers guidelines for the treatment of primary vesicoureteral reflux in children, based on the available data.

Methods.—The Panel performed systematic review of the literature on vesicoureteral reflux published from 1965 to 1994. The outcomes data on 7 different forms of treatment were analyzed: intermittent antibiotic therapy; bladder training; continuous antibiotic prophylaxis; antibiotic prophylaxis plus bladder training; antibiotic therapy, bladder training, and anticholinergic agents for dysfunctional voiding; open surgery; and endoscopic surgery. The analysis focused on probability of reflux resolution, chances of pyelonephritis and scarring, and treatment-related complications. The Panel made treatment recommendations on the basis of the scientific evidence and expert opinion.

Results.—Few of the recommendations were based solely on scientific evidence of a beneficial effect on health outcomes. For most children with vesicoureteral reflux, the Panel recommended continuous antibiotic prophylaxis. There was no evidence to support the use of urethral dilation and internal urethrotomy, or the use of cystoscopic examination to predict the resolution of reflux. The data supported the use of urodynamic studies in patients with symptoms of voiding dysfunction, but not in those with a normal voiding pattern. The Panel advised clinicians to communicate to parents the known risks and benefits of the available treatment options, including which are based on opinion or experience vs. scientific evidence. Noting the scarcity of direct evidence to support one treatment over another, the Panel recommended that patient and parent preferences play an important role in treatment decisions. The benefits of antibiotics to maintain continuous urine sterility appeared to outweigh the potential adverse effects.

The Panel recommended surgery for patients with grade III or greater reflux who do not have spontaneous resolution. Surgery is rarely, if ever, indicated in lower grades of reflux. However, there was scant evidence to support this recommendation. More aggressive treatment was recommended for girls, based on their higher risk for urinary tract infection. The Panel also recommended more aggressive treatment for grade V reflux, based on the opinion that it is less likely to resolve over time, and for patients who have renal scarring when reflux is diagnosed. For children with voiding dysfunction, the Panel suggested that anticholinergics and bladder training could be added to antibiotic prophylaxis. Noting the lower success rate of surgery in children with voiding dysfunction, the Panel recommended assessment for voiding dysfunction at the initial evaluation.

Discussion.—Recommendations for the management of primary vesicoureteral reflux in children are presented, based on a thorough review of the literature. Few of the recommendations are based purely on scientific evidence of health benefit, however. The investigators cite some key areas for future research, including the reflux-associated risk of renal scarring associated with urinary tract infection and the mechanism thereof.

▶ This is must reading for all urologists. Treatment recommendations are based on peer-reviewed outcomes data. Most children can be safely started on antibiotic prophylaxis with a very low risk of scarring while on prevention. The median resolution time of 3.5 years for grade III reflux is longer than previously reported. The final decision regarding surgery or antibiotic prevention is still largely determined by parent and patient preference.

D.E. Coplen, M.D.

The Characteristics of Primary Vesico-Ureteric Reflux in Male and Female Infants With Pre-natal Hydronephrosis
Yeung CK, Godley ML, Dhillon HK, et al (Great Ormond Street Hosp for Children NHS Trust, London)
Br J Urol 80:319–327, 1997

23–2

Introduction.—Pediatric urological debate is seen concerning infants with primary vesicoureteric reflux detected after a pre-natal diagnosis of hydronephrosis. It is still unknown to what extent developmental anomalies contribute to reflux-associated nephropathy. Previous studies have noticed a preponderance of boys and of dilated upper urinary tracts, while, within older groups of children, there is a preponderance of females and not of upper urinary tract dilatation. Babies with vesicoureteric reflux were assessed to determine the relationships among kidney damage, severity of vesicoureteric reflux, and gender.

Methods.—There were 155 infants, who had a mean age of 8.7 weeks, with vesicoureteric reflux. Two hundred thirty-six reflux units were analyzed for relationships among severity of reflux, presence of focal and generalized types of kidney damage on image, exposure to urinary tract infection, and gender. Another group of 29 males without vesicoureteric reflux were compared to this group for bladder wall thickness determined from US.

Results.—The same proportion of males and females were affected by bilateral vesicoureteric reflux. The majority of kidneys that were exposed to vesicoureteric reflux were normal (67%). Of the 78 abnormal kidneys, 53 had a generalized damage and 71 (91%) had severe grades IV and V reflux that predominantly affected males. Males were almost exclusively affected by grade V reflux. Mild reflux (grades I–III) was seen in 78% of female units as compared to 46% of male units and was independently associated with normal kidneys. For males with vesicoureteric reflux, the mean bladder wall thickness was significantly greater than for males with vesicoureteric reflux and for males without vesicoureteric reflux.

Conclusion.—There was an identification of 2 patterns of vesicoureteric reflux that were distinct but not exclusive. One affected mostly females and a proportion of males, and was a mild reflux associated with normal kidneys. The other almost exclusively affected males and was a severe reflux combined with kidney damage.

▶ This is an excellent retrospective analysis of reflux detected because of antenatally identified hydronephrosis. Many of the kidneys with high-grade reflux have either focal or generalized scarring indicative of a primary developmental abnormality. Male infants have a much higher incidence of high-grade reflux than females. The resolution rate is similar in both sexes, but the resolution rate of greater than 40% in grades IV and V is much higher than commonly cited for older children with similar grades. If the kidneys are normal at presentation and the infant remains infection free on prevention, surgery is usually not required for antenatally detected reflux.

D.E. Coplen, M.D.

Are Younger Children at Highest Risk of Renal Sequelae After Pyelonephritis?

Benador D, Benador N, Slosman D, et al (Cantonal Univ Hosp, Geneva)
Lancet 349:17–19, 1997   23–3

Objective.—Pyelonephritis is common in infants and children, and often leads to irreversible renal parenchymal lesions. Previous studies have suggested that the risk of permanent renal damage is greatest for infants less than 1 year old and lowest for those older than 5 years. This belief has led to age-based differences in treatment, even though renal scarring does

TABLE 2.—Findings of Repeat Scintigraphy

	Age (years)			All ages (n=108)
	<1	1–5	>5	
Children with renal scars	20/50 (40%)	31/36 (86%)	14/22 (64%)	65 (60%)
Children with partial reversible lesions	13/50 (26%)	18/36 (50%)	9/22 (41%)	40 (37%)
Renal scars in children with a first urinary-tract infection	20/47 (43%)	26/31 (84%)	8/10 (80%)	54/88 (61%)

(Courtesy of Benador D, Benador N, Slosman D, et al: Are younger children at highest risk of renal sequelae after pyelonephritis? *Lancet* 349:17–19, 1997. Copyright by The Lancet Ltd., 1997.)

occur in older children. Scintigraphy was used to study the frequency of renal sequelae of pyelonephritis in children of varying age groups.

Methods.—The prospective study included 201 children, aged 0 to 16 years, hospitalized with probable pyelonephritis and a positive urine culture. Each patient received 1 to 3 weeks of antibiotic treatment. During the acute urinary tract infection, the children were studied by technetium-99m-dimercaptosuccinic acid (DMSA) scintigraphy and US. They also had voiding cystourethrography at least 6 weeks after the end of antibiotic treatment. If renal parenchymal lesions appeared on scintigraphy, the study was repeated after at least 2 months. The age-related risk of renal sequelae was calculated by age group. There were 199 infants less than 1 year old, 47 children aged 1 to 5 years, and 35 children and adolescents older than 5 years.

Results.—The frequency of renal lesions during the acute infection was 55% in the infants under 1 year, 79% in the children aged 1 to 5 years, and 69% in the children older than 5 years. Scintigraphy was repeated an average of 3 months later in 108 of these 127 children (Table 2). The frequency of renal scarring on repeat examination was 40% in the infants under 1 year, 86% in the children aged 1 to 5 years, and 64% in the children older than 5 years. Vesicoureteric reflux was present in 36% of these children. Overall, 88 children with an initial documented urinary tract infection had repeat scintigraphy. The frequency of renal scarring was 43% in infants under 1 year, 84% in children aged 1 to 5 years, and 80% in children older than 5 years.

Conclusions.—This prospective study finds that renal sequelae are not less frequent in older children than in infants with pyelonephritis. The major factor involved in renal parenchymal damage appears to be the infectious process itself, irrespective of age. Prevention of renal sequelae is a key objective in the management of pyelonephritis. Treatments to prevent such sequelae will benefit all children, regardless of age.

New Renal Scarring in Children Who at Age 3 and 4 Years Had Had Normal Scans With Dimercaptosuccinic Acid: Follow Up Study
Vernon SJ, Coulthard MG, Lambert HJ, et al (Victoria Infirmary, Newcastle Upon Tyne, England; Univ of Newcastle Upon Tyne, England)
BMJ 315:905–908, 1997   23–4

Introduction.—In the presence of vesicoureteric reflux, renal scars may be caused by a urinary tract infection, particularly in very young children. However, the age beyond which there is no further risk of developing a first scar remains uncertain, and there is evidence that older children with normal kidneys have little risk of a scar developing. The current protocol is to provide no follow-up to children with normal US results and normal results on scanning with dimercaptosuccinic acid after the fourth birthday. This protocol was tested for its safety by having families with children who had normal scan results when aged 3 or 4 years to bring them back for repeat scanning 2–11 years later.

Methods.—Repeat scans were given to children who originally were scanned when they were 3 years old (209 children) or 4 years old (220 children) 2–11 years later. The original scans were US and dimercaptosuccinic acid scans for children with normal results with a urinary tract infection.

Results.—More than 80% of children had repeat scanning and the rest were believed by their general practitioner or parent not to have had another urinary infection. In the 3- and 4-year-old groups, the rate of further infections since the original scan was similar. In the 3-year-old group, it was 27% and in the 4-year-old group, it was 31%. Repeat scanning was not performed in only a few children known to have had further urinary tract infections. In the 3-year-old group, 1.4% did not have repeat scans, and in the 4-year-old group, 1.8% did not. At repeat scanning, 2.4% of the 3-year-olds had new kidney scars and none of the 4-year-olds had new kidney scars. Those who had scars were younger than 3.4 years when scanned originally.

Conclusion.—There is a 1 in 40 risk of development of a scar after the third birthday in children with a urinary tract infection but unscarred kidneys, and after the fourth birthday, the risk drops to even 0. In many children, the need for urinary surveillance is much reduced.

▶ It is commonly believed that the renal parenchyma is less susceptible to infection and scarring in older children. However, the first study (Abstract 23–3) shows a significant risk of scarring in children greater than 5 years of age as determined by dimercaptosuccinic acid scan. Although it is difficult to distinguish changes of acute pyelonephritis from pre-existing scars, the incidence was as high as 80% in children who had their first documented urinary tract infection. The incidence of scarring was the same in children with and without reflux.

The second study (Abstract 23–4) evaluates the incidence of new scars in children who previously had normal scan results. In contrast to the first article, the incidence of new scars was very small, but the patient populations are different because the first studied acute pyelonephritis and the second evaluated largely asymptomatic children (25% to 30% had infection with or without fever). About 1 in 40 children risk development of a new scar without obvious urinary tract symptoms.

Children are at greatest risk for renal scarring after acute pyelonephritis. Renal scarring does not appear to be related to age and predisposing anatomical abnormalities.

D.E. Coplen, M.D.

Urinary Beta$_2$-Microglobulin as a Marker for Vesicoureteral Reflux

Assadi FK (Thomas Jefferson Univ, Philadelphia; The Alfred I duPont Inst, Wilmington, Del)
Pediatr Nephrol 10:642–644, 1996   23–5

Background.—A major cause of end-stage renal disease and hypertension in young adults is renal scarring associated with vesicoureteral reflux (VUR) and urinary tract infection (UTI) in childhood. Efforts to decrease the incidence and severity of renal scarring are aimed at early diagnosis, appropriate imaging, and effective treatment of UTI in patients at risk. The utility of urinary β_2-microglobulin (β_2 M) measures as a screening test to detect tubular dysfunction associated with VUR was reported.

Methods.—Fifty-six children with various grades of reflux and 39 children without reflux matched for age and gender were assessed. Bladder urine was acquired at vesicoureterography.

Findings.—Mean urinary β_2 M/creatinine (Cr) ratio was 1.82 µg/mg Cr in the refluxing group, compared with 0.54 µg/mg Cr in the nonrefluxing group (Fig 1). Patients with grade IV and V reflux had significantly greater urinary β_2 M/Cr values than children without reflux. None of the children with grade I, II, or III reflux had a urinary β_2 M/Cr ratio exceeding 0.92 µg/mg Cr. There were no significant differences among the mean β_2 M/Cr ratio for grade I, II, or III refluxers or nonrefluxers.

Conclusions.—Urinary β_2 M/Cr ratios are elevated in children with high-grade reflux. Such measures may be of use for detecting tubular damage early in patients with VUR.

▶ Beta$_2$-microglobulin is a small-molecular weight protein that is filtered by the glomerulus but efficiently reabsorbed (99%) by the proximal tubules. Elevated urinary levels are indicative of fetal renal injury. This study shows elevated levels in children with high grades of VUR. It is hard to imagine that all these children have renal scars, but if they do, this would be an easier method of detection than the gold standard dimercaptosuccinic acid. If they do not have scars, this would imply that high grades of reflux cause renal tubular injury which is different from scarring associated with pyelonephritis.

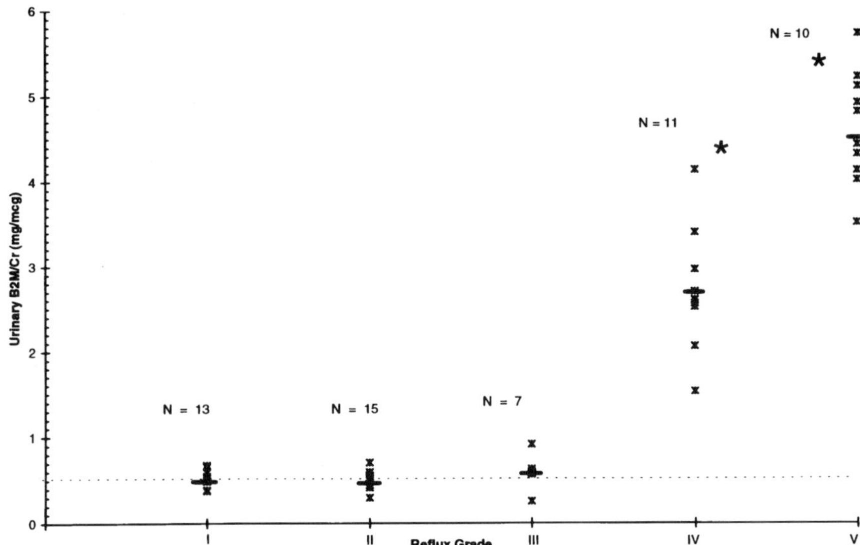

FIGURE 1.—Scattergram plotting the urinary beta$_2$-microglobulin/creatinine ratios (β_2M/Cr) against reflux grade in patients with vesicoureteral reflux. *Dense horizontal lines* depict mean values observed in each group of patients. *Broken line* depicts the upper limit of normal for control subjects. *n* is number of patients studied in each group (several patients had the same value, giving the appearance of fewer than total scatter). * $P < 0.01$ vs. control subjects. (Courtesy of Assadi FK: Urinary beta$_2$-microglobulin as a marker for vesicoureteral reflux. *Pediatr Nephrol* 10:642–644, 1996. Copyright Springer-Verlag.)

We also do not know if these levels return to normal after resolution of reflux (either spontaneously or surgically).

D.E. Coplen, M.D.

Intermittent Trimethoprim-Sulfamethoxazole in Children With Vesico-ureteral Reflux

Hori C, Hiraoka M, Tsukahara H, et al (Fukui Med School, Matsuoka, Japan)
Pediatr Nephrol 11:328–330, 1997   23–6

Background.—Low-dose trimethoprim-sulfamethoxazole (TMP-SMZ) is often used as prophylaxis for recurrent urinary infection in adults. Previous research has indicated that, in adults, delivering the same total dose intermittently 3 times a week is as effective as giving the same dose daily. This article examines whether intermittent dosing (every 2 days) with TMP-SMZ is as beneficial as daily dosing in preventing recurrent urinary infection in children with ureteral reflux.

Methods.—The study involved 35 children (24 boys, 11 girls) 1 month to 9 years old (median, 5 months), who had vesicoureteral reflux; bilateral reflux was present in 18 patients. Thus, the 53 ureters were classified as grade I in 2 ureters, grade II in 16, grade III in 19, grade IV in 14, and grade V in 2. After the urinary infections cleared, prophylactic TMP-SMZ (1 mg/kg TMP, 5 mg/kg SMZ) was administered at bedtime every other day. TMP-SMZ was given for 6 to 50 months (mean, 23 months), and urine samples were routinely assessed throughout the period.

Findings.—Recurrences were noted in none of the boys, but in 2 of the girls. These 2 girls (both over 3 years old) had 7 recurrences, all due to *Escherichia coli*, and urodynamic evaluation revealed that both girls had unstable bladders. Thus, the total recurrence rate for all girls was 0.027 per patient month. Two children (2 and 5 months old) who were undergoing chemoprophylaxis developed transient neutropenia (< 1,000/µL), but this resolved spontaneously. No leukocytopenia, thrombocytopenia, or abnormal serum transaminase or creatinine levels were noted.

Conclusions.—Despite a high preponderance of grades III and IV reflux in these patients, every-other-day dosing with low-dose TMP-SMZ was effective in preventing recurrent urinary infection. The finding of a higher recurrence rate in girls was similar to previous reports. Patient compliance was good and no significant side effects occurred. Given these encouraging findings, further studies will focus on the proper dosage for intermittent low-dose TMP-SMZ prophylaxis in children with ureteral reflux.

▶ Preventive antibiotics effectively prevent recurrent infections in children with vesicoureteral reflux. Daily prevention is associated with a lower incidence of renal scars than antimicrobial administration only when infection develops. Preventive antibiotics are usually administered daily, using one third to one half the therapeutic dose. The potential benefits of decreasing the dose and frequency include decreased antimicrobial resistance and dosage-related side effects, including leukopenia, thrombocytopenia, and thyroid dysfunction. The authors show the efficacy of an every-other-day dosing schedule. The only breakthrough infections were in 2 girls with significant voiding dysfunction. My usual practice is to increase the dose of TMP-SMZ to a maximum of 5 mL, and this effectively prevents infection in older children regardless of their weight.

D.E. Coplen, M.D.

Ciprofloxacin Safety in a Pediatric Population

Jick S (Boston Univ)
Pediatr Infect Dis J 16:130–134, 1997   23–7

Introduction.—Ciprofloxacin, a fluoroquinolone antibacterial agent, is used to treat many infections, particularly those that are resistant to other antimicrobials. It has mostly been prescribed for adults, but in some instances, it has been prescribed for pediatric patients. A previous study indicated that quinolones may cause arthropathic effects in major weight-bearing synovial joints in animals and pediatric patients. The lack of published quinolone-induced joint toxicity in children was evaluated and the risk of musculoskeletal disorders associated with exposure to this drug was estimated in a retrospective cohort study.

Methods.—There were more than 1,700 patients 17 years of age or younger who received at least 1 ciprofloxacin prescription in a 5-year period, and who were examined for an adverse event, defined as an event that required physician referral or hospitalization, and that occurred within 45 days of receiving a prescription for ciprofloxacin.

Results.—Within the patient group, 5% had cystic fibrosis, and no patient with cystic fibrosis had newly diagnosed arthritis. Only 5 patients received 5 or more ciprofloxacin prescriptions. No newly diagnosed acute arthritis or serious liver or kidney disease was found in this population receiving ciprofloxacin. Ciprofloxacin therapy, however, may have exacerbated a patient's hemolytic-uremic syndrome.

Conclusion.—There were no serious or unusually high rates of any adverse events with ciprofloxacin usage in a pediatric population, including joint toxicity. However, this group had only 35 patients who received 5 or more prescriptions, indicating that long-term continuous use is limited in this group.

▶ Because quinolones cause dose-dependent arthritis in the weight-bearing joints of animals, they are rarely used in the pediatric population. Quinolones were initially used in children with cystic fibrosis and chronic pulmonary infections. In the initial compassionate use study, there was a 1.5% incidence of arthralgias that resolved without intervention.[1] In this review of more than 1,700 patients, no adverse joint effects were reported after short courses of therapeutic ciprofloxacin. The lower incidence in this review may be related to the fact that only adverse events that required physician referral or hospitalization were counted and the patients were observed for only 45 days. Regardless, short-course therapy in selected children with symptomatic bacteriuria sensitive only to quinolones is probably appropriate.

D.E. Coplen, M.D.

Reference

1. Hampel B, Hullmann R, Schmidt H: Ciprofloxacin in pediatrics: Worldwide clinical experience based on compassionate use—safety report. *Pediatr Infect Dis J* 16:127–129, 1997.

Voiding Dysfunction After Bilateral Extravesical Ureteral Reimplantation

Lipski BA, Mitchell ME, Burns MW (Children's Hosp and Med Ctr, Seattle)
J Urol 159:1019–1021, 1998   23–8

Introduction.—An effective method of reflux repair is the modified Lich-Gregoir extravesical reimplantation. There have been reports of voiding dysfunction after bilateral extravesical ureteral reimplantation. Patients who had standard and minimized dissection bilateral extravesical reimplantation were reviewed to clarify postoperative risk and duration of transient voiding dysfunction. It was also determined whether minimizing the dissection was effective at reducing postoperative voiding dysfunction.

Methods.—Thirty-three children who had bilateral extravesical ureteral reimplantation for reflux were retrospectively reviewed. The review included preoperative and postoperative radiologic studies, and postoperative postvoid residuals. Eleven of the 33 children had ureteroneocystostomy using a modified Lich-Gregoir technique with ureteral advancement. A modified procedure, in which the detrusor dissection was minimized and the obliterated umbilical artery was preserved, was performed in the remaining 22 of 33 patients. Similar preoperative characteristics were seen in both groups. A comparison was conducted between the 2 groups to determine postoperative surgical success and signs of voiding dysfunction.

Results.—An average of 5.9 ± 3.1 days passed before patients were able to void at least half of the bladder volume. Successful postoperative Foley catheter or suprapubic tube removal occurred after an average length of 7.4 ± 4.2 days. Eventually, all children were able to void adequately. In 97% of the ureters, reflux was cured, according to the results of postoperative voiding cystourethrograms. No postoperative vesicoureteral obstruction was seen. No significant difference in the length of time necessary to void was seen. There were also no significant differences in the duration of catheterization or operative success between the standard vs. limited detrusor dissection procedures.

Conclusion.—For repairing reflux without ureteral obstruction, extravesical ureteral reimplantation is an effective method, but it can result in a high rate of transient postoperative urinary retention, even when detrusor dissection is minimized.

▶ Urinary retention after bilateral extravesical ureteral reimplantation is a devastating complication. In this series, while all children were able to void eventually, 2 patients required intermittent catheterization for 2 months postoperatively and 1 patient was catheterized for 3 months. Minimizing detrusor dissection did not seem to alter the incidence of voiding dysfunction. Short-term patient morbidity is decreased with the extravesical approach, and the procedure effectively corrects reflux, but parents must be informed of this potential short-term problem.

D.E. Coplen, M.D.

Polytetrafluoroethylene Giant Granuloma and Adenopathy: Long-term Complications Following Subureteral Polytetrafluoroethylene Injection for the Treatment of Vesicoureteral Reflux in Children

Aragona F, D'Urso L, Scremin E, et al (Univ of Padua, Italy)
J Urol 158:1539–1542, 1997   23–9

Background.—Subureteral polytetrafluoroethylene injection (STING) is often used in children as a bulking agent to treat vesicoureteral reflux. This application has come into question, however, with evidence that polytetrafluoroethylene particles can cause local granuloma formation and even migrate. These authors report 3 cases of long-term complications after STING in children, and review the literature on this topic.

Methods.—Over 3 years, 2 boys and 1 girl (4, 7, and 6 years old, respectively) who had received STING to treat vesicoureteral reflux either 2, 3, or 4.5 years earlier were evaluated because of disease recurrence. At the current evaluation, all 3 had grade III vesicoureteral reflux that was bilateral in the 4-year-old boy and occurred on the left side in the other 2 patients. All 3 underwent open surgery to determine why the vesicoureteral reflux recurred.

Findings.—The 4-year-old boy had an enlarged pelvic lymph node that contained many multinucleated foreign-body giant cells. The 7-year-old boy underwent pelvic node biopsy, which revealed polytetrafluoroethylene adenopathy. The 6-year-old girl underwent ureteroneocystostomy, at which time a hard nodular mass was found firmly adherent to the ureteral wall. Histologic examination revealed a foreign-body giant-cell reaction with birefringent polytetrafluoroethylene particles.

Conclusions.—All 3 of these patients showed polytetrafluoroethylene particles in the pelvic nodes that were causing a heavy multinucleated foreign-body reaction. Comparisons of these findings with literature reports are complicated by the fact that not all reports include information on the size of the polytetrafluoroethylene particles or on how much of the polytetrafluoroethylene paste was injected. It may be that larger particle sizes (60–80 µm in diameter) and a smaller injection volume into more vascularly isolated spaces might be associated with less migration and granuloma formation. Nonetheless, the current findings indicate that polytetrafluoroethylene injection should probably be avoided in children because of its associated adenopathy and tendency to migrate.

▶ Subureteric Teflon injection durably cures more than 70% of vesicoureteral reflux. However, there is considerable debate over its safety. Proponents feel that local inflammation is related to volume and injection technique and argue that particle migration does not or should not occur. This paper clearly shows migration of Teflon particles to regional lymph nodes and intense granulomatous inflammation. These characteristics make the use of Teflon in children debatable.

D.E. Coplen, M.D.

The Use of the Detrusorrhaphy for Vesico-Ureteric Reflux: The Way Forward?
Steinbrecher HA, Rangecroft L (Royal Victoria Infirmary, Newcastle upon Tyne, England)
Br J Urol 79:971–974, 1997   23–10

Introduction.—The Cohen intravesical technique has been widely accepted as the gold standard for ureteral reimplantation, but urologists in the United Kingdom continue to employ the extravesical detrusorrhaphy technique for patients with vesicoureteral reflux (VUR). A prospective and retrospective analysis examined outcome of all detrusorrhaphies carried out for simple single-system VUR at a single institution over a 4-year period.

Methods.—Twenty-nine patients (43 renal units) were analyzed in 2 groups: those undergoing asynchronous bilateral procedures (2 patients) and unilateral procedures (15 patients) (group 1), and those undergoing synchronous bilateral procedures (12 patients) (group 2). All patients underwent detrusorrhaphy with ureteral advancement, as described by Zaontz et al. (1987). Patients had a mean age at operation of 54 months; the mean follow-up was 17 months for group 1 and 5 months for group 2. Data examined included duration of anesthesia, catheterization, and postoperative stay, postoperative complications, and outcome. Success was defined in both operative and clinical terms.

Results.—Twenty-six patients had urinary tract infections, which were recurrent in 13, and 3 had antenatal hydronephrosis related to VUR postnatally. The mean duration of anesthesia was 69 minutes in group 1 and 80 minutes in group 2. All patients were catheterized urethrally; the mean duration of catheterization was 3 days in group 1 and 5 days in group 2. Hospital stay ranged from 2 to 16 days overall; the mean stay was 3 days for group 1 and 6 days for group 2. Fourteen patients had postoperative complications, the most common of which were urinary tract infections (5), hematuria (3), and urinary retention (2). One patient required operative conversion to bilateral Cohen ureteral reimplantation. Operative and clinical success rates were similar within and between groups. Two of 17 patients in group 1 did not have their reflux cured with surgery and were still symptomatic. There were 4 failed bilateral procedures in group 2; all 4 patients remained symptomatic postoperatively.

Conclusion.—When performed unilaterally, detrusorrhaphy may be an appropriate surgical treatment for VUR. Its success rate in such cases is comparable to that of other operative procedures. Patients undergoing synchronous bilateral procedures, however, had a lower success rate and more serious complications.

▶ Extravesical reimplantation is now routinely performed at many centers. Whether it is as successful and less morbid than intravesical reimplants is unclear. The most distressing complication with this approach is postoperative urinary retention. This occurred in 2 patients and required intermittent catheterization for up to 2 months after surgery. The 67% (bilateral) and 88% (unilateral) success rate is certainly less than the 97% to 99% reported for intravesical reimplantation. Intravesical reimplants can be safely performed without ureteral or urethral catheters, and the majority of patients go home within 48 hours of surgery.

D.E. Coplen, M.D.

24 Cryptorchidism

Paternity After Bilateral Cryptorchidism: A Controlled Study
Lee PA, O'Leary LA, Songer NJ, et al (Univ of Pittsburgh, Pa)
Arch Pediatr Adolesc Med 151:260–263, 1997   24–1

Objective.—Although fertility after bilateral cryptorchidism is reduced, 13% to 62% of married men have reported fathering children. An epidemiologic study compared paternity among men with former bilateral cryptorchidism, men with former unilateral cryptorchidism, and a control group.

Methods.—Paternity was statistically compared among married and cohabiting men with bilateral cryptorchidism ($n = 73$), men with unilateral cryptorchidism ($n = 450$), and a control group ($n = 518$). Lifestyle factors, including drug use, smoking history, alcohol consumption, mumps or sexually transmitted diseases, and occupational exposure to hazardous materials, were recorded.

Results.—Men with former bilateral cryptorchidism were almost 10 times less likely to father children than were men in the other 2 groups. Lifestyle factors had no significant effect on paternity. The testicular position before surgery did not appear to be related to subsequent paternity. The age at orchiopexy and fertility were not related.

Conclusion.—Married and cohabiting men with former bilateral cryptorchidism were almost 10 times less likely to father children. The age at orchiopexy and the position of the testes at surgery did not appear to have an effect on fertility.

▶ Paternity after bilateral cryptorchidism is notably decreased compared with that in both the general population and those with unilateral cryptorchidism. This does not appear to be influenced by the age at orchiopexy, although the average in this series was 8 years old. Testicular biopsy data would support early orchiopexy, although this has not been proved with long-term paternity studies such as this. The study also does not show an influence of preoperative testicular position. This is valuable information that can be discussed with families.

D.E. Coplen, M.D.

Treatment With a Luteinizing Hormone-releasing Hormone Analogue After Successful Orchiopexy Markedly Improves the Chance of Fertility Later in Life

Hadžiselimović F, Herzog B (Basler Children's Hosp, Basel, Switzerland; Inst for Andrology, Liestal, Switzerland)
J Urol 158:1193–1195, 1997

24–2

Introduction.—Possible impaired fertility later in life is the principal reason why cryptorchidism must be rectified as early as possible. Severe infertility in adulthood often results in boys with cryptorchidism with a paucity of germ cells (less than 0.2 germ cells per tubular cross-section).

Methods.—Spermiograms of young adults who had cryptorchidism as boys and received hormonal treatment were analyzed and compared with those of young adults who did not receive hormonal treatment. A low dose of buserelin was given to patients after successful orchiopexy to counteract the paucity of priming hormones. Ten patients had unilateral or bilateral cryptorchidism and a severe paucity of germ cells. The spermiograms of these patients were analyzed when the patients became young adults and were compared with those of 23 controls. The controls had cryptorchidism

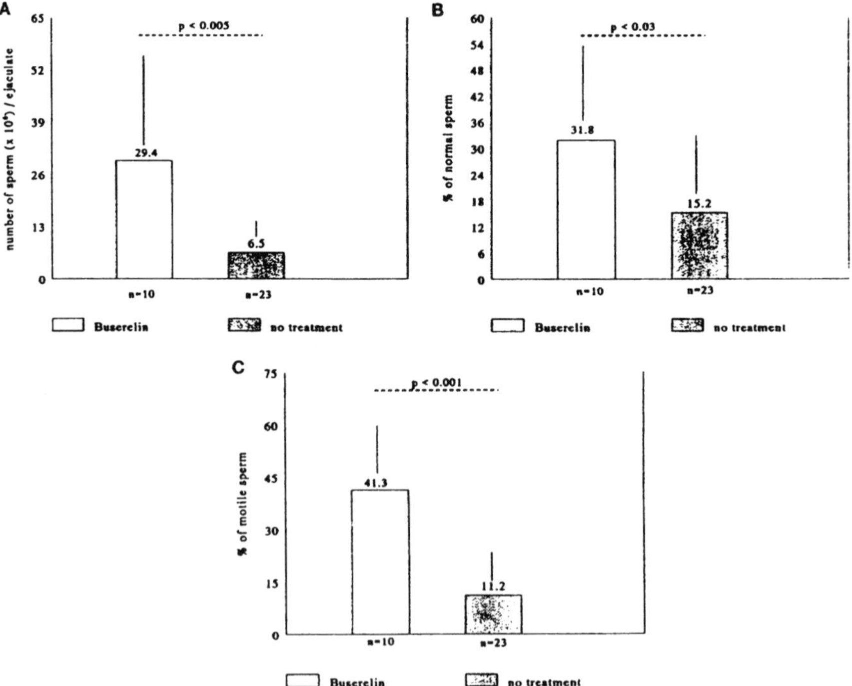

FIGURE.—**A,** total sperm count. **B,** normal sperm forms. **C,** sperm motility. (Courtesy of Hadžiselimović F, Herzog B: Treatment with a luteinizing hormone-releasing hormone analogue after successful orchiopexy markedly improves the chance of fertility later in life. *J Urol* 158:1193–1195, 1997.)

with a comparable severe paucity of germ cells, but they did not receive hormonal treatment.

Results.—Hormonal treatment with the luteinizing hormone-releasing hormone analogue buserelin corrected germ cell deficiency; however, it was not known how long this effect lasted. Significantly improved spermiograms were seen in patients who received hormonal therapy after orchiopexy when compared with those in the control group (Figure). The number of spermatozoa was increased, the motility was improved, and the number of normal forms of spermatozoa was increased with treatment with buserelin.

Conclusion.—A long-lasting, positive effect on germ cells seems to result with the administration of buserelin as a nasal spray every other day for 6 months after successful orchiopexy. In patients treated with buserelin, the prognosis of fertility has been greatly enhanced.

▶ A subset of males with cryptorchidism have an endocrinopathy that impairs transformation of gonocytes into fetal spermatogonia. In this study, all men had testicular biopsies performed at the time of orchiopexy that showed a marked diminution of germ cells per tubule. This is a very select group, because historically 60% of men with a history of unilateral cryptorchidism have a normal semen analysis and 90% achieve paternity. Treatment appears to increase sperm counts, but there were only 10 patients in this study, and the count is not necessarily related to eventual paternity. The greatest promise for this therapy may be in the group with bilateral cryptorchidism.

D.E. Coplen, M.D.

Late Presentation of Cryptorchidism: The Etiology of Testicular Reascent

Rabinowitz R, Hulbert WC Jr (Univ of Rochester, NY)
J Urol 157:1892–1894, 1997   24–3

Introduction.—Little has been published regarding spontaneous testicular reascent after surgical treatment for cryptorchidism. Some reports described descended testes that subsequently ascended and required surgical correction. A 2-year experience with orchiopexy and ascended testes was reviewed retrospectively.

Results.—One hundred three boys with 115 undescended testes had orchiopexy in a 2-year period. Multiple confirmations of previous testicular descent were recorded in 21 of the boys. Forty percent had a nurse or physician parent, and 40% were examined in the office or with general anesthesia by a pediatric urologist or pediatric surgeon. Surgery was performed at ages 5–14 years, an average of 2 years after the initial presentation with reascent. Testicular descent did not result in 5 patients given human chorionic gonadotropin. A patent processus vaginalis was present in 12 of 23 patients. Most boys had the testis located in the superficial inguinal pouch. In all of the boys, the gubernacular attachment was in an abnormal location, and in half of the boys, it was ectopic.

Conclusion.—The cause of this condition is a missed diagnosis at a younger age. Findings associated with reascended testes show that the testis does not reascend, but is undescended and almost completely descended. The diagnosis becomes more obvious with somatic growth as the distance between the terminal portion of the gubernaculum of the apparently descended testis and the scrotum increases. Through puberty, periodic physical examination should be conducted to confirm intrascrotal testicular location.

▶ Does the retractile testicle retract and become a truly undescended testicle? Rarely, if ever. In most late presentations, the testis is in the superficial ectopic pouch. Early in life, the testis is almost descended. However, the distance between the ectopic gubernacular attachment and the dependent portion of the scrotum increases with somatic growth. Because of this possibility, testicular descent needs to be confirmed periodically.

D.E. Coplen, M.D.

The Vanishing Testis: Anatomical and Histological Findings
Merry C, Sweeney B, Puri P (Our Lady's Hosp for Sick Children, Dublin)
Eur Urol 31:65–67, 1997   24–4

Introduction.—Vanishing testis, which appears to be a different entity from testicular maldescent or cryptorchidism, is strongly suggested by the presence of a vas deferens and vessels lying side by side along the normal course of testicular descent. Although some studies report that testicular tissue is not found in this condition, viable testicular remnants have been observed on histologic analysis of blind-ending cord structure in up to 20% of vanishing testis. This issue was considered in a review of 105 cases of vanishing testes.

Methods.—The records of 2,509 boys with 3,064 undescended testes were reviewed. Exploration in the 691 (23%) impalpable testes revealed 144 (21%) cases of absent testis. Operative findings were reviewed to determine whether cases of absent testis represented testicular agenesis or vanishing testis. Vanishing testis was diagnosed when the vas deferens and vessels lay side by side but ended blindly.

Results.—Thirty-nine (27%) of absent testes were classified as complete agenesis of testis and 105 (73%) were determined to be vanishing testis. The latter condition was bilateral in 5 boys and equally distributed in the remaining 95 (50 on the left and 45 on the right). Only 2 of the 100 boys had associated anomalies. The site of blind-ending cord structures was intra-abdominal in 21%, inguinal canal in 59%, superficial inguinal ring in 18%, and scrotum in 2%. Testicular tissue was found in 4 of the 47 cases for which histologic information was available.

Discussion.—The incidence of vanishing testis was found to be much higher than the incidence of true congenital absence of testis in boys with nonpalpable testes. Vanishing testis is thought to be caused by an in utero vascular accident, such as torsion. The finding of testicular tissue in 4 patients suggests that inguinal exploration should be performed to prevent the risk of future malignancy in patients with cord structures entering the internal ring.

▶ Antenatal testicular torsion is more common than agenesis. In 80% of cases, the blind-ending vessels are distal to the internal ring. Because germinal elements may persist, either laparoscopic dissection with excision of cord elements or inguinal exploration should be performed when cord structures cross the internal ring.

D.E. Coplen, M.D.

25 Myelomeningocele/ Incontinence

Neurogenic Bladder Dysfunction Due to Myelomeningocele: Neonatal Versus Childhood Treatment
Wu HY, Baskin LS, Kogan BA (Univ of California, San Francisco)
J Urol 157:2295–2297, 1997   25–1

Objective.—Among newborn infants with myelomeningocele and neurogenic bladder dysfunction, urodynamic studies can evaluate the risk for upper urinary tract deterioration. However, there is debate as to whether treatment should be given early, when upper tract deterioration occurs, or when continence becomes a socially important issue. Acting from a preventive philosophy, the authors have practiced aggressive treatment starting as early as possible. They evaluated the effects of this approach on renal and bladder outcome.

Methods.—The analysis included 46 infants (31 girls, 15 boys) with myelomeningocele and neurogenic bladder dysfunction in whom urodynamic studies indicated a high risk for renal deterioration. In this group, treatment included clean intermittent catheterization starting in the first year of life. Their renal and bladder outcomes were compared with those of 52 children in whom treatment was delayed until after 4 years of age. Mean follow-up was 83 months in the early-treatment group and 59 months in the delayed-treatment group. Average age at last follow-up was 85 and 143 months, respectively.

Results.—The 2 groups had similar renal and bladder function to start with; more than one fourth had hydronephrosis, and nearly half had trabeculation or reflux at voiding cystourethrography. There were no differences in urinary infection rate, need for prophylactic antibiotics, rate of improvement in hydronephrosis, trabeculation, reflux, or bladder compliance. Reflux improved spontaneously in 55% of patients. Persistent hydronephrosis developed in 13% of the early-treatment group and 14% of the delayed-treatment group. However, just 11% of patients in the early-treatment group required bladder augmentation during the first year of life, compared with 27% of patients in the delayed-treatment group. Overall incontinence rates were comparable (Table 2).

TABLE 2.—Early vs. Late Treatment: Clinical Outcomes

	No. Pts. (%)	
	Treatment at Ages 0 to 11 Mos. (46 pts.)	Treatment at Ages Greater Than 47 Mos. (52 pts.)
Infection:*		
Asymptomatic bacteriuria	6 (13)	7 (14)
Symptomatic urinary tract infection	21 (46)	27 (52)
Pyelonephritis	5 (11)	3 (6)
Antibiotic prophylaxis†	9 (20)	9 (17)
Renal sonography:†		
Deterioration	1 (2)	1 (2)
Improvement	8 of 14 (57)	6 of 13 (46)
Persistent abnormality	6 (13)	7 (14)
Voiding cystourethrography:†		
New trabeculation	2 (4)	3 (6)
Improvement of trabeculation	2 of 10 (20)	3 of 12 (25)
Persistent trabeculation	8 of 10 (80)	9 of 12 (75)
New reflux	1 (2)	0
Improvement of reflux	2 of 9 (22)	4 of 12 (33)
Persistent reflux	2 of 9 (22)	5 of 12 (42)
Cystometrography:†		
New onset high pressure	0	1 (2)
No improvement in compliance (excluding pts. with augmentation)	5 (12)	4 (11)
Surgery:*		
Vesticostomy	3 (7)	4 (8)
Augmentation	5 (11)	14 (27)‡
Reimplantation	5 (11)	3 (6)
Artificial sphincter	1 (2)	5 (10)
Incontinence†	18 (39)	20 (38)
Noncompliance†	10 (22)	20 (39)

*Patient history.
†At last follow-up.
‡P < 0.05.
(Courtesy of Wu HY, Baskin LS, Kogan BA: Neurogenic bladder dysfunction due to myelomeningocele: Neonatal versus childhood treatment. *J Urol* 157:2295–2297, 1997.)

Conclusions.—The findings support the use of early urologic treatment in newborn infants with myelomeningocele and neurogenic bladder dysfunction who are at high risk for urologic deterioration. Early treatment with clean intermittent catheterization may help avert irreversible bladder dysfunction and the need for bladder augmentation. Patient compliance is better as well, and there may be psychological benefits.

▶ The primary urologic goal in the management of the newborn with myelomeningocele is renal preservation. The upper tracts are at risk in those infants with increased outlet resistance. Clean intermittent catheterization and anticholinergics, cutaneous vesicostomy, and perhaps alpha-blockade with phenoxybenzamine can be used to accomplish this goal in this subset of patients. This nonrandomized series showed a lower augmentation rate when clean intermittent catheterization was initiated earlier in life. However, the patients treated after 4 years of age were significantly older at the last follow-up, and the younger group may have subsequent deterioration. The protective mechanism of clean intermittent catheterization with respect to bladder compliance is unclear. Is it the pharmacologic bladder relaxation, bladder emptying at low pressure, or both? Surprisingly, although treatment was initiated at a later time, the older group did not have a higher incidence of hydronephrosis, renal deterioration, and such.

D.E. Coplen, M.D.

Reproductive Understanding, Sexual Functioning and Testosterone Levels in Men With Spina Bifida

Decter RM, Furness PD III, Nguyen TA, et al (Pennsylvania State Univ, Hershey)

J Urol 157:1466–1468, 1997   25–2

Introduction.—Although the number of patients with spina bifida who reach adulthood has been increasing, few studies have examined the sexual functioning of men with this condition. A questionnaire administered to a group of men with myelodysplasia sought to determine patient educational level, understanding of reproductive physiology, and sexual functioning.

Methods.—Study participants were 57 men aged 18 to 55 (median age, 28.6) who were being followed up at a multidisciplinary clinic. Forty-four agreed to blood tests for measurement of serum testosterone. Questionnaires were administered at the time of a regular clinic visit.

Results.—Most (84%) patients had a 12th grade or higher education. School classes were reported by 58% as their source of knowledge about sexual reproduction; 72% were able to accurately describe the basic concepts of reproductive physiology. Overall, 72% said that they had penile erections and 53% ejaculated. Both erection and ejaculation were more consistently present in men with lesions at lower neurologic levels. Men with ventriculoperitoneal shunts had lower rates of erections and ejaculations than those without the shunts (61% and 30% vs. 88% and 83%, respectively). Attempted sexual intercourse was reported as successful in 35%, and 8 men (14%) fathered children. All men who achieved paternity were ambulatory and without a ventriculoperitoneal shunt at the time of conception; all but 1 had L5 or sacral level lesions (Table). Testosterone levels were normal in 39 of the 44 men who had serum levels measured (mean, 507.6 ng/dL). One of the men who fathered a child had below normal (151 ng/dL) level of serum testosterone.

Discussion.—Many men with spina bifida have an understanding of reproductive physiology and are able to have erections and ejaculate. Despite reproductive capabilities, however, only a third of the patients interviewed for this study had attempted intercourse and only 14% had fathered children. Serum testosterone levels showed a normal distribution,

TABLE.—Lesion Level and Sexual Functioning in Men With Spina Bifida

Lesion Level	No. Pts.	Erection Achieved	Ejaculation Achieved	No. Pts. (%) Sexual Intercourse Attempted	Paternity Attempted	Paternity Achieved
Thoracic	12	6 (50)	1 (17)	0 (0)	0	0
L1–2	3	3 (100)	2 (67)	1 (33)	0	0
L3	13	9 (69)	5 (38)	2 (15)	1 (8)	1 (8)
L4	11	7 (64)	6 (55)	3 (27)	0 (0)	0
L5	8	6 (75)	6 (75)	5 (63)	5 (63)	2 (25)
Sacral	10	10 (100)	10 (100)	9 (90)	5 (50)	5 (50)
Totals	57 (100)	41 (72)	30 (53)	20 (35)	11 (19)	8 (14)

(Courtesy of Decter RM, Furness PD III, Nguyen TA, et al: Reproductive understanding, sexual functioning and testosterone levels in men with spina bifida. *J Urol* 157:1466–1468, 1997.)

and erection and ejaculation were achieved even by men with more severe lesions.

▶ Sexual function in men with spina bifida is affected by the physical and cognitive limitations of the disability and psychological and social impact of the condition. Erectile capability is related to the neurologic level as shown by Rigi-scan determination.[1] In this review, the high level of sexual understanding is clearly related to their educational level (84% high school graduates). Most of the men had lumbosacral abnormalities while men with a thoracic level had not attempted intercourse. This information should be an encouragement for the parents of an ambulatory male with spina bifida.

D.E. Coplen, M.D.

Reference

1. Sandle AD, Worley F, Leroy EC, et al: Sexual function and erection capability among young men with spina bifida. *Dev Med Child Neurol* 38:823–829, 1996.

Bladder Rehabilitation, the Effect of a Cognitive Training Programme on Urge Incontinence

Vijverberg MAW, Elzinga-Plomp A, Messer AP, et al (Univ Hosp for Children and Youth 'Het Wilhelmina Kinderziekenhuis', Utrecht, The Netherlands)
Eur Urol 31:68–72, 1997
25–3

Background.—The term "urge incontinence" is applied to children with a medical history of urologic or nephrologic problems, usually with recurrent urinary tract infections with or without vesicoureteral reflux. Unpleasant experiences during voiding can lead a child to withhold micturition, and the bladder muscle reacts with overactivity and then hypertrophy. In most such cases, daytime wetting is a manifestation of the "urge syndrome." The target for treatment should be daytime wetting and the incorrect way of voiding. Ninety-five children took part in a 10-day inpatient program that used biofeedback methods to overcome urge incontinence.

Methods.—The study group included 9 boys and 86 girls with a mean age of 9.9 years. All had a long history of daytime wetting and recurrent urinary bladder infections, with no improvement after 1 year of medical therapy. Based upon urodynamic studies, children were categorized as having urge syndrome and urge incontinence, true dysfunctional voiding, or lazy bladder syndrome. The latter group of 11 children was excluded from the study. Evaluations were conducted 6 months after completion of the biofeedback program.

Results.—The program involves instructions on "how" to urinate, learning to react adequately to urge signals from the bladder, and a conscious attempt by the child to obtain a standard micturition frequency of 6 voidings per day. At 6 months, 65 children (68.4%) had a good result, 12 (12.6%) had an average result, and 18 (19.0%) showed virtually no improvement. Nine of those who failed to improve were too young, but fared better when they entered the program again after 1.5 years. Psychological treatment was recommended for 4 of the remaining children who failed to improve with biofeedback.

Discussion.—Children who were aged 9 or older had a higher success rate than younger children, but there was no relation between severity of the abnormal urodynamic pattern and the outcome of biofeedback training. Overall, however, the program was successful in helping most children to overcome urge incontinence.

▶ This manuscript describes a labor-intensive approach to the treatment of urge incontinence. The best results were achieved in children older than 9 years because any behavioral modification program requires patient understanding and compliance. This program used a 10-day hospitalization; however, but in my experience, a voiding diary, timed voiding, and treatment of fecal soiling and constipation result in significant improvement in most patients without the use of medications or biofeedback.

D.E. Coplen, M.D.

Oral Desmopressin as a New Treatment Modality for Primary Nocturnal Enuresis in Adolescents and Adults: A Double-blind, Randomized, Multicenter Study
Janknegt RA, Zweers HMM, Delaere KPJ, et al (Univ Hosp Maastricht, The Netherlands; Twenteborg Hosp, Almelo, The Netherlands; Hosp The Wever, Heerlen, The Netherlands; et al)
J Urol 157:513–517, 1997   25–4

Background.—Nocturnal enuresis occurs in people of all ages, but because of the social impact, it is often more problematic for adolescents and adults. Desmopressin delivered in a nasal spray has been successful in treating this condition, but the aerosolized version does have limitations

TABLE 3.—Responses for the Entire Study Population

| | Nasal Spray | Tablets (double-blind) | | Open Label at 400 µg. (wks.) | | |
		200 µg.	400 µg.	1–4	5–8	9–12
Total No. pts.	66	31	32	53	51	51
Response:*						
Complete	31 (47)	7 (23)	12 (37)	29 (55)	29 (57)	26 (51)
Partial	30 (45)	13 (42)	13 (41)	17 (32)	16 (31)	17 (33)
None	5 (8)	11 (35)	7 (22)	7 (13)	6 (12)	8 (16)

No. Pts. (%)

*_Complete response_, ≥90% decrease in wet nights compared to baseline; _partial response_, ≥50% but < 90% decrease in wet nights compared to baseline but still not dry; _no response_, < 50% decrease in wet nights compared to baseline.

(Courtesy of Janknegt RA, Zweers HMM, Delaere KPJ, et al: Oral desmopressin as a new treatment modality for primary nocturnal enuresis in adolescents and adults: A double-blind, randomized, multicenter study. _J Urol_ 157:513–517, 1997.)

(e.g., when the patient has a cold). These authors evaluated the efficacy of an oral formulation of desmopressin in adolescents and adults who had a proven response to the desmopressin nasal spray.

Methods.—A total of 90 patients (53 men and 37 women, 12 to 45 years old) with nighttime-only involuntary voiding were eligible for the study. None was taking drugs likely to interact with desmopressin. The study was divided into 4 phases. In phase 1, patients with nocturnal enuresis received 2 weeks of treatment with 20 µg of desmopressin nasal spray. Those who responded with at least a 50% decrease in the number of wet nights per week proceeded to phase 2. In phase 2, after a 1-week washout period, patients were randomized to 200 or 400 µg of desmopressin tablets for 4 weeks. Phase 3 consisted of a 2-week washout period. Then in phase 4, patients took 400 µg of desmopressin tablets for 12 weeks. Any patient who became dry during the washout period was withdrawn from the study. Follow-up continued for 2 weeks after the end of treatment.

Findings.—Of the initial 90 patients, only 66 proceeded to phase 2, and dropouts and withdrawals continued throughout the study. In phase 2, both doses of desmopressin significantly decreased the number of wet nights per week compared with baseline, although no difference in effect was found between the higher and lower doses. Furthermore, no difference in effect was found between the oral doses in phase 2 and the nasal spray in phase 1. During phase 4, whereas the decrease in the number of wet nights per week remained the same in the group that had taken 400 µg in phase 2, those who had taken the 200-µg dose in phase 2 and were then escalated to the 400-µg dose in phase 4 experienced a significant further decrease in the number of wet nights per week. In phase 4, the response rate to 400 µg of desmopressin was between 84% and 87%. Overall responses are listed in Table 3. Side effects were reported by 4 patients (dizziness, edema, change in mood, headache), and both doses of desmopressin tablets were well tolerated as reported by 96% of patients and 94% of physicians.

Conclusions.—The oral desmopressin tablets were as effective as the nasal spray in controlling nocturnal enuresis. Both the 200- and the 400-µg desmopressin tablets significantly decreased the number of wet nights per week from baseline values. In particular, a desmopressin dose escalation from 200 to 400 µg resulted in further improvement during the 12-week last phase. Thus, the 400-µg desmopressin dose is preferred, although the dose may need to be titrated in individual patients to assure the optimal dose for that patient.

▶ The much larger dose of oral desmopressin is not associated with an increased incidence of hyponatremia, edema, or other side effects. The oral preparation may be easier to administer or transport, but absorption may be variable as with the nasal preparations. A larger oral dose may be required to achieve the 50% complete success rate of nasal desmopressin. The oral preparation is not yet approved for nocturnal enuresis in the United States.

D.E. Coplen, M.D.

26 Congenital Anomalies

The Importance of Accurate Diagnosis and Early Close Followup in Patients With Suspected Multicystic Dysplastic Kidney
Minevich E, Wacksman J, Phipps L, et al (Univ of Cincinnati, Ohio)
J Urol 158:1301–1304, 1997   26–1

Introduction.—In infants, the most common form of cystic renal disease is multicystic dysplasia. The ability to diagnose multicystic dysplastic kidney has improved with recent refinements in diagnostic studies, such as renal ultrasound and radionuclide imaging. It has been well established that conservative treatment is preferred for children with unequivocal multicystic dysplastic kidney who have a stable or regressive pattern of disease during close follow-up. However, if the condition worsens, early nephrectomy is a viable option. Three children with suspected multicystic dysplastic kidney who had surgical exploration were studied.

Methods.—Surgical exploration was done on 3 patients with suspected multicystic dysplastic kidney. Eight months later, 1 child who had a large retroperitoneal mass suggestive of neuroblastoma did not comply with follow-up. Three months later, another patient had a growing renal cystic mass that was suggestive of a multilocular cyst. The remaining patient had a cystic nephroma suspected at 2 months of follow-up.

Results.—Extensive stage III Wilms' tumor was seen in the patient with suspected neuroblastoma. Segmental multicystic dysplastic kidney of the lower pole of an ipsilateral duplicated system was found in the child with a suspected multilocular cyst. Mesoblastic nephroma was confirmed by the National Wilms' Tumor Study Pathology Center in the patient in whom cystic nephroma was suspected.

Conclusion.—Multicystic dysplastic kidney should be unequivocally diagnosed early in life. During the first year of life, the urologists should make the initial radiologic diagnosis and follow up with renal ultrasound every 3–4 months. If the diagnosis becomes equivocal at any point or if compliance is a cause of concern, surgical exploration is indicated.

▶ Multicystic dysplastic kidneys are now followed up conservatively. These 3 cases point out the importance of making an unequivocal diagnosis. Renal scans should be obtained when the ultrasound does not have the "typical" appearance, and follow-up ultrasounds should be obtained in the first year of life to assure a stable or diminishing pattern.

D.E. Coplen, M.D.

Can Careful Ultrasound Examination of the Urinary Tract Exclude Vesicoureteric Reflux in the Neonate?

Avni EF, Ayadi K, Rypens F, et al (Erasme Hosp, Brussels, Belgium)
Br J Radiol 70:977–982, 1997   26–2

Introduction.—The detection of numerous uropathies has resulted from the widespread use of obstetric ultrasound. However, there is still controversy over the best way to evaluate fetal uropathies. A voiding cystourethrography at birth is recommended by some for every patient with a uropathy detected in utero, while others consider such a procedure unnecessary. A review of neonates with known vesicoureteric reflux was conducted to determine whether a normal-appearing urinary tract coexists with vesicoureteric reflux and whether an unnecessary voiding cystourethrography can be avoided with a normal ultrasound examination.

Methods.—A review was conducted of the ultrasound features of 35 neonates with known vesicoureteric reflux. Signs that have been shown to result from or to be associated with vesicoureteric reflux were used for criteria: pelvic dilatation above 7 mm on a transverse scan, caliceal or ureteral dilatation, pelvic or ureteral wall thickening, absence of the corticomedullary differentiation, and signs of renal dysplasia. Among the 35 neonates, 57 refluxing renal units were found. In 22, vesicoureteric reflux was bilateral.

Results.—At least 1 ultrasound anomaly that would have prompted voiding cystourethrography was seen in 50 of 57 refluxing renal units (87.7%). In 29 refluxing renal units (50.9%), pelvic dilatation above 7 mm was present. In 24 refluxing renal units, caliceal dilatation was present, with the dilatation involving the calices but not the renal pelvis in 7 units. In 15 refluxing renal units, ureteral dilatation was seen. In 7 refluxing renal units, pelvic or ureteral wall thickening was seen. In 32 refluxing renal units, corticomedullary differentiation was absent (56.1%). In 19 refluxing renal units, ultrasound signs of dysplasia were found. In 7 refluxing renal units in 6 patients, no ultrasound anomaly was found (12.3%). A careful and meticulous ultrasound examination of the neonatal urinary tract allows the detection of more than 87% of refluxing renal units by showing at least 1 sonographic abnormality.

Conclusion.—A vesicoureteric reflux does not usually coexist with a normal-appearing urinary tract on ultrasound, and in such cases, a voiding cystourethrography is not necessary.

▶ The authors try to determine factors predictive of reflux in neonates with prenatally detected hydronephrosis. In 13% of cases, none of the 7 ultrasound criteria was abnormal. Unfortunately, only neonates who had reflux were evaluated, so it is impossible to determine the sensitivity of each variable. Most series show that only one third of infants with greater than 7-mm dilation have reflux. It is clear that ultrasound should not include just renal pelvic measurement, since calicectasis or distal ureteral dilation can be the only ultrasound abnormality in infants with reflux.

D.E. Coplen, M.D.

Long-term Results of Percutaneous Endopyelotomy in the Treatment of Children With Failed Open Pyeloplasty

Capolicchio G, Homsy YL, Houle A-M, et al (Montreal Children's Hosp; Hôpital St Justine, Montreal; Royal Victoria Hosp, Montreal)
J Urol 158:1534–1537, 1997   26–3

Introduction.—For children with primary ureteropelvic junction obstruction, open pyeloplasty has an overall success rate of better than 90%. For patients who need a repeat operation, percutaneous endopyelotomy may be an alternative with lower morbidity, as experience with adult patients suggests. The cases of 9 children undergoing percutaneous endopyelotomy after failed open pyeloplasty were reported.

Methods.—The patients (median age, 7 years) were operated on over a 10-year period. All had previously undergone Anderson-Hynes pyeloplasty for congenital ureteropelvic junction obstruction. Endopyelotomy was performed at a median of 7.5 months after the failed open surgery. The endopyelotomy technique consists of retrograde placement of a guide wire into the renal pelvis, creation of percutaneous nephrostomy access, and cold-knife endopyelotomy. Balloon dilation was used in some patients. Indwelling 4.6F to 7F double-pigtail stents were left in place for 6 weeks. The results were assessed in terms of normalization or improvement of renographic diuretic washout time, stability of split renal function at follow-up, improvement of hydronephrosis, and absence of symptoms.

Results.—Endopyelotomy was performed in a median operative time of 240 minutes. The percutaneous procedure was successful in all patients but 1. All 8 patients with successful operations were symptom free at an average follow-up of 5.6 years. Endopyelotomy had to be repeated in 1 patient after 4 years. Complications included 1 case of urinary tract infection, 1 of pneumonia, and 1 of bleeding requiring blood transfusion.

Conclusion.—For children in whom open pyeloplasty has failed, percutaneous antegrade endopyelotomy offers a safe and effective alternative to repeated open surgery. In this study, the results were durable over a mean follow-up of nearly 6 years. This procedure is performed infrequently; therefore, it should always be done by an experienced endoscopist in a pediatric referral center.

▶ This report, showing that antegrade endopyelotomy is safe and efficacious in the management of secondary ureteropelvic junction obstruction, confirms previous study findings with long-term follow-up. There was 1 late failure 5 years after endopyelotomy. This rarely happens after open pyeloplasty in children; however, these patients may require longer follow-up. For failed pyeloplasty, antegrade endopyelotomy should be the initial approach.

D.E. Coplen, M.D.

27 Posterior Urethral Valves

Proximal Urinary Diversion in the Management of Posterior Urethral Valves: Is It Necessary?
Tietjen DN, Gloor JM, Husmann DA (Univ of Texas, Dallas; Mayo Clinic, Rochester, Minn)
J Urol 158:1008–1010, 1997
27–1

Introduction.—Early decompression of the bladder via catheter drainage and serial assessment of renal function is the classic management protocol for infants with posterior urethral valves. The subsequent change in serum creatinine levels is used to ascertain the effectiveness of upper tract decompression. In the 15% of patients in whom creatinine levels fail to normalize after adequate lower urinary tract decompression, it is believed that a thick-walled bladder is the cause of relative ureterovesical junction obstruction. Some say that renal dysplasia is reflected by persistent elevations in serum creatinine levels after bladder decompression, and that these patients do not need high diversion. The percent of patients who had renal insufficiency after supravesical urinary diversion was determined. The incidence of fixed ureterovesical junction obstruction in those who had proximal urinary diversion was ascertained.

Methods.—Twenty-six patients with posterior urethral valves were treated with supravesical urinary diversion. At birth, the mean gestational age was 35 weeks. Persistently high serum creatinine levels were present (median, 2.5 mg/dL) after initial decompression via an indwelling catheter (median, 7 days). The median creatinine level was 1.3 mg/dL at 1 month after proximal urinary diversion. The median nadir creatinine level was 1.0 mg/dL at 1 year. Fixed ureterovesical junction obstruction was found in 2 of 52 renal units (4%) with the Whitaker test in all 26 patients at reconstruction.

Results.—Renal dysplasia was seen in 44 of 52 renal units (85%) with renal biopsy. End-stage renal disease developed in 11 patients (42%) after a median follow-up of 9 years.

Conclusion.—Renal biopsy invariably demonstrates areas of renal dysplasia in neonates with posterior urethral valves who have proximal urinary diversion for fixed ureterovesical junction obstruction. Despite proximal diversion, end-stage renal disease frequently develops. The necessity of supravesical urinary diversion is brought into question.

▶ Incision is the preferred initial treatment for urethral valves. The difficult clinical dilemma is what to do with an infant with a persistently elevated or rising creatinine level after incision. In the absence of significant acidosis or sepsis, the infant should initially be observed since the creatinine level will often normalize during 2–3 weeks. If the level does not normalize, significant dysplasia or obstruction may be present. Unfortunately, Whitaker tests were not done at the time of diversion in this study, so we don't know if diversion initiated detrusor atrophy that resulted in a low incidence of ureterovesical junction obstruction. An appropriate compromise in this subset of valve patients may be percutaneous nephrostomy placement with diversion if the creatinine level decreases and the Whitaker test is positive.

D.E. Coplen, M.D.

28 Pediatric Penis

Severe Hypospadias With Genital Ambiguity: Adult Outcome After Staged Hypospadias Repair
Miller MAW, Grant DB (Great Ormond Street Hosp for Children, London)
Br J Urol 80:485–488, 1997   28–1

Background.—Hypospadias is a common congenital malformation in males, and can vary greatly in severity. The most extreme form is severe perineoscrotal hypospadias with genital ambiguity. Because little information exists on the long-term follow-up of males with this condition, these authors examined almost 20 years of case records to provide follow-up data on the results of corrective surgery.

Methods.—Review of medical records identified 33 men with perineoscrotal hypospadias and genital ambiguity. Genetic analysis revealed a 46,XY karyotype in 21 patients, a 45,X/46,XY karyotype in 7, and true hermaphroditism in 5. All 33 patients had undergone staged surgical repair for hypospadias while children, with a median of 3 surgical procedures (range, 2–8). Questionnaires were sent to all patients to determine demographics, medical history, sexual function, urologic function, and general medical and psychological well-being. Additionally, all patients were asked if they would submit to a physical examination.

Findings.—Of the 33 patients identified, 19 returned a completed questionnaire (age range, 17.7–36.6 years). Twelve of the 19 had experienced intercourse, with 6 having done so in the previous 3 months. Whereas 15 patients believed that their erections and orgasms were satisfactory, only 7 said that their ejaculation was normal. Spraying of the urinary stream was reported by 9 men. Four respondents said their quality of life and psychological well-being had suffered because of their condition, and 2 showed evidence of mild depression. Physical examinations were performed on 9 men (age range, 17–29 years), which revealed urethral fistula in 2 patients, a history of acute urinary retention in 2 patients, and a history of chronic renal failure with renal transplantation in 1 patient.

Conclusions.—Men who underwent staged surgical correction of severe perineoscrotal hypospadias with genital ambiguity continued to experience problems with micturition and ejaculation. Erectile function, however, was usually normal. Most patients reported no significant decrease in their psychological well-being resulting from their surgery. Nonetheless, appropriate counseling should be offered as these patients mature, to make sure they understand the nature of their condition.

▶ This is an important follow-up study of men with "corrected" severe hypospadias. Seven had mixed gonadal dysgenesis and 5 were true hermaphrodites, and it is unclear how this influenced the sexual outcomes. A spraying urinary stream and weak ejaculation were the most common complaints, while most patients were satisfied with the quality of erection and orgasm. There did not appear to be any significant psychological concerns in these patients, but selection bias may exist because men with the worst problems may not have completed the questionnaire. It is clear, on the basis of this study, that men with severe hypospadias require follow-up after puberty.

D.E. Coplen, M.D.

Defects of the Testosterone Biosynthetic Pathway in Boys With Hypospadias
Aaronson IA, Cakmak MA, Key LL (Med Univ of South Carolina, Charleston)
J Urol 157:1884–1888, 1997
28–2

Introduction.—Previous studies reported that approximately 5% of boys with severe hypospadias but fully descended testes have an identifiable disorder of testosterone biosynthesis. Using recently published data on steroid levels in normal boys and microassay methods that allow accurate measurement of steroid concentration, investigators examined the incidence of defects in 3 enzymes in boys with proximal hypospadias.

Methods.—The study group included 29 boys ranging in age from 11 months to 13 years (mean, 3 years 10 months) and 1 adult. All had hypospadias, fully descended testes, and a 46,XY karyotype. Testes were confirmed to be normal by histologic examination in 19 cases; in the remaining 10 cases, testes that were normal in position, size, and consistency were presumed to be histologically normal. Testes in the adult were smaller and softer than normal, but he refused biopsy. Fasting blood was drawn for investigation of 3 enzymes on the testosterone biosynthetic pathway: 3β-hydroxysteroid dehydrogenase, 17α-hydroxylase, and 17,20-lyase. Twelve boys underwent adrenocorticotropic hormone stimulation.

Results.—Eight of 30 patients had basal steroid concentrations and precursor-to-product ratios in the normal range. Values were equivocal in 7 patients, some of whom were in the upper limit of the normal range. Findings were clearly abnormal in 15 (50%) cases. Pure 3β-hydroxysteroid dehydrogenase deficiency was present in 7, pure 17,20-lyase deficiency in 4, a combination of 3β-hydroxysteroid dehydrogenase deficiency and 17,20-lyase deficiency in 3, and a combination of 3β-hydroxysteroid dehydrogenase deficiency and 17α-hydroxylase deficiency in 1. Six of the patients with 3β-hydroxysteroid dehydrogenase deficiency had at least 2 affected pathways. Adrenocorticotropic hormone stimulation yielded varied effects, with widening of the precursor-to-product ratios in some boys and narrowing in others.

Conclusion.—Because 3β-hydroxysteroid dehydrogenase occupies a gateway position on the testosterone biosynthesis pathway, any deficiency of this enzyme is likely to lead to hypospadias. A defect in the enzyme was present in more than a third of the boys in this study. There was also a high incidence of 17,20-lyase deficiency, but only 1 of 30 was deficient in 17α-hydroxylase. Overall, findings support the hypothesis that hypospadias results from fetal endocrinopathy and suggest that enzymes in the adrenal glands may be affected independently.

▶ The phallus is formed between the eighth and twelfth week of gestation. Hypospadias is almost always an isolated anatomical abnormality. The majority of hypospadias is probably the result of abnormal androgen production and not secondary to androgen receptor abnormalities.[1] Clinically this is apparent because the hypospadias phallus enlarges at puberty in nearly all cases.

In this study, 50% of males with proximal hypospadias had testosterone biosynthetic defects. These enzymatic defects were not as pronounced as present in adrenogenital syndrome. Given the known increased familial incidence of hypospadias and the inheritance of biosynthetic defects, the potential for future antenatal therapy to prevent some severe hypospadias exists.

D.E. Coplen, M.D.

Reference

1. Sutherland RW, Wiener JS, Hicks JP, et al: Androgen receptor gene mutations are rarely associated with isolated penile hypospadias. *J Urol* 156:828–831, 1996.

Skin Flap Closure by Dermal Laser Soldering: A Wound Healing Model for Sutureless Hypospadias Repair
Kirsch AJ, Duckett JW, Snyder HM, et al (Children's Hosp of Philadelphia)
Urology 50:263–272, 1997   28–3

Objective.—There have been many attempts at sutureless surgery in an attempt to reduce the inflammatory response, maintain luminal continuity, and simplify technically difficult procedures such as urethra, nerve, vascular, or vas deferens repair. In hypospadias repair, laser tissue soldering (LTS) using the diode laser and human albumin-hyaluronate-indocyanine green solder is safe and effective in providing an immediate and leak-free closure. The mechanisms of laser welding and tissue soldering remain unclear. A rat skin model was used to study the physiology, histology, and immunohistochemistry of wound healing after LTS relative to suturing.

Methods.—Dorsal skin flaps were raised and bisected in Sprague-Dawley rats. The wounds were then closed by suturing from a dermal approach, closed by LTS, or left open. Healing was evaluated at intervals up to 21 days. Tensiometric analysis and examination of wound architecture were performed after surgery. Temperatures in the resting skin and in laser-exposed skin with and without solder were measured in the deep dermis, in the superficial striated muscle layer, and within the solder. Temperatures were measured as mean peak levels over a 1-minute laser activation time.

Results.—Continuous suturing took a mean of 5 minutes, compared with about 8 minutes for either LTS or discontinuous suturing. There were 2 seromas in the sutured group and 1 partial wound dehiscence in both the sutured and LTS groups. For the first 5 days after LTS, tensile strength was significantly increased, but was comparable to that observed 7 and 10 days after suturing. Immediately after LTS, tensile strength was comparable to that of a wound allowed to heal for 7 days. By 14 days, wounds that were left open and those closed by LTS were stronger than those closed by suturing. Wounds closed by LTS showed no signs of thermal injury or foreign-body reaction. All LTS-treated wounds showed dermal incorporation of solder by 21 days. With laser activation of solder, temperature increased to 65.0°C in the deep skin and 70°C in the superficial skin, vs. 101°C within the solder.

Conclusions.—This rat skin flap model shows that sutureless LTS offers increased tensile strength for up to 7 days after closure. Tensile strength is greater within 3 days. Using the technique followed in this experiment, LTS does not seem to alter the normal wound-healing process. Increased wound strength arises from the solder-tissue interaction initially and then from extracellular matrix infiltration of solder. The authors suggest that this technique may permit sutureless surgery for hypospadias repair using skin flaps.

▶ This is an excellent histologic and biomechanical evaluation of tissue soldering and wound healing. Advantages include minimal tissue handling, watertight closure, early re-epithelialization, increased early tensile strength, absence of a foreign-body reaction, and decreased scar formation. While soldering took longer than suturing in this model, it will probably have an important role in complex laparoscopic reconstructions.

D.E. Coplen, M.D.

Efficacy and Safety of Lidocaine-Prilocaine Cream for Pain During Circumcision
Taddio A, Stevens B, Craig K, et al (Hosp for Sick Children, Toronto; Univ of Toronto; Univ of British Columbia, Vancouver; et al)
N Engl J Med 336:1197–1201, 1997   28–4

Background.—Despite evidence that the procedure causes intense pain in the neonate, physicians do not use analgesia when performing circumcision. There is a need for an analgesic that is safe, effective, and simple to use in this situation. Five percent lidocaine-prilocaine cream was evaluated for use in reducing the pain of circumcision in newborns.

Methods.—The double-blind, randomized, controlled trial included 68 full-term male neonates undergoing circumcision. Thirty-eight received 2.5% lidocaine/2.5% prilocaine cream over the penis under an occlusive dressing 60–80 minutes before the procedure. The others received placebo. Pain during the procedure was assessed by behavior cues, i.e., facial actions, crying time, as well as the physiologic measures of heart rate and blood pressure. Plasma lidocaine, prilocaine, and the prilocaine metabolite o-toluidine were measured after treatment.

Results.—The 2 groups were similar in gestational age, birth weight, and other demographic characteristics. Pain appeared to be less in the infants receiving lidocaine-prilocaine, as evidenced by less facial activity, lesser crying times, and lesser increases in heart rate. Facial activity was reduced by 12% to 49% at various stages of the procedure, crying time was reduced, and an increase in heart rate was 10 beats/min less. The groups were similar in their blood methemoglobin concentrations. Sixty-one percent of the lidocaine-prilocaine group had detectable lidocaine in plasma, and 55% had detectable prilocaine.

Conclusions.—Application of lidocaine-prilocaine cream is an effective and safe treatment for reducing pain in newborns undergoing circumcision. It provides a simple alternative to nerve block and should be considered for routine use.

▶ EMLA is a mixture of lidocaine and prilocaine that is useful as a topical anesthetic. Systemic absorption of the prilocaine can potentially lead to methemoglobinemia in neonates. This study confirms the safety of EMLA in neonates undergoing circumcision. The analgesic efficacy and therapeutic benefit to the infant is less clear, as the magnitude of pain relief varied during the procedure. The authors state, "the neonates in the lidocaine-prilocaine group still had pain, albeit at an attenuated level." A dorsal nerve block or circumferential infiltration of lidocaine is more effective but does require an increased level of physician expertise.[1]

D.E. Coplen, M.D.

Reference

1. Lenhart JG, Lenhart NM, Reid A, et al: Local anesthesia for circumcision: Which technique is most effective? *J Am Board Fam Pract* 10:13–19, 1997.

29 Pediatric Reconstruction

Transverse Retubularized Ileum: Early Clinical Experience With a New Second Line Mitrofanoff Tube
Gerharz EW, Tassadaq T, Pickard RS, et al (Univ College London)
J Urol 159:525–528, 1998   29–1

Introduction.—Reconstructive urologists are seeking modifications of the Mitrofanoff principle to reduce long-term complications such as stomal stenosis. Surgeons need alternative options if the vermiform appendix, as the catheterizable tube of choice, is not available. A universally appli-

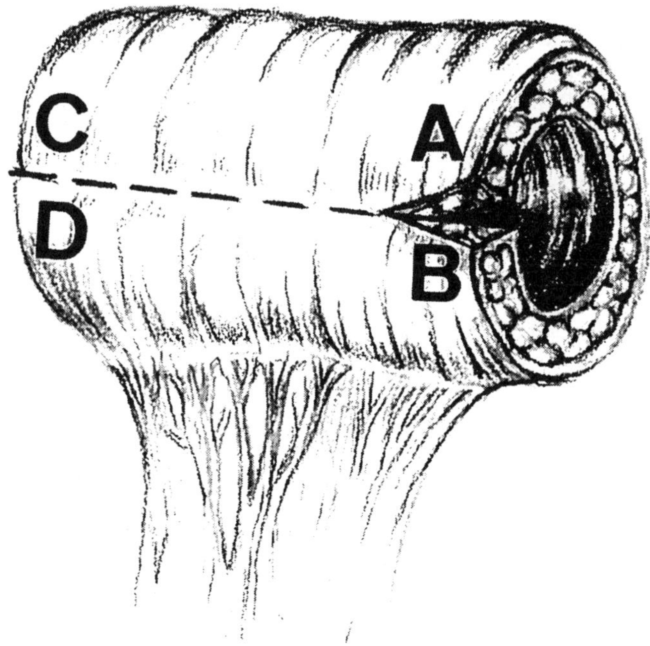

FIGURE 1.—Ileal segment 2–2.5 cm long is excised and opened longitudinally about 1 cm from mesentery. (Courtesy of Gerharz EW, Tassadaq T, Pickard RS, et al: Transverse retubularized ileum: Early clinical experience with a new second line Mitrofanoff tube. *J Urol* 159:525–528, 1998.)

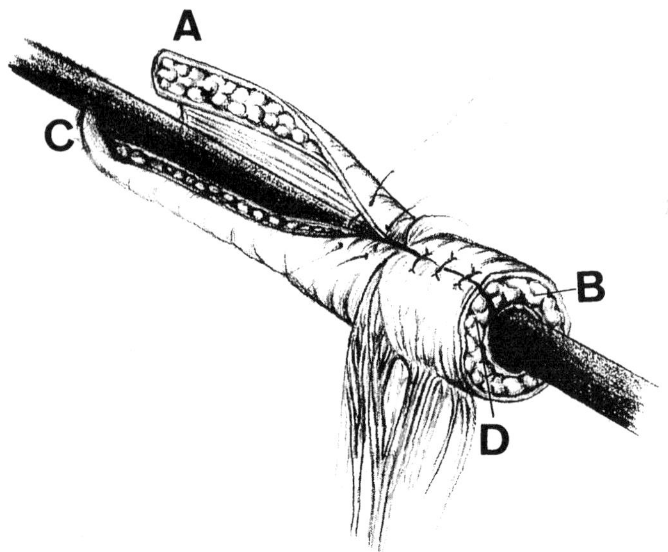

FIGURE 3.—Retubularization in transverse direction using interrupted sutures (4-zero chromic catgut or 5-zero polydioxanone). (Courtesy of Gerharz EW, Tassadaq T, Pickard RS, et al: Transverse retubularized ileum: Early clinical experience with a new second line Mitrofanoff tube. *J Urol* 159:525–528, 1998.)

cable, reliable, and reproducible alternative procedure with a low rate of complications has not yet been found. Early clinical experience with a new technique that uses a reconfigured ileal tube was reviewed.

Methods.—Nine children, ages 1–16, and 7 adults, ages 18–56, with various abnormalities of the lower urinary tract were treated with a new technique of channel formation for intermittent catheterization. In primary reconstruction of the lower urinary tract and in revision procedures, the new method was used. There was an excision of an ileal segment 2 cm long (Fig 1). At about 1 cm from the mesentery, the bowel wall was opened longitudinally. There was retubularization of the resulting rectangle with a 14F catheter in a transverse direction (Fig 3). The native bladder, augmented bladder, or an intestinal reservoir was used to implant the longer portion of the tube submucosally. The stoma was formed by the shorter portion. A double tube was created in 4 patients.

Results.—Complete continence day and night, with easy catheterization after surgery, was seen in 13 patients (81%). Continuous leakage required reimplantation of the intact ileal tube to achieve continence in 2 patients with tunnel failure. Adjustment of the interval of catheterization obviated minor leakage with bladder fullness in an 11-year-old boy.

Conclusion.—This straightforward technique is an excellent second-choice use of the Mitrofanoff principle because of the advantages of constant availability, minimal loss of bowel, relative simplicity (high tube motility, no mesentery interfering with implantation), minimized risk of stone formation (no staples), reliable continence (no leak point), and easy catheterization (longitudinal folds).

▶ The retubularized ileum avoids many of the catheterization problems associated with tapered ileum. The length of the short small-bowel segment removed is the circumference of the new channel. The mesentery is in the middle of the tube, so reimplantation and creation of the stoma are easier than with a tapered ileum. This is an excellent option when the appendix or ureter is unavailable.

D.E. Coplen, M.D.

Combined Mitrofanoff and Antegrade Continence Enema Procedures for Urinary and Fecal Incontinence

Mor Y, Quinn FMJ, Carr B, et al (Great Ormond Street Hosp, London)
J Urol 158:192–195, 1997   29–2

Introduction.—Congenital abnormalities, trauma, or previous operations may lead to functional abnormalities of both the urinary and gastrointestinal tracts. Thus, fecal incontinence or intractable constipation can coexist with wetting. Between 1989 and 1995, a Mitrofanoff conduit and a channel for antegrade continence enemas were constructed in 18 children with double incontinence or urinary incontinence and intractable constipation.

Patients and Methods.—The patients, 9 boys and 9 girls, ranged in age from 2 to 18 years (average age, 8.4) and had a variety of underlying abnormalities. Six were wheelchair bound at the time of surgery. Both procedures were performed simultaneously in 13 patients. In the remaining 5 cases, the Mitrofanoff conduit and antegrade continence enema procedures were performed 17 to 46 months apart. The appendix was used to construct the enema channel in 8 cases and the Mitrofanoff channel in 5 cases. In 2 cases, the appendix was long enough for both procedures, but in 3 cases, it was missing or unsuitable. Alternative sources of channels were the cecal flap, ileum, ureter, and detrusor tube. Stomas were constructed with a triangular posterior V skin flap or multiple skin flaps according to the V.Z.Q. technique. In 13 patients, the stomas were in close proximity in the right lower abdominal quadrant.

Results.—Except for 1 abscess near an antegrade continence enema stoma, convalescence was generally uneventful in these children. In 10 cases, dilation or minor revisions were required, and repeat operations for reconstruction of antegrade continence enema channels or for a detrusor tube Mitrofanoff channel were performed in 3 cases. Fifteen patients (83%) are clean or rarely soil and all of their stomas are continent. Three of the 15 have a catheter in situ because their stomas are difficult to catheterize. Enemas are performed every 24 to 72 hours and require approximately 30 minutes to complete. Two of the failures resulted from closing of the channels; the third patient had severe constipation necessitating colostomy.

Conclusion.—Many doubly incontinent patients can be treated successfully with construction of a channel for an antegrade continence enema and a Mitrofanoff conduit. Although 12 of 18 patients became clean and dry, more than half required revision surgery. Success is also dependent on the child's motivation.

▶ Fecal soiling and intractable constipation commonly coexist with urinary incontinence in the spina bifida population. This can often be managed with a combination of dietary changes, enemas, and digital stimulation. However, if this is not addressed at the same time as urinary abnormalities, then the patient will not have any significant improvement in social accommodation. The continent appendicocecostomy (Malone) has been developed as an isolated fecal continence adjunct or in combination with urinary tract reconstruction. Simultaneous use of the appendix for both cecal and bladder stomas has been described but was possible in only 2 of 18 patients in this series. Stomal stenosis occurred in only 1 of 10 patients when the appendix was used in the continence enema. Stomal stenosis occurred in 5 of 7 patients where a cecal flap was utilized for the enema stoma. Thus, if alternative Mitrofanoff channels are not available for the bladder, there are significant complications with the antegrade continence enema. In these situations, consideration should be given to the use of a button cecostomy using a gastrostomy button.[1]

D.E. Coplen, M.D.

Reference

1. Kalidasan V, Elgabroun MA, Guiney EJ: Button caecostomy in the management of faecal incontinence. *Br J Surg* 84:694, 1997.

Female Epispadias

Mollard P, Basset T, Mure PY (Hôpital Debrousse, Lyon, Cedex, France)
J Urol 158:1543–1546, 1997
29–3

Background.—Epispadias is very rare in females. These authors report the diagnostic findings, treatments, and outcomes in 10 females with epispadias.

Methods.—The 10 female patients ranged in age from 3 to 16 years old. All were completely incontinent, and 9 of 10 had reflux. All had a bifid clitoris and each had half a hemipreputial fold. The mons pubis was depressed, with thin skin and no hair in the medial part. The labia majora and minora were separated anteriorly, often with poor development of the labia minora. Interpubic length fell between 25 and 30 mm in 8 of the patients, and was 45 mm in a 6-year-old and 6 cm in a 9-year-old. The urethra was short and patulous, and the bladder neck was large and incompetent. All patients underwent antireflux surgery and bladder neck reconstruction similar to that used for exstrophy surgery, with optional genital reconstruction. These 3 procedures were performed as a 2-step procedure (separated by 2 to 9 years) in 3 patients and as a 1-step procedure (simplified cervicoplasty) in 4 patients. Two patients refused the genital reconstruction, and 1 patient had a very difficult course that eventually required complete reconstruction via transureteroureterostomy. Follow-up ranged from 1 to 18 years.

Findings.—Complete continence was achieved in 8 of the 10 patients by 1 year after surgery. The patient with the most difficult course continues to have occasional minimal leakage at night, but during the day is completely dry. One girl who remained incontinent underwent endoscopic silicone injection and a posterior bladder neck plasty; the incontinence persists, but is improving. None of the 10 patients require intermittent catheterization. Genital reconstruction generally gave acceptable results, although the labia minora continue to be asymmetric and the glans of the clitoris appears split.

Conclusions.—Bladder neck reconstruction provided overall satisfactory continence, and genital reconstruction gave overall acceptable results. The authors now typically use a 1-stage combined perineal and abdominal approach (á la Hendren) with a simplified bladder neck reconstruction once the child turns 5 years old and can follow toilet instructions.

▶ Female epispadias is associated with pubic diastasis, a short patulous urethra, and an open bladder neck. It is very rare, but the presence of a bifid clitoris is diagnostic. Historically, as in this series, correction was delayed. However, as part of the spectrum of the bladder exstrophy complex, the condition is most successfully treated with a neonatal repair, and these children should be referred at birth to a pediatric urology center. When epispadias is treated at birth, a formal bladder neck reconstruction as described in this paper may not be required.

D.E. Coplen, M.D.

Urethral Lengthening With Anterior Bladder Wall Flap (Pippi Salle Procedure): Modifications and Extended Indications of the Technique
Pippi Salle JL, McLorie GA, Bägli DJ, et al (Hosp de Clinicas de Porto Alegre, Brazil; Hosp Crianca Conceicao, Brazil; The Hosp for Sick Children, Toronto)
J Urol 158:585–590, 1997   29–4

Introduction.—Surgical treatment of urinary incontinence in patients with neurogenic bladder or bladder exstrophy often leads to urinary retention and the need for clean intermittent catheterization for emptying the bladder. The method of urethral reconstruction presented here, a modification of the author's original technique, achieves urethral lengthening with an anterior bladder wall flap.

Methods.—The patients, 10 girls and 7 boys with a mean age of 9.3 years, underwent bladder neck reconstruction for urinary incontinence.

The 13 patients with neurogenic bladder had a low leak point pressure and remained incontinent using anticholinergics and intermittent catheterization; 2 had undergone unsuccessful operations. Nine patients with neurogenic bladder underwent the original procedure using a midline anterior bladder wall flap. The 4 patients with bladder exstrophy were treated with the modified procedure using an anterolateral bladder wall flap. An extended flap of distal mucosa was used in the remaining 4 cases to avoid ureteral reimplantation. Bladder augmentation was used in 13 cases (detubularized ileum in 10 and detubularized colon in 3). Modifications in the original lengthening procedure, used in the last 7 patients, include a widened base to the urethral flap, a lateralized flap in those with previous bladder surgery, and discontinuation of ureteroneocystostomy as a routine part of the repair.

Results.—With a mean follow-up of 25.6 months, continence was achieved in 12 (70%) patients who remained dry for more than 4 hours between catheterizations. Three of the remaining patients were incontinent and 2 were dry for 1 to 2 hours between catheterizations. Continence was achieved by 9 of 13 with neurogenic bladder, 3 of 4 with exstrophy, and 6 of 7 boys. Children aged 7 years or older were able to achieve self-catheterization. There were 2 cases of urethrovesical fistula; 1 was closed successfully.

Conclusion.—In most of these patients with insufficient bladder outlet resistance, urethral lengthening with an anterior bladder wall flap offered good continence. Catheterization was able to be accomplished by the children or their parents in 14 of 17 cases. Modifications of the original procedure were successful in 6 of 7 cases.

▶ Because catheterization of anterior detrusor tube urethral lengthenings (Kropp or Tanagho) is sometimes difficult, the Pippi Salle technique was developed. All of these flap valve procedures are dependent upon catheterization for bladder emptying. This procedure leaves the posterior wall intact, eliminating potential irregularities that make catheterizations difficult. Although 20% of the children are still wet, this is not surprising because complete dryness is very difficult to achieve in the patient with a neurogenic bladder and a low leak point pressure.

D.E. Coplen, M.D.

Subject Index

A

Adenocarcinoma
prostate (*see* Cancer, prostate)
Adenopathy
polytetrafluoroethylene, after
subureteral polytetrafluoroethylene
injection for vesicoureteral reflux,
in children, 292
Adhesion
molecule CD44, cell, expression, and
incidence of seminoma in
cryptorchid boys and infertile men,
274
Adolescent
enuresis in, primary nocturnal, oral
desmopressin for, 307
Adrenal, 41
lesions, MRI differentiation of
pheochromocytoma from other
lesions, 7
masses in patients with malignancies,
comparison of two algorithms and
their associated charges in
evaluation of, 5
myelolipoma, natural history and
treatment of, 41
Adrenocortical
oncocytoma, case reports, 42
African blacks
prostate cancer in, 184
Age
decreases nitric oxide
synthase-containing nerve fibers in
penis (in rat), 269
female, effect on pregnancy rate in male
infertility, 235
as prognostic factor for squamous
carcinoma of penis, 245
Agency for Health Care Policy and
Research guidelines
for prostate hyperplasia, benign,
adherence to, 140
Aging
impact on penile hemodynamics in
normal responders to
pharmacological injection, 263
Algorithms
in evaluation of adrenal masses in
patients with malignancies,
comparison of two and their
associated charges, 5
Allergic
nephropathy associated with
norfloxacin and ciprofloxacin
therapy, 11

Allium sativum
treatment for transitional cell carcinoma
(in mice), 118
Allograft (*see* Transplantation)
Alpha-1 inflatable penile prosthesis
Mentor, for impotence, safety and
efficacy outcome of, 264
Alprostadil (*see* Prostaglandin, E$_1$)
American Cancer Society
guidelines for early detection of prostate
cancer, 160
National Prostate Cancer Detection
Project, observations on early
detection of prostate cancer from,
166
AMS 700 series
inflatable penile prostheses, long-term
mechanical reliability of, 264
Anastomosis
level, effect on outcome of end-to-side
epididymovasostomy, 231
vesicourethral, rectus fascial sling
suspension after radical
prostatectomy, 192
Anatomical
findings in vanishing testis, 300
Androgen
blockade, combined, bicalutamide *vs.*
flutamide in, for advanced prostate
cancer, clinical benefits of, 201
Angiography
CT, helical, for examination of living
renal donors, 54
Anomalies
congenital, 311
Antibiotics
prophylactic, for primary vesicoureteral
reflux, in children, 283
Antibody
hepatitis B surface antigen-negative,
hepatitis B core antibody-positive
donors, risk of transplanting
kidneys from, 63
Antigen
Bard bladder tumor antigen test in
detection of bladder cancer, 155
Fas, intrarenal expression during acute
and/or chronic rejection of renal
allografts, 81
hepatitis B surface antigen-negative,
hepatitis B core antibody-positive
donors, risk of transplanting
kidneys from, 63
prostate-specific (*see* Prostate, -specific
antigen)

E

Author Index

A